A Color Handbook

Pediatric Clinical Ophthalmology

Scott E. Olitsky, MD

Chief of Ophthalmology
Children's Mercy Hospital
Kansas City, MO, USA

Professor of Ophthalmology
University of Missouri, Kansas City School of Medicine
Clinical Associate Professor of Ophthalmology
University of Kansas School of Medicine
Kansas City, MO, USA

Leonard B. Nelson, MD

Co-Director Pediatric Ophthalmology
Associate Professor of Ophthalmology and Pediatrics
Jefferson Medical College of Thomas Jefferson University
Philadelphia, PA, USA

Pediatric Ophthalmology Service
Wills Eye Institute,
Philadelphia, PA, USA

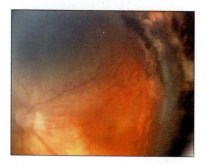

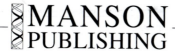

MANSON
PUBLISHING

Copyright © 2012 Manson Publishing Ltd

ISBN: 978-1-84076-151-1

A CIP catalogue record for this book is available from the British Library.

For full details of all Manson Publishing titles please write to:
Manson Publishing Ltd, 73 Corringham Road, London NW11 7DL, UK.
Tel: +44(0)20 8905 5150
Fax: +44(0)20 8201 9233
Website: www.mansonpublishing.com

Commissioning editor: Jill Northcott
Project manager: Paul Bennett
Copy editor: Ruth Maxwell
Book design and layout: DiacriTech, Chennai, India
Colour reproduction: Tenon & Polert Colour Scanning Ltd, Hong Kong
Printed by: New Era Printing Company Ltd, Hong Kong

Contents

Preface 6

Editors and Contributors . . .7
Abbreviations 9

**Chapter 1 Functional
anatomy** **11**
Kammi Gunton
Introduction 12
Orbit and external eye 12
Extraocular muscles 14
Anterior segment 17
Posterior segment 19

**Chapter 2 Ocular
examination in infants
and children** **21**
Rudolph S. Wagner
Introduction 22
Ocular examination 22
   The 'red reflex' 23
   Assessment of vision and
   visual acuity 23
   Cover test for
   strabismus 28
   Light reflex testing 29
   Color vision testing 30
   Assessment of
   stereoacuity 30
   Ophthalmoscopy 31
Vision screening 31
   Photoscreening 32
   Autorefraction 32
   Visual evoked potential . . .32

**Chapter 3 Retinopathy of
prematurity** **33**
David K. Coats and Ashvini Reddy

Chapter 4 Amblyopia **43**
*Robert W. Arnold, Scott E. Olitsky,
and David K. Coats*

**Chapter 5 Strabismus
disorders** **51**
*Scott E. Olitsky and Leonard B.
Nelson*
Strabismus 52
Comitant strabismus 54
   Congenital esotropia 54
   Accommodative
   esotropia 56

   Congenital exotropia 57
   Intermittent exotropia . . .57
Incomitant strabismus 58
   Third cranial nerve palsy . .58
   Fourth nerve palsy 59
   Sixth nerve palsy 60
Strabismus syndromes 61
   Duane's syndrome 61
   Brown's syndrome 62
   Monocular elevation
   deficiency (MED) 62
   Möbius syndrome 64

Chapter 6 Conjunctiva **65**
Steven J. Lichtenstein
Introduction 66
Conjunctivitis 68
Bacterial conjunctivitis 69
Viral conjunctivitis 74
Herpes conjunctivitis 76
Giant papillary
   conjunctivitis 77
Allergic conjunctivitis 78
Vernal keratoconjunctivitis . . .80
Phlyctenular keratoconjunctivitis
   (phlyctenulosis) 82
Ophthalmia neonatorum 83

Chapter 7 Cornea **85**
Brandon D. Ayres
Introduction 86
Congenital corneal
   opacity 86
   Embryology 86
   Peters anomaly 86
   Sclerocornea 87
   Congenital dermoid 88
   Birth trauma 88
   Congenital hereditary
   endothelial dystrophy 89
   Congenital hereditary
   stromal dystrophy 90
   Posterior polymorphous
   membrane dystrophy 90
Metabolic diseases 91
   Mucopolysaccharidosis . . .91
   Hurler's syndrome
   (MPS I-H) 92
   Scheie's syndrome
   (MPS I-S) 92

   Hunter's syndrome
   (MPS II) 92
   Morquio's syndrome
   (MPS IV A and B) 93
   Maroteaux–Lamy syndrome
   (MPS VI A and B) 93
   Sly's syndrome
   (MPS VII) 93
   Idiopathic
   mucopolysaccharidoses . . .93
   Mucolipidosis 93
   Sialidosis (ML I) 93
   I-Cell disease (ML II) 93
   Pseudo-Hurler dystrophy
   (ML III) 94
   ML IV 94
Miscellaneous metabolic
   diseases 94
   Fabry's disease 94
   Cystinosis 94
   Tyrosinemia 95
Infectious diseases 95
   Herpes simplex
   virus (HSV) 95
   Congenital syphilis 96
   Rubella 96

Chapter 8 Lens disorders . .**97**
Richard P. Golden
Introduction 98
Structural lens
   abnormalities 98
   Aphakia 98
   Spherophakia
   (microspherophakia) 98
   Coloboma 98
   Subluxation
   (ectopia lentis) 98
   Lenticonus 99
   Persistant fetal
   vasculature 99
Cataracts 100
   Nuclear cataracts 100
   Lamellar cataracts 100
   Anterior polar cataracts . .100
   Posterior polar cataracts . .100
   Sutural cataracts 102
   Anterior subcapsular
   cataracts 102
   Posterior subcapsular
   cataracts 102

Cerulean (blue-dot)
  cataracts 102
  Complete cataracts 102
Etiology of cataracts 104
  Genetic and metabolic
  diseases 104
  Trauma 106
  Medication and
  toxicity 106
  Maternal infection 107
Diagnosis of cataracts 108
Management/treatment of
  cataracts 108
  Visual significance 108
  Surgery 109
  Aphakia 110
  Pseudophakia 111
  Amblyopia 111
Cataract prognosis 112

Chapter 9 Glaucoma 113
Daniel T. Weaver
Introduction 114
Diagnosis of pediatric
  glaucoma 114
  Ocular examination 117
Differential diagnosis of
  pediatric glaucoma 118
Primary infantile
  glaucoma 119
Juvenile open-angle
  glaucoma 120
Primary pediatric glaucoma
  associated with systemic
  disease 121
  Lowe's syndrome 121
  Sturge–Weber
  syndrome 121
  Neurofibromatosis 122
Pediatric glaucoma associated
  with ocular anomalies . . .123
  Axenfeld–Rieger
  syndrome 123
  Aniridia 124
  Peters anomaly 125
Secondary childhood
  glaucoma 126
  Trauma 126
  Neoplasia 126
  Uveitis (iritis) 126
  Glaucoma following pediatric
  cataract surgery 127
  Other causes of secondary
  glaucoma in children . . .127

Treatment of pediatric
  glaucoma 128
  Drug treatment 128
  Surgical management . . .129
Summary 130

**Chapter 10 Retinal
diseases 131**
*Vicki M. Chen and Deborah K.
VanderVeen*
Introduction 132
Coats' disease 132
Leber's congenital
  amaurosis 134
X-linked congenital stationary
  night blindness 136
Achromatopsia 138
Stargardt disease 140
Best's disease 142
Persistent fetal vasculature . .144
X-linked juvenile
  retinoschisis 146
Albinism 148
Retinal dystrophies with
  systemic disorders
  (ciliopathies) 149

Chapter 11 Uveitis 151
Gregory Ostrow
Introduction 152
Common clinical features . .152
Classification 154
Anterior uveitis 155
  Juvenile idiopathic
  arthritis 155
  Juvenile
  spondyloarthropathies . .156
  Sarcoidosis 156
  Herpetic iridocyclitis . . .157
Intermediate uveitis 158
Posterior uveitis 158
  Toxoplasmosis 158
  Toxocariasis 159
  Vogt–Koyanagi–Harada
  syndrome 160
  Sympathetic ophthalmia .160
Masquerade syndromes 162
  Retinoblastoma 162
  Leukemia 162

**Chapter 12 Diseases of the
optic nerve 163**
Paul H. Phillips
Introduction 164

Optic nerve hypoplasia 164
Morning glory disc
  anomaly 168
Optic disc coloboma 169
Peripapillary staphyloma . . .170
Congenital tilted disc 170
Optic pit 172
Myelinated retinal
  nerve fibers 172
Papilledema 174
Pseudopapilledema 175
Optic disc drusen 176

**Chapter 13 Disorders of the
lacrimal system 177**
Donald P. Sauberan
Introduction 178
Dacryocele 178
Nasolacrimal duct
  obstruction 180
Lacrimal sac fistula 182
Decreased tear
  production 183
Dacryoadenitis 184

Chapter 14 The eyelids . . .185
Srinivas Iyengar
Introduction 186
Anophthalmia/
  microphthalmia 186
Cryptophthalmos and
  ankyloblepharon 186
Coloboma of the eyelid 186
Blepharoptosis 187
Epicanthal folds and
  euryblepharon 188
Lagophthalmos 188
Lid retraction 188
Ectropion, entropion, and
  epiblepharon 189
Blepharospasm 189
Blepharitis 189
Hordeolum 190
Chalazion 190
Tumors of the eyelid 190
Preseptal and orbital
  cellulitis 191
Herpes simplex, molluscum
  contagiosum, and verruca
  vulgaris 191
Allergic conjunctivitis 192
Trauma 192
Summary 192

Chapter 15 Ocular manifestations of systemic disorders **193**
Merrill Stass-Isern and Laurie D. Smith

Introduction 193
Cystinosis 194
Marfan's syndrome 196
Homocystinuria 198
Wilson's disease 200
Fabry disease 201
Osteogenesis imperfecta ...202
The mucopolysaccharidoses .204
Sickle cell disease 208
Albinism 210
Congenital rubella 216

Chapter 16 Oculoneurocutaneous syndromes ('phakomatoses') **217**
Jerry A. Shields and Carol L. Shields

Introduction 218
  Genetics 218
  Malignant potential 218
  Formes frustes 218
Tuberous sclerosis complex (Bourneville's syndrome) 218
Neurofibromatosis (von Recklinghausen's syndrome) 222
Retinocerebellar hemangioblastomatosis (von Hippel–Lindau syndrome) 226
Racemose hemangiomatosis (Wyburn-Mason syndrome) 229
Encephalofacial cavernous hemangiomatosis (Sturge–Weber syndrome) 230
Oculoneurocutaneous cavernous hemangiomatosis 232
Organoid nevus syndrome 233

Chapter 17 Neuro-ophthalmology **235**
Jane C. Edmond

Introduction 236
Cortical visual impairment ..236
Migraine headache 237
Congenital motor nystagmus 238

Spasmus nutans 239
Opsoclonus 239
Horner's syndrome 240
Congenital ocular motor apraxia 241
Myasthenia gravis 242

Chapter 18 Ocular tumors **243**
Carol L. Shields and Jerry A. Shields

Introduction 244
Clinical signs of childhood ocular tumors 244
  Eyelid and conjunctiva ..244
  Intraocular tumors 244
  Orbital tumors 245
Diagnostic approaches 245
  Eyelid and conjunctiva ..245
  Intraocular tumors 245
  Orbital tumors 246
Therapeutic approaches 246
  Eyelid and conjunctiva ..246
  Intraocular tumors 246
  Orbital tumors 246
Eyelid tumors 246
  Capillary hemangioma ..246
  Facial nevus flammeus ..248
  Kaposi's sarcoma 248
  Basal cell carcinoma 248
  Melanocytic nevus 248
  Neurofibroma 248
  Neurilemoma (schwannoma) 249
Conjunctival tumors 249
  Introduction 249
  Choristomatous conjunctival tumors 249
  Epithelial conjunctival tumors 253
  Melanocytic conjunctival tumors 254
  Vascular conjunctival tumors 256
  Xanthomatous conjunctival tumors 257
  Lymphoid/leukemic conjunctival tumors 258
  Non-neoplastic lesions that simulate conjunctival tumors 258
  Conclusions 258
Intraocular tumors 259
  Retinoblastoma 259
  Retinal capillary hemangioma 264

Retinal cavernous hemangioma 265
Retinal racemose hemangioma 265
Astrocytic hamartoma of the retina 266
Melanocytoma of the optic nerve 266
Intraocular medulloepithelioma 266
Choroidal hemangioma .266
Choroidal osteoma 266
Uveal nevus 268
Uveal melanoma 268
Congenital hypertrophy of retinal pigment epithelium 270
Leukemia 270
Orbital tumors 271
  Dermoid cyst 271
  Teratoma 271
  Capillary hemangioma ..271
  Lymphangioma 272
  Juvenile pilocytic astrocytoma 272
  Rhabdomyosarcoma ...272
  Granulocytic sarcoma ('chloroma') 272
  Lymphoma 272
  Langerhan's cell histiocytosis 272
  Metastatic neuroblastoma 273

Chapter 19 Ocular trauma **275**
Denise Hug

Introduction 276
Eyelid 276
Open globe 278
Ocular surface injury 280
Intraocular trauma 282
Iridodialysis 282
Cataract 284
Retina 284
Optic nerve injury 286
Orbital fracture 286
Other orbital injury 288
Child abuse 289
  Shaking injury 289

References and bibliography **291**

Index **313**

Preface

This color handbook was conceived to fill a need for pediatricians and primary care physicians not completely met by existing encyclopedic treatises on pediatric ophthalmology. Our intent was to write a clinically oriented, cohesive text that reviewed the signs, symptoms, and treatment of common ocular diseases and disorders in infants and children. Ocular disorders are of major significance because they often provide clues to the presence not only of systemic diseases but also of other congenital malformations. The recognition, understanding, early treatment and, ultimately, prevention of ocular diseases in childhood will have lasting and gratifying effects for all physicians who care for affected children.

We thank all of our contributing authors for their knowledge and assistance in the preparation of this book. In addition, we are grateful to the publishers at Manson Publishing for their guidance and patience in the production and completion of this book. Lastly, no book in the field of pediatric ophthalmology could exist today without acknowledging the memory of two outstanding pediatric ophthalmologists, Drs Marshall Parks and Robison Harley, who helped establish this subspecialty and paved the way for all of us in this field.

Scott E. Olitsky, MD
Leonard B. Nelson, MD

Contributors

EDITORS

Scott E. Olitsky, MD
Chief of Ophthalmology
Children's Mercy Hospital
Kansas City, MO, USA

Professor of Ophthalmology
University of Missouri, Kansas City School of
    Medicine
Clinical Associate Professor of Ophthalmology
University of Kansas School of Medicine
Kansas City, MO, USA

Leonard B. Nelson, MD
Co-Director Pediatric Ophthalmology
Associate Professor of Ophthalmology and
    Pediatrics
Jefferson Medical College of Thomas Jefferson
    University
Philadelphia, PA, USA

Pediatric Ophthalmology Service
Wills Eye Institute
Philadelphia, PA, USA

CONTRIBUTORS

Robert W. Arnold, MD
Pediatric Ophthalmology and Strabismus
    Ophthalmic Associates
Anchorage, AK, USA

Brandon D. Ayres, MD
Cornea Service, Wills Eye Institute
Jefferson Medical College of Thomas Jefferson
    University
Philadelphia, PA, USA

Vicki M. Chen, MD
Assistant Professor of Ophthalmology
Pediatric Ophthalmology & Motility Disorders
New England Eye Center
The Floating Hospital for Children at Tufts
    Medical Center
Boston, MA, USA

David K. Coats, MD
Baylor College of Medicine
Texas Children's Hospital
Houston, TX, USA

Jane C. Edmond, MD
Associate Professor of Ophthalmology and
    Pediatrics
Baylor College of Medicine
Texas Children's Hospital
Houston, TX, USA

Richard P. Golden, MD
Clinical Assistant Professor of Ophthalmology
The Ohio State University College of Medicine
Nationwide Children's Hospital
Columbus, OH, USA

Kammi Gunton, MD
Assistant Surgeon
Pediatric Ophthalmology Service
Wills Eye Institute
Philadelphia, PA, USA

Denise Hug, MD
Associate Professor of Ophthalmology
Children's Mercy Hospitals and Clinics
University of Missouri, Kansas City School of
    Medicine
Kansas City, MO, USA

Srinivas Iyengar, MD
Oculoplastic Surgery Fellow
Eyesthetica
Santa Monica, CA, USA

Steven J. Lichtenstein, MD, FAAP
Associate Clinical Professor
Department of Surgery & Pediatrics
University of Illinois College of Medicine at
    Peoria & Chicago
Illinois Eye Center, Peoria, IL, USA

Gregory Ostrow, MD
Director
Pediatric Ophthalmology and Adult
    Strabismus Service
Scripps Clinic
San Diego, CA, USA

Paul H. Phillips, MD
Professor
Pediatric Ophthalmology and Strabismus,
    Neuro-Ophthalmology
University of Arkansas for Medical Sciences
Arkansas Children's Hospital
Little Rock, AR, USA

Ashvini Reddy, MD
Baylor College of Medicine
Texas Children's Hospital
Houston, TX, USA

Donald P. Sauberan, MD
Eye Surgical Associates
Lincoln, NE, USA

Jerry A. Shields, MD
Director
Ocular Oncology Service
Wills Eye Institute
Philadelphia, PA, USA

Consultant in Ocular Oncology
Children's Hospital of Philadelphia, &
    Professor of Ophthalmology
Jefferson Medical College
Thomas Jefferson University
Philadelphia, PA, USA

Carol L. Shields, MD
Associate Director
Ocular Oncology Service
Wills Eye Institute
Philadelphia, PA, USA

Consultant in Ocular Oncology
Children's Hospital of Philadelphia, &
    Professor of Ophthalmology
Jefferson Medical College
Thomas Jefferson University
Philadelphia, PA, USA

Laurie D. Smith, MD, PhD, FAAP
    Diplomate, ABMG
Clinical and Biochemical Geneticist
Section of Dysmorphology
Clinical Genetics & Metabolism
Department of Pediatrics
Children's Mercy Hospitals & Clinics
Kansas City, MO, USA

Assistant Professor
University of Missouri
Kansas City School of Medicine
Kansas City, MO, USA

Merrill Stass-Isern, MD
Associate Professor of Ophthalmology
Children's Mercy Hospitals and Clinics
University of Missouri
Kansas City School of Medicine
Kansas City, MO, USA

Rudolph S. Wagner, MD
Clinical Associate Professor of Ophthalmology
    & Director of Pediatric Ophthalmology
Institute of Ophthalmology & Visual Sciences
University of Medicine & Dentistry of New
    Jersey
New Jersey Medical School
Newark, NY, USA

Deborah K. VanderVeen, MD
Children's Hospital Boston
Harvard Medical School
Boston, MA, USA

Daniel T. Weaver, MD
Pediatric Ophthalmologist
Chair, Department of Ophthalmology
Billings Clinic
Billings,
MT, USA

AAP American Academy of Pediatrics
ACE angiotensin-converting enzyme
AD autosomal dominant
ADHD attention deficit hyperactivity disorder
AHP anomalous head position
AIDS acquired immune deficiency syndrome
AKC atopic keratoconjun ctivitis
AOM acute otitis media
A-RS Axenfeld–Rieger syndrome
AR autosomal recessive
AV arteriovenous
CA-MRSA community aquired methicillin-resistant *Staphylococcus aureus*
CBS cystathionine beta synthase
CHED congenital hereditary endothelial dystrophy
CHRP congenital hypertrophy of the retinal pigment epithelium
CHSD congenital hereditary stromal dystrophy
CIN conjunctival intraepithelial neoplasia
CNS central nervous system
CSNB congenital stationary night blindness
CT computed tomography
CVI cortical visual impairment
DNA deoxyribonucleic acid
DVD dissociated vertical deviation
ECF-A eosinophil chemotactic factor of anaphylaxis
EGA estimated gestational age
ELISA enzyme-linked immunosorbent assay
EOG electro-oculography
ERG electroretinography
ESRD end-stage renal disease
FNAB fine-needle aspiration biopsy
GABA gamma aminobutyric acid
GAG glycosaminoglycan
GPC giant papillary conjunctivitis
GPI glycosylphosphatidyl inositol
HA-MRSA hospital acquired methicillin-resistant *Staphylococcus aureus*
HBID hereditary benign intraepithelial dyskeratosis
HIV human immunodeficiency virus
HSV herpes simplex virus
HZV herpes zoster virus
ICE iridocorneal endothelial (syndrome)
ICP intracranial pressure
ICRB International Classification of Retinoblastoma

IGF-1 insulin-like growth factor 1
IOL intraocular lens
IOOA inferior oblique muscle overaction
IOP intraocular pressure
IUGR intrauterine growth retardation
JIA juvenile idiopathic arthritis
JRA juvenile rheumatoid arthritis
LCA Leber's congenital amaurosis
MED monocular elevation deficiency
MIC minimum inhibitory concentration
ML mucolipidosis
MMP matrix metalloproteinase
MPS mucopolysaccharidosis
MRI magnetic resonance imaging
MRNF myelinated retinal nerve fiber
MRSA methicillin-resistant *Staphylococcus aureus*
MSSA methicillin-sensitive *Staphylococcus aureus*
MTHFR methylene tetrahydrofolate reductase
NF neurofibromatosis
NSAID nonsteroidal anti-inflammatory drug
OCT optical coherence tomography
OI osteogenesis imperfecta
ONCCH oculoneurocutaneous cavernous hemangiomatosis
ONCS oculoneurocutaneous syndromes
ONS organoid nevus syndrome
PAC perennial allergic conjunctivitis
PAM primary acquired melanosis
PCG primary congenital glaucoma
PEVP pattern-evoked potential
PFV persistant fetal vasculature
PHPV persistent hyperplastic primary vitreous
PMMA polymethylmethacrylate
PPD purified protein derivative
PPMD posterior polymorphous membrane dystrophy
PSR proliferative retinopathy
ROP retinopathy of prematurity
RP retinitis pigmentosa
RPE retinal pigment epithelium
SAC seasonal allergic conjunctivitis
SLE systemic lupus erythematosus
SLRP small leucine-rich proteoglycan
SW Sturge–Weber syndrome
TORCHS toxoplasmosis, rubella, cytomegalovirus, herpes simplex, and syphilis
TRIC trachoma inclusion conjunctivitis agent

TSC tuberous sclerosis complex
UBM ultrasound biomicroscopy
VDRL Venereal disease Research Laboratory
VECP visually evoked cortical potential
VEGF vascular endothelial growth factor
VEP visual evoked potential
VHL von Hippel–Lindau syndrome
VKC vernal keratoconjunctivitis
VKH Vogt–Koyanagi–Harada syndrome
VMA vanillylmandelic acid
VMD2 vitelliform macular dystrophy type 2
WHO World Health Organization
WM Wyburn-Mason syndrome
XLRS X-linked juvenile retinoschisis

Functional anatomy

Kammi Gunton, MD

- **Introduction**

- **Orbit and external eye**

- **Extraocular muscles**

- **Anterior segment**

- **Posterior segment**

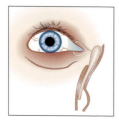
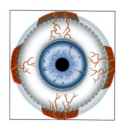
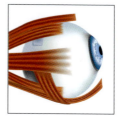
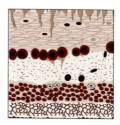

Introduction

This chapter reviews the basic anatomy of the eye, with emphasis on any differences in the pediatric eye. In addition, attention is directed to the functional relevance of the anatomy. The areas covered will include the orbit and external eye, extraocular muscles, anterior segment, and posterior segment.

Orbit and external eye

Each orbit is a pear-shaped bony cavity that tapers posteriorly to form the optic canal. Its volume is approximately 30 mL and it measures approximately 40 mm in an adult.[1] The presence of the globe or an implant is required to continue the bony expansion of the orbit in childhood. The bony orbit is composed of four walls: the roof (frontal bone and lesser wing of the sphenoid), the lateral wall (zygomatic bone and greater wing of the sphenoid), the floor (maxillary, zygomatic, and the palatine bones), and the medial wall (ethmoid, lacrimal, maxillary, and sphenoid bones) (**1**). The thinnest walls of the orbit are the lamina papyracea in the ethmoid bone and the posterior—medial portion of the maxillary bone in the floor. With blunt trauma, these bones easily break allowing for decompression of the globe rather than rupture.

The eyelids provide the external covering for the globe. They contain a dense, fibrous tissue called the tarsus that provides the rigidity of the lids. The orbicularis oculi muscle innervated by the facial nerve allows eyelid closure. The levator palpebrae supplied by cranial nerve III, along with Mueller's muscle innervated by the sympathetic system, opens the eyelids. The levator palpebrae inserts on the anterior surface of the tarsal plate, making the eyelid crease in

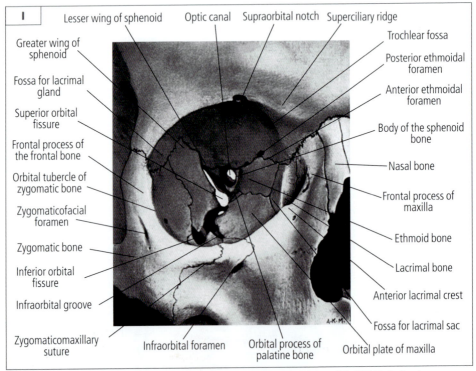

1 Bony orbit. (Reproduced with permission from Catalano RA, Nelson LB (1994). *Pediatric Ophthalmology: A Text Atlas.* Appleton & Lange, Norwalk.)

the upper lid. Congenital fibrosis of the levator palpebrae results in congenital ptosis. Meibomian glands are located in the eyelid and produce the oily layer in the tear film. Blockage of these openings results in formation of a chalazion. Finally, the orbital septum is connective tissue that forms a barrier between the anterior orbital structures such as the skin, and the deeper orbital structures. The septum attaches to the orbital rim, the levator aponeurosis, and the lower lid retractors. Penetration of the septum by infection differentiates preseptal cellulitis (anterior to the septum) from orbital cellulitis.

The lacrimal system is responsible for maintaining the moisture of the external eye. Tears play a vital role in the health and protection of the cornea and conjunctiva. The tear film consists of three layers: an outer lipid layer, a middle aqueous layer, and an inner mucus layer. The meibomian glands secrete the oily layer as previous discussed. The lacrimal gland and the accessory lacrimal glands secrete the middle aqueous layer. The lacrimal gland is located in the superotemporal quadrant of the orbit in the lacrimal gland fossa of the frontal bone.[2] The gland is divided into two parts by the aponeurosis of the levator palpebrae muscle: a larger orbital portion and a palpebral portion. The secretory ducts of the lacrimal gland empty into the superior cul-de-sac approximately 5 mm above the tarsal border. All ducts pass through the palpebral lobe. Damage to the palpebral portion will significantly impact on the secretory function. The facial nerve supplies the lacrimal gland. In addition, the accessory lacrimal glands of Krause and Wolfring are located within the superior cul-de-sac (**2**).

The drainage system for the tears begins with the eyelids pumping the tears towards the puncta which are small outpouchings located 6 mm from the medial angle of the eyelids

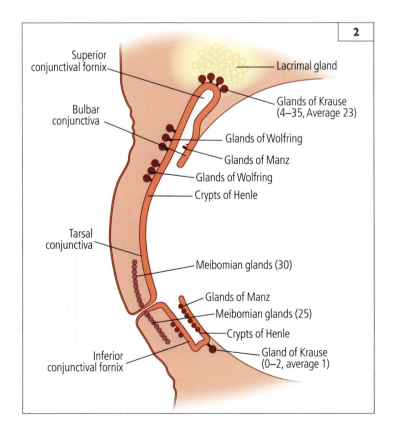

2 Location of lacrimal glands and secretory glands.

Superior conjunctival fornix

Lacrimal gland

Glands of Krause (4–35, Average 23)

Bulbar conjunctiva

Glands of Wolfring

Glands of Manz

Glands of Wolfring

Crypts of Henle

Tarsal conjunctiva

Meibomian glands (30)

Glands of Manz

Meibomian glands (25)

Crypts of Henle

Inferior conjunctival fornix

Gland of Krause (0–2, average 1)

(medial canthus). The puncta are openings approximately 0.5 mm in diameter in each eyelid. Fluid drains through them into a canaliculus which moves perpendicular to the eyelid for 2 mm, then follows the eyelid contour for 8–10 mm until the upper and lower portions fuse to form the common canaliculus. The valve of Rosenmuller separates the common canaliculus from the lacrimal sac, preventing reflux of tears. The lacrimal sac is approximately 10 mm long, located within the lacrimal sac fossa at the level of the middle meatus in the nose. The fundus of the sac extends only 3–5 mm above the medial canthus. Tears pass through the nasolacrimal duct, which lies within the maxillary bone. The duct courses laterally and posterior to empty into the nose under the inferior turbinate. The valve of Hasner is a mucosal fold that lies at the distal end of the nasolacrimal duct to prevent the nasal contents from entering the nasolacrimal sac. It is the most common site of blockage in congenital nasolacrimal duct obstruction (**3**).

Extraocular muscles

Six extraocular muscles are responsible for the motility of the eye (*Table 1*). The seventh extraocular muscle is the levator palpebrae, which has already been discussed. All the muscles originate in a circular arrangement at the apex of the bone surrounding the optic canal, called the annulus of Zinn, except the inferior oblique muscle.[3] The optic nerve, cranial nerves III and VI, and the ophthalmic artery also pass through the annulus of Zinn to enter the orbit. The four rectus muscles course anteriorly to insert on their respective quadrant of the eye: medial rectus, lateral rectus, superior and inferior rectus. The medial rectus inserts closest to the limbus (5.5 mm), followed by the inferior rectus (6.0 mm), then the lateral rectus (7.0 mm), and finally the superior rectus (7.7 mm). The imaginary line connecting these insertions is called the spiral of Tillaux (**4**). The width of the insertions measures approximately 9–10 mm. The rectus muscles are 37 mm in length with tendons ranging from

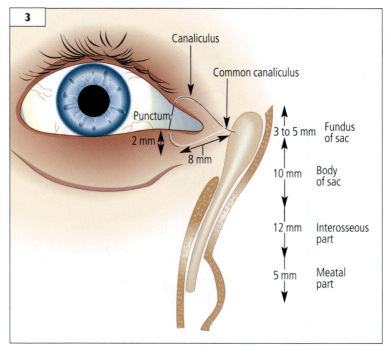

3 The lacrimal system.

Canaliculus

Common canaliculus

Punctum

2 mm

8 mm

3 to 5 mm — Fundus of sac

10 mm — Body of sac

12 mm — Interosseous part

5 mm — Meatal part

3 mm (medial rectus) to 7 mm (lateral rectus). A portion of each rectus muscle also inserts onto connective tissue anchored to the bony orbit called a pulley. These pulleys play an important role in stabilizing the rectus muscles and the globe relative to the orbit during contractions.[4] They also prevent slippage of the muscles in extreme positions of gaze. The pulleys contain smooth muscle which contracts to change the location of the pulley. Diseases of the pulleys may contribute to incomitant deviations such as A and V patterns.[5]

Two muscles insert obliquely on the eye. In the superior quadrant, the superior oblique originates at the annulus of Zinn and is reflected back to the eye through its pulley the trochlea, which is attached to the frontal bone. The superior oblique inserts under the superior rectus muscle posterior to the equator. It is approximately 40 mm in length with a 20 mm tendon. Its insertion measures between 7 and 18 mm in width. The inferior oblique muscle originates from the anterior margin of the maxillary bone lateral to the nasolacrimal

Table 1 Functions of the extraocular muscles

Muscle	Primary	Secondary	Tertiary
Medial rectus	Adduction	–	–
Lateral rectus	Abduction	–	–
Superior rectus	Elevation	Intorsion	Adduction
Inferior rectus	Depression	Extorsion	Adduction
Superior oblique	Intorsion	Depression	Abduction
Inferior oblique	Extorsion	Elevation	Abduction

Modified from Nelson LB, Catalano RA (1989). *Atlas of Ocular Motility*. Philadelphia, Saunders, p. 21, with permission.

4 Spiral of Tillaux.

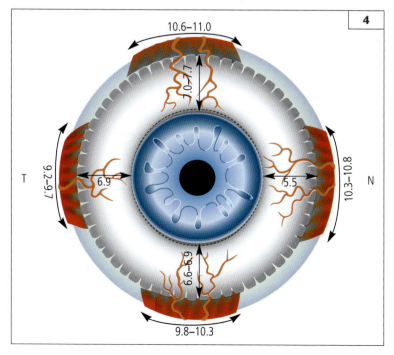

groove. It heads posteriorly, laterally, and superiorly to insert posterior to the equator in the inferotemporal quadrant. The inferior oblique is the shortest of the extraocular muscles, measuring 37 mm, with almost no tendon. Its insertion is 5–14 mm wide (**5**).

Cranial nerve III innervates the majority of the extraocular muscles, and all the intraocular muscles. A single nucleus of the III nerve innervates both levator palpebrae muscles. This is the only muscle with bilateral innervations from one nucleus. The fibers of the III nerve divide into a superior division, which supplies the levator palpebrae and superior rectus and the inferior division, which supplies the medial rectus, inferior rectus, and the inferior oblique. The parasympathetic innervation of the iris sphincter responsible for miosis of the pupil also travels with the inferior division of the III nerve, with the nerve to the inferior oblique. The IV cranial nerve supplies the ipsilateral superior oblique muscle, and the VI cranial nerve supplies the ipsilateral lateral rectus. The blood supply to the anterior eye comes from the lateral and medial branches of the ophthalmic artery. These vessels divide into anterior ciliary arteries. Each rectus muscle carries two anterior ciliary arteries, except the

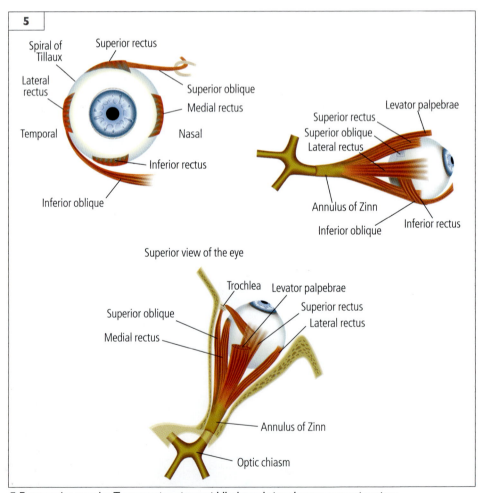

5 Extraocular muscles. Top: anterior view; middle: lateral view; bottom: superior view.

lateral rectus, which has only one ciliary artery. Disinserting more than two rectus muscles carries the risk of compromising the anterior circulation of the eye.

Anterior segment

The cornea is the transparent, outermost layer of the eye and is responsible for two-thirds of the eye's refractive power. The average corneal diameter of a child's eye is 12 mm vertically and 11 mm horizontally. There is a linear increase in corneal diameter during the prenatal period to result in an average diameter of 9.7–10.0 mm horizontally at 40 weeks gestation.[6] During the first year of life, there continues to be a rapid rate of growth of approximately 0.14 mm per month. The growth rate then slows or stops, with no further growth detected after 6 years of age.[7]

The central cornea thickness is an average of 512 μm and increases in the periphery to 1.0 mm.[8] The cornea contains the highest concentration of nerve endings per area, but remains avascular for transparency. There are three layers in the cornea: the endothelium, stroma, and epithelium. The inner endothelial cells pump fluid from the stroma to maintain the transparency of the cornea. Underlying the endothelial cells is a basement membrane called Descemet's membrane. Tightly arranged lamellae of collagen with minimal keratocytes make up the stroma. The regular arrangement allows for transparency. The outer layer of the cornea provides a barrier function (**6**).

The sclera is the nontransparent, more rigid outer layer of the eye. Changes in the arrangement and type of collagen give it the characteristic white color. The posterior sclera is almost twice as thick as the anterior sclera, but has only 60% of the stiffness of the anterior sclera.[9] The sclera is thinnest just posterior to the insertions of the rectus muscles (0.3 mm). Transport of drugs across the sclera is dependent on its hydration level. The degree of hydration of the sclera differs with age, varying with the crosslinking and interweave of the collagen fibers.[10] The axons of the ganglion cells of the retina exit through a sieve-like opening in the sclera called the lamina cribrosa. These fibers will form the optic nerve.

6 Corneal structure.

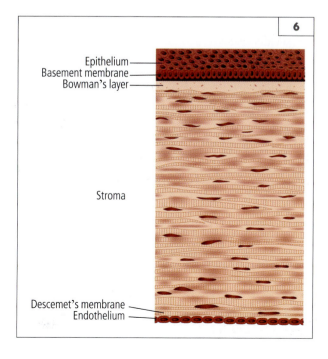

Epithelium
Basement membrane
Bowman's layer

Stroma

Descemet's membrane
Endothelium

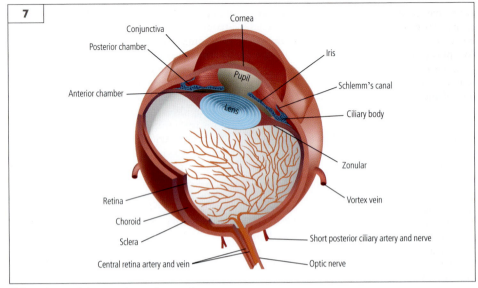

7 Structures of the anterior and posterior segment.

The transition between the cornea and the sclera is called the limbus (7). This region is the source of the stem cells for both the corneal and conjunctival epithelium. The cornea is reliant on the conjunctiva and fluid from within the eye (anterior chamber) for moisture, nutrition, and immune protection. The conjunctiva is a mucus membrane that covers the sclera (bulbar conjunctiva) and the inner eyelids (palpebral conjunctiva). The tight fold between the bulbar conjunctiva and the palpebral conjunctiva is called the fornix. Foreign bodies are limited in their migration into the orbit by the conjunctiva. The conjunctiva is well vascularized and contains numerous lymphoid cells[11] in addition to goblet cells to provide mucin to the tear film. The conjunctiva also secretes electrolytes and water into the aqueous layer. Growth factors, androgens, and direct innervations regulate the conjunctival secretions into the tear film.[12,13]

Underlying the cornea is the anterior chamber of the eye. This aqueous-filled cavity measures approximately 3 mm in depth. New devices allow more precise quantification and better imaging into the iridocorneal angle within the anterior chamber. These include anterior segment optical coherence tomography (OCT) and classic ultrasound biomicroscopy (UBM).[7,14] The majority of the aqueous fluid is resorbed at the anterior chamber angle, although 10% exits through scleral absorption. The anterior chamber angle is made up of the trabecular meshwork, which extends from the sclera spur to the termination of Descemet's membrane called Schwalbe's line. Fluid egresses through this meshwork of thin, fibrocellular sheets to gather in the canal of Schlemm.

The anterior chamber ends at the iris. The iris sphincter and dilator muscles control the amount of light that can enter the eye through the pupil. The dilator muscle is innervated by the sympathetic system, and the sphincter muscle is innervated by the parasympathetic system.[15] The color of the iris is dependent on the amount of melanin within the stroma. Absence of melanin makes the iris appear whitish blue. The area between the iris and the anterior surface of the lens and zonules is called the posterior chamber. Its volume is approximately 0.06 mL.[16] The ciliary body is a ring of tissue that extends from the sclera at the limbus to the anterior extent of the retina called the ora serrata. This ciliary body is further divided into the pars plicata, which is a 2 mm zone that contains smooth muscle and the ciliary processes and the pars plana, which lies more posteriorly. The ciliary processes in the pars plicata are connected to the lens zonules (annular ligament of Zinn). When the ciliary muscle contracts the entire structure moves inward and anteriorly. This relaxes the zonules, which in turn releases the tension on the lens, allowing for accommodation. Aqueous is also secreted by the ciliary body from the nonpigmented cells along the apex. Pigmented epithelial cells continue posterior in the ciliary body, which will eventually merge with the retinal pigment epithelium. The pars plana is approximately 4 mm wide and extends from the pars plicata to the termination of the retina, which is called the ora serrata. The ora serrata is located approximately 6 mm from the limbus. The pars plana is the safety location for the injection of intravitreal medications.

Posterior segment

The retina is formed from neuroectoderm and forms the innermost layer of the posterior eye. The sensory retina is a highly specialized, multi-layered arrangement.[17] There are nine layers within the retina: three layers of nuclei, three layers of fibers, two limiting membranes, and the outer segments of the rods and cones[18] (**8**). The most anterior layer is the nerve fiber layer made up of the axons of the ganglion cells. These axons will join to form the optic nerve and exit through an opening in the sclera. Ganglion cells respond to impulses from bipolar cells, which receive their signals from the rods and cones. Amacrine cells located within the inner plexiform layer of the retina further modulate the signal sent to the ganglion cells. Other cells which modulate the signal and support the structures within the retina include

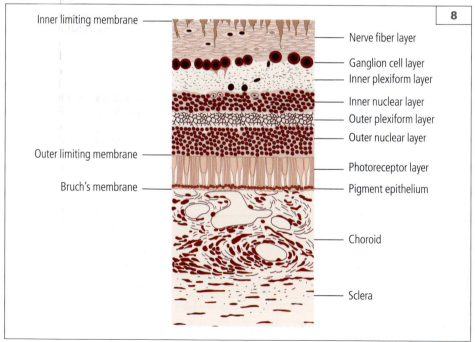

Inner limiting membrane

8

Nerve fiber layer

Ganglion cell layer
Inner plexiform layer

Inner nuclear layer
Outer plexiform layer
Outer nuclear layer

Outer limiting membrane

Photoreceptor layer

Bruch's membrane

Pigment epithelium

Choroid

Sclera

8 Layers of the retina.

horizontal cells in the outer plexiform layer as well as Müller cells. Underlying the sensory retina is a layer of pigmented cells called the retinal pigment epithelium. The basal lamina of this layer forms Bruch's membrane. The apical portion extends in villous processes to surround the outer segments of the rods and cones. The function of the retinal pigment epithelium is to absorb excess light that has entered the eye, metabolize vitamin A and rhodopsin, support the metabolic functions of the rods and cones, and form the blood—retinal barrier. The richly vascular choriocapillaris underlies the retinal pigment epithelium. It supplies the outer half of the retina as well as the retinal pigment epithelium. The inner retina is supplied by the central retinal artery. Separation of the retina from the retinal pigment epithelium is called a retinal detachment.

The retina is further divided into sections by geography. The macular region is approximately 4.5 mm in diameter. It is further located within the temporal vascular arcades. Cones are the predominate structure. Within the macula is a 1.5 mm depression called the fovea. There is absence of the other layers of the retina, so that light falls on the cone outer segments. This area provides the best visual resolution in the eye (**9**).

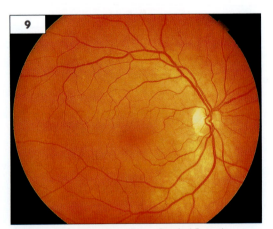

9 Normal human retina. (From Strobel S *et al. Paediatrics and Child Health – The Great Ormond Street Colour Handbook,* Manson Publishing.)

Ocular examination in infants and children

Rudolph S. Wagner, MD

- **Introduction**

- **Ocular examination**
  The 'red reflex'
  Assessment of vision and visual acuity
  Cover test for strabismus
  Light reflex testing
  Color vision testing
  Assessment of stereoacuity
  Ophthalmoscopy

- **Vision screening**
  Photoscreening
  Autorefraction
  Visual evoked potential

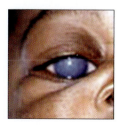
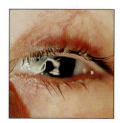
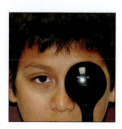
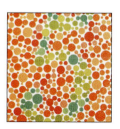

Introduction

Proper performance of the pediatric eye examination is both a challenging and rewarding experience. Abnormal visual experiences early in life may have devastating and long-lasting effects. The pediatrician plays an important role in identifying those patients who may need consultation with an ophthalmologist. The screening process may utilize only simple tools and techniques or can take advantage of some of the new technological advances presently available to help achieve optimal results, particularly regarding vision screening and ophthalmoscopy. The importance of recognition of any ocular abnormalities that require referral cannot be overemphasized.

Ocular examination

The performance of an eye examination in an infant or young child requires flexibility in approach and a willingness to modify the sequence of the examination according to the age and cooperative ability of the child. Nevertheless, there are essential aspects of the examination such as the testing for a 'red reflex' during the neonatal period. The pediatrician must determine what information is critical to achieve an accurate diagnosis in the individual child, and then complete an examination and determine treatment or referral options. Early detection and prompt treatment of ocular disorders in children are critical since infants are susceptible to the development of deprivation amblyopia in cases of unilateral visual axis obstruction, and nystagmus as a result of bilateral visual deprivation.

A chief complaint and a detailed history of the present illness are obtained from the parents or guardian. This should also be obtained from the verbal child, as this may also provide useful information. This time is also useful for attempting to establish good rapport with the child. As in any examination, information as to past medical history, including birth weight, allergies, and medications taken is essential. Familial history is particularly important in suspected multisystem and genetic disorders.

General inspection of the child's overall appearance and body habitus may provide an immediate diagnosis in some specific syndromes. Obvious external features such as ptosis, blepharophimosis, and lid and iris colobomas should be noted. Signs of conjunctival discharge and vascular injection may indicate infection or intraocular inflammation. Corneal edema or opacification may indicate congenital glaucoma (**10**). Palpation of the lacrimal sac area may produce a mucoid discharge from the puncta, indicating a nasolacrimal duct obstruction (**11**). The pupils

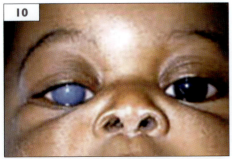

10 Corneal opacity in the right eye secondary to acute corneal edema in congenital glaucoma.

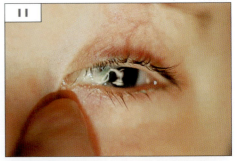

11 Expression of mucoid discharge from the lacrimal puncta in an infant with a congenital nasolacrimal duct obstruction.

can be checked for reactivity to light and near targets and for the presence of an afferent pupillary defect. The latter is diagnosed with a swinging flashlight test. As the light is directed from the normal eye to the eye with the afferent defect in the visual pathway, both pupils will dilate. This indicates an abnormality in the afferent limb of the pupillomotor response.

The 'red reflex'

Every child should receive his/her first eye exam in the newborn nursery. Evaluation for a normal red reflex in the newborn eye can help to eliminate several potentially vision-, and even life-threatening, ocular disorders. Red reflex testing can also be performed at any time later in life.

The 'red reflex' test is best performed in a room with the lights turned down. The examiner looks through a direct ophthalmoscope and initially focuses on each pupil from a distance of about 12–18 inches (30–45 cm). It is also useful to focus on both pupils simultaneously from a distance of 24–36 inches (60–90 cm). The examiner should observe a bright reddish-yellow or a light gray reflex in more darkly pigmented eyes. It is important that the reflex appears symmetric and is not blunted or dull. Linear or diffuse dark spots with a surrounding bright reflex may indicate a partial corneal or lenticular opacity. Absence of a reflex may indicate a total lenticular opacity. A white reflex or leukocoria may be seen in eyes with retinoblastomas or large chorioretinal colobomas. Performance of the simultaneous red reflex test or Bruckner Test may detect asymmetric reflexes that could indicate amblyogenic factors such as differences in refractive error between the eyes. It is not necessary to dilate the pupils pharmacologically to appreciate a red reflex. As mentioned, dulling the room lights is very useful. If pupillary dilation is desired it is safest to use 2.5% phenylephrine drops.[1]

It is important that the pediatrician records his/her observations from the red reflex exam performed during the first 3 months of life and at other visits up to 3 years of age.

Assessment of vision and visual acuity

Recently, emphasis has been placed on vision screening being performed by pediatricians and other primary health care providers. They have been instructed to screen both for visual acuity and for ocular alignment using either a unilateral cover test at 3 m (10 feet) or a Random-dot-E stereo test at 40 cm (630 seconds of arc). The age-specific guidelines developed by the American Academy of Pediatrics, Section on Ophthalmology, are listed in *Table 2* (overleaf).

With the possible exception of red reflex testing in infants, the single most important aspect of the pediatric eye examination is the assessment of visual acuity in each eye. Most significant ocular disease will produce a reduction of visual acuity in one or both eyes.

Infants begin to smile to a human face around 6 weeks of age and follow objects in the environment starting around 8 weeks.[2] Clinically, one can stimulate a child's interest in a colorful toy or object and observe his or her fixation behavior. Under binocular conditions the child is observed for the presence of nystagmus or torticollis. It is well recognized that children with good vision in only one eye may function and behave as well as a child with excellent binocular visual acuity. Therefore, it is imperative to assess the vision independently in each eye. Fixation of each eye can be evaluated by the 'CSM' formula: (1) central, if not eccentric; (2) steady; and (3) maintained, if the fixation does not revert to the fellow eye as in a strabismic child.

Table 2 Eye examination guidelines*

Ages 3–5 years

Function	Recommended tests	Referral criteria	Comments
Distance visual acuity	Snellen letters Snellen numbers Tumbling E HOTV Picture tests: – Allen figures – LEA symbols	**1.** Fewer than 4 of 6 correct on 20 ft (6 m) line with either eye tested at 10 ft (3 m) monocularly (i.e. less than 10/20 or 20/40) OR **2.** Two-line difference between eyes, even within the passing range (i.e. 10/12.5 and 10/20 or 20/25 and 20/40)	**1.** Tests are listed in decreasing order of cognitive difficulty; the highest test that the child is capable of performing should be used; in general, the tumbling E or the HOTV test should be used for children 3–5 years of age and Snellen letters or numbers for children 6 years and older **2.** Testing distance of 10 ft (3 m) is recommended for all visual acuity tests **3.** A line of figures is preferred over single figures **4.** The nontested eye should be covered by an occluder held by the examiner or by an adhesive occluder patch applied to the eye; the examiner must ensure that it is not possible to peek with the nontested eye
Ocular alignment	Cross cover test at 10 ft (3 m)	Any eye movement	Child must be fixing on a target while cross cover test is performed
	Random-dot-E stereotest at 16 inch (40 cm)	Fewer than 4 of 6 correct	
	Simultaneous red reflex test (Bruckner test)	Any asymmetry of pupil color, size, brightness	Direct ophthalmoscope used to view both red reflexes simultaneously in a darkened room from 2–3 ft (0.6–0.9 m); detects asymmetric refractive errors as well
Ocular media clarity (cataracts, tumors, etc)	Red reflex	White pupil, dark spots, absent reflexes	Direct ophthalmoscope, darkened room. View eyes separately at 12–18 inch (30–45 cm); white reflex indicates possible retinoblastoma

6 years and older

Function	Recommended tests	Referral criteria	Comments
Distance visual acuity	Snellen letters Snellen numbers Tumbling E HOTV Picture tests: – Allen figures – LEA symbols	**1.** Fewer than 4 of 6 correct on 15 ft (4.5 m) line with either eye tested at 10 ft (3 m) monocularly (i.e. less than 10/15 or 20/30) OR **2.** Two-line difference between eyes, even within the passing range (i.e. 10/10 and 10/15 or 20/20 and 20/30)	**1.** Tests are listed in decreasing order of cognitive difficulty; the highest test that the child is capable of performing should be used; in general, the tumbling E or the HOTV test should be used for children 3–5 years of age and Snellen letters or numbers for children 6 years and older **2.** Testing distance of 10 ft (3 m) is recommended for all visual acuity tests

Table 2 Eye examination guidelines* (*continued*)

		6 years and older	
Function	Recommended tests	Referral criteria	Comments
			3. A line of figures is preferred over single figures
			4. The nontested eye should be covered by an occluder held by the examiner or by an adhesive occluder patch applied to the eye; the examiner must ensure that it is not possible to peek with the nontested eye
Ocular alignment	Cross cover test at 10 ft (3 m)	Any eye movement	Child must be fixing on a target while cross cover test is performed
	Random-dot-E stereotest at 16 inch (40 cm)	Fewer than 4 of 6 correct	
	Simultaneous red reflex test (Bruckner test)	Any asymmetry of pupil color, size, brightness	Direct ophthalmoscope used to view both red reflexes simultaneously in a darkened room from 2–3 ft (0.6–0.9 m); detects asymmetric refractive errors as well
Ocular media clarity (cataracts, tumors, etc)	Red reflex	White pupil, dark spots, absent reflexes	Direct ophthalmoscope, darkened room. View eyes separately at 12–18 inch (30–45 cm); white reflex indicates possible retinoblastoma

*Assessing visual acuity (vision screening) represents one of the most sensitive techniques for the detection of eye abnormalities in children. The American Academy of Pediatrics Section on Ophthalmology, in cooperation with the American Association for Pediatric Ophthalmology and Strabismus and the American Academy of Ophthalmology, has developed these guidelines to be used by physicians, nurses, educational institutes, public health departments, and other professionals who perform vision evaluation services.

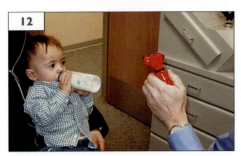

12 Child's attention is obtained with a toy.

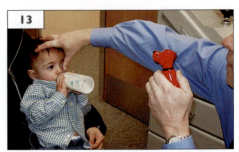

13 Examiner covers the left eye and observes the child's ability to maintain fixation with the right eye.

The examiner covers one eye (usually with the hand, thumb, or occluder) and notes whether the infant looks steadily at a light or fixation target. The eye is then uncovered. (**12, 13**). A strabismic patient who strongly prefers the eye just uncovered will switch fixation to that eye. A child with poor vision in the absence of strabismus may react strongly to occlusion of the better-seeing eye. The anxiety and avoidance maneuvers precipitated by the occlusion may provide evidence of poor visual acuity in the uncovered eye.

Cross-fixation may be observed in infants with large angle esotropia and equal visual acuity. These children find it more convenient to follow objects to their right with the esotropic left eye and *vice versa*. This produces an apparent diminished ability to abduct either eye and a pseudoparesis of the lateral rectus muscles. Temporary occlusion of either eye or rotating the baby in a chair on an adult's lap will usually demonstrate that abduction is present.

This part of the examination is best performed during the initial part of the evaluation of the child, as it requires good cooperation from the child and can be fatiguing to both the patient and doctor. In many cases, the infant or child is brought to the pediatric ophthalmologist specifically for this evaluation. The earliest age that objective visual acuity testing with input from the child can be accomplished is approximately 2.5–3 years of age. It is always useful to measure visual acuity binocularly since this reflects how the child is seeing in normal viewing conditions. It is well recognized that children with latent nystagmus (nystagmus that is present when one eye is covered) may see dramatically better binocularly than with either eye individually. Furthermore, in the binocular state, compensatory head postures for nystagmus with a null zone or torticollis from paralytic strabismus can be appreciated. In fact, occlusion of one eye may eliminate a compensatory face position in some cases of paralytic strabismus. This finding may help to distinguish an ocular from a nonocular cause of torticollis.[3]

Distance visual acuity is most useful and ideally should be measured at 6 m (20 feet). Instruments and charts can be calibrated for distances down to 3 m (10 feet) to accommodate smaller examination rooms. There are a number of symbols or optotypes available. Line tests with 0.1 log unit differences between the lines should be used.[4] Picture charts or symbols such as HOTV are useful for children who have not learned to recognize the standard Snellen letters or numbers. The HOTV test consists of a wall chart composed only of Hs, Os, Ts, and Vs. The child is provided with a card containing a large H, O, T, and V and is asked to indicate or match the correct symbol visualized at distance. Most practitioners do not use the tumbling-E (or illiterate-E) test since many preschool children find it confusing. The LH or Lea optotypes are very useful for vision screening (**14**). These optotypes, which include a circle, apple, square, and house, all blur to a circle beyond the child's threshold acuity.[5]

Visual acuity measured at 0.33 m (13 inches) is not an essential part of the pediatric eye examination although assessment of the near point of accommodation is useful. Other than an unusual child with accommodative insufficiency, there are very few conditions in which a child will have normal distance acuity with subnormal near acuity. Single optotype visual acuity cards used at near fixation or standard near cards should be reserved for situations in which distance acuity testing is not possible. Pathologic vision loss diminishes acuity both for near and distance, therefore near visual acuity testing is appropriate in emergency situations.

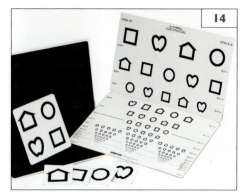

14 Visual acuity testing chart using 'Lea' optotypes.

Presentation of a full line of optotypes eliminates the crowding phenomenon present in many amblyopic eyes. Children with amblyopia will be able to recognize smaller optotypes when presented individually. Whatever 'eye chart' is used, care must be taken to occlude the nontested eye totally (**15, 16**). Children frequently peek around the hand-held occluder and must be monitored carefully (**17**). It may be useful to occlude the eye with a strip of inexpensive 5 cm (2-inch) tape (e.g. 3M-Micropore) (**18**). Those experienced in assessing visual acuity in the preschool verbal age group understand the individual variability and necessity of being flexible in examination technique. A great deal of effort is often expended in persuading the child to allow the occlusion and subsequently coaxing from him or her, an appropriate response. The time and effort are necessary, however, and the ability to assess the visual acuity accurately in this age group is the prerequisite of a good eye examination.

15 The right eye is occluded to test the visual acuity in the left eye.

16 The occluder is now placed before the left eye.

17 A child with poor vision may 'peek' around the occluder, invalidating the results.

18 Tape is placed over the right eye to ensure visual acuity of the left eye is being measured.

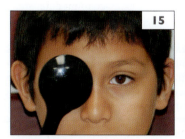

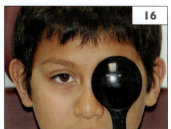

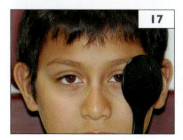

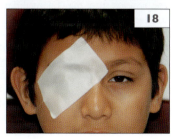

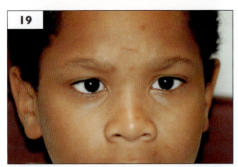

19 A child with right esotropia is observed during attempted binocular fixation prior to the cover test.

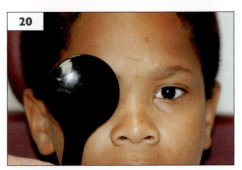

20 The right eye is covered and the left eye observed for movement. There is no change in position.

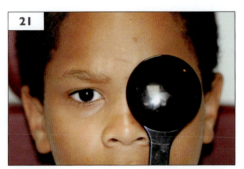

21 The left eye is now occluded and the right eye observed. Previously esotropic right eye has now abducted to the orthophoric primary position. (Compare with the right eye position in 10.)

Cover test for strabismus

Implicit to cover testing is the ability of each eye, in turn, to be capable of central (foveal) fixation when the fellow eye is covered. If organic disease (cataracts, cloudy media, and so on) or functional conditions (eccentric fixation) prevent central fixation with either eye, cover testing may be invalidated.

Placement of the occluder should be minimally traumatic to the child. The traditional black paddle is handy but, if rejected, the examiner's hand or thumb dropped from above may provide a more familiar, less threatening cover.

Fixation targets should be used to provide an accommodative stimulus. Vision charts at 3 m (10 feet) and at 0.33 m (13 inches) work well in older preschool and school-age children. Small interesting pictures are useful for obtaining near fixation in smaller children. Younger preschool children can be offered toys, movies, and the like, with accommodative detail and story content to enhance interest.

The cover test is performed by having the patient look at an accommodative target under binocular viewing conditions. The examiner places an occluder over one eye, while watching the fellow eye for a shift in fixation (19, 20). A shift is evidence that the uncovered eye was not regarding the target with its fovea while both eyes were viewing. This deviation is called heterotropia or, if the direction is specified, exotropia, esotropia, or hypertropia.

Heterotropia is a manifest deviation because it exists (is manifest) under normal or casual seeing circumstances, i.e., with both eyes viewing. Because the patient begins the test with both eyes viewing, the cover test examines a binocular circumstance.

If no shift occurs, heterotropia may still exist. If the occluder was placed in front of the deviating eye, the fellow eye would already be fixed on the target, and no shift would be expected. Obviously in most cases the examiner already knows which eye is deviating because one eye is directed at the object of regard and the other is not. However, in small-angle deviations this is often not obvious, and it is sometimes hard to be sure that the child is regarding the object intended.

To complete the test, the patient must be returned to binocular viewing for at least several seconds so that fusion (binocular vision) can be accomplished if this potential exists. The fellow eye is covered in the same manner as the first (**21**). The sequence is: (1) cover one eye, observing the fellow eye; (2) uncover that eye for a few seconds; and (3) cover the second eye while observing the first eye. The sequence should be repeated to make sure that a subtle, rapid switch in fixation did not take place unnoticed during the binocular interval. Many strabismus patients can readily alternate fixation, and if a switch occurs during the test, the examiner might be placing the occluder before the deviating eye each time.

ALTERNATE COVER TEST

The alternate cover test is performed by moving the occluder directly from one eye to the other without allowing an interval for binocular viewing. Fusion is suspended throughout the test. If no ocular shift occurs as the occluder is moved directly from one eye to the other, the eyes are truly aligned, i.e. orthophoric. Even with fusion suspended, the foveas are in the position to regard the target without having to shift. However, if a shift does occur, a deviation exists. If the deviation is corrected by fusion, i.e. if the deviating eye moves into alignment under binocular conditions, the deviation is said to be latent and is called a heterophoria (or phoria, for short). It should be apparent that the alternate cover test does not diagnose a phoria by itself but depends on the findings of the cover test.

ALTERNATIVE METHODS OF DETECTING STRABISMUS

When cover testing is impossible because of organic disease, eccentric fixation, or lack of cooperation, other estimates of ocular deviations can be made. In infants and exceptionally uncooperative patients, Hirschberg estimates may have to be done. A light source is directed at both eyes. The number of millimeters that the light reflex is decentered from the pupillary axis is approximated. This measurement can then be used to give an estimate of the magnitude of the misalignment that is present.

Light reflex testing

When performing light reflex testing, it is imperative to have the light in the same line as the examiner's viewing eye. In fact, it is a good idea to hold the muscle light touching the examiner's cheek as a reminder and to frequently repeat the measurement.

Angle kappa is the angle formed by the pupillary axis and the visual axis. The pupillary axis is a line passing through the center of the pupil perpendicular to the cornea. The optical axis is the line connecting the optical centers of the cornea and the lens. The visual axis is the line of sight, connecting the fovea and the fixation point. The angle kappa is formed at the intersection of the pupillary and visual axes at the center of the entrance pupil. When the optical axis and the visual axis do not coincide, angle kappa is present. Clinically this erroneously demonstrates a strabismus with a corneal light reflex test. In general, a positive angle kappa is found in most children. This means that the corneal light reflex is not centered but is located slightly nasal to the center of the pupil. A large positive angle kappa simulates an exotropia. Of course barring eccentric fixation, a cover test will distinguish a positive angle kappa from a manifest exotropia.[6]

Versions or binocular eye movement should be checked in the nine diagnostic or cardinal positions of gaze. Examination of the oblique positions can be done by gross observation as the patient follows a near target into these positions. If versions are not full, ductions (single eye movements) should be tested in all fields of action of the individual eye. Recognition and quantification of duction

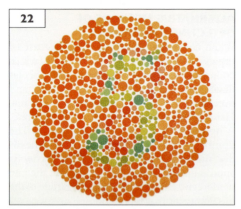

22 Example of the color plates used in Ishihara testing.

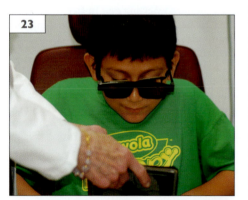

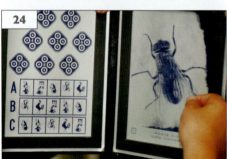

23, 24 Child wearing polarized lenses attempts to pick up the stereo image of a fly.

deficits are important in diagnosing paretic and restrictive extraocular muscle disorders.

It is not uncommon for patients with congenital esotropia to have limited abduction. Physicians other than ophthalmologists frequently interpret this as sixth cranial nerve paralysis, even to the point of ordering unnecessary radiologic procedures. Patching of one and then the other eye usually results in improvement of ductions within hours or days at most. Even without patching, ductions improve with age in these patients. If the child does not allow manual covering of each eye, occluder patches will frequently work. Noisy targets (such as jangling keys) held at close range work best to produce fixation and following by the child.

Color vision testing

The H-R-R pseudoisochromatic plates are an excellent test series, since they examine for yellow—blue as well as red—green defects and provide a rough quantitative capability. The directions enclosed with this test are explicit and will not be reviewed here. The test is dependent on the child knowing numbers (**22**). There is a form of the Ishihara color test available that utilizes the shapes of a circle and square in place of numbers. These tests do not discriminate *anopes* (total color defectives) from *anomalies* (partial color defectives) but are useful for screening.

Assessment of stereoacuity

Stereoacuity is probably the most fundamental sensory test, widely used in vision screening. Stereoacuity of 60 seconds of arc or better correlates with bifoveal fusion (the ability to use both foveas simultaneously). A score below 67 seconds virtually proves bifoveal fixation that approaches the highest level of stereoacuity.[7]

The Titmus (or stereo Fly) test is used frequently (**23, 24**). The test is sensitive to light and a better score can be obtained by assuring good illumination. The test is also sensitive to the distance maintained from the eyes, which must be respected if accuracy is desired. Allowing the child to touch the test will deface it sooner, but the improved cooperation is well worth the expense of replacement.

Showing the house fly test picture to a 2- to 6-yearold will frequently produce a giggly or frightened response, especially if he has been told he's wearing 'magic' glasses. This can be taken as evidence that the fly appears as three dimensional. Ask the patient to pick up the wings with his fingers. It is also useful to ask the child to place his finger under the wing. As a credibility check, the examiner may turn the book sideways so that the fly cannot be seen stereoscopically (the disparity is now vertical).

A positive response to the larger figures proves at least peripheral fusion (good but not perfect binocular vision). A response below 67 seconds of arc (7, 8, and 9 on the circle test) proves bifoveal fusion. Of course, it would be possible for a patient with bifoveal fixation to test less than 67 seconds by failing to understand the test or becoming bored with it.

An alternative method of testing stereoacuity at near fixation is the Random-dot-E test, manufactured by Stereo Optical Company, Inc. (Chicago, IL). This test is recommended for use in screening for ocular misalignment (see *Table 2*).

Ophthalmoscopy

This part of the eye examination is usually performed last and is not always possible to do. Visualization of the retina and optic nerve with a direct ophthalmoscope or similar device provide useful information. It can be combined with, or substituted for, the red reflex test in older cooperative children.

In addition to or in place of the use of the classic direct ophthalmoscope, the PanOptic ophthalmoscope can be used. This instrument provides a panoramic view of the fundus which is five times larger than that seen with a standard direct ophthalmoscope. The greater working distance between the examiner and the child may result in improved cooperation during this difficult part of the eye exam.

Vision screening

In an ideal world, every child would be seen regularly by an eye doctor trained in the evaluation and treatment of diseases that occur in children. However, this is neither practical nor affordable. Therefore, the ability to screen children effectively for vision problems is important. The American Academy of Pediatrics (AAP) recognizes that the pediatrician plays a vital role in screening children for vision problems. This screening process may use many of the examination techniques discussed previously. The AAP also recognizes that the development and testing of innovative tools to help facilitate vision screening, especially in preverbal or nonverbal children, can lead to increased efficiency and better outcomes. The AAP encourages additional research on all vision screening devices with the ultimate goal of eliminating preventable childhood blindness and treatable visual disability.[8]

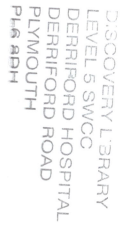

Photoscreening

Photoscreening cameras have become widely available for detecting amblyogenic factors. They have been found to be useful for pediatricians and others interested in screening preverbal children.[4] These cameras typically utilize eccentric flash photorefraction. The most commonly used device (MTI photoscreener) provides an instant two meridian photograph of the retinal reflex on Polaroid film (25).[9] With a properly taken photograph, strabismus, asymmetric and abnormal refractive errors, and media opacities are detected. These cameras may prove useful for mass vision screening programs. Some require ophthalmologists to interpret the photographs. This technology provides an accurate, reliable method of detecting amblyogenic factors in children without pharmacologic pupillary dilation. The major limitation of these cameras is the frequency of off-center fixation (29%), which requires a second photograph to be taken. This becomes less likely as the photographer becomes more experienced in using the camera.

Autorefraction

Autorefractors are also commonly used for preschool vision screening. The Welch Allyn SureSight™ detects and measures abnormal readings automatically in 5 seconds. It is operated at a nonthreatening distance of 14 inches (35 cm). It detects abnormalities in refractive errors such as abnormal amounts of hyperopia, myopia, and astigmatism. It can detect anisometropia or unequal refractive error between the two eyes, which is a common etiology of amblyopia. However, it will not assess ocular alignment. Small angles of strabismus could lead to significant amblyopia.

Visual evoked potential

Pattern-evoked potential (PEVP) testing has demonstrated that infant visual acuity reaches normal levels at 6 months of age.[10] This electrophysiologic test can be used clinically to record and monitor visual acuity in young children. PEVP testing, however, requires sophisticated equipment and specially trained technicians to obtain accurate results.

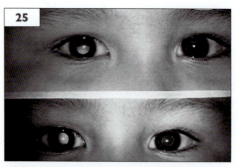

25 Polaroid screening photograph showing asymmetric pupillary reflex in child with anisometropia (unequal refractive errors in the eyes).

Retinopathy of prematurity

David K. Coats, MD and Ashvini Reddy, MD

DEFINITION/OVERVIEW

Retinopathy of prematurity (ROP) is an important cause of potentially preventable blindness in children. It is a vasoproliferative disorder of the retina that primarily affects severely premature infants. Blindness is considered a top priority by the World Health Organization (WHO) for several key reasons. The number of 'blind years' is extraordinarily high for a person blinded in infancy, and is associated with staggering emotional, social, and economic costs to the affected child, the child's family, and society at large. Many causes of blindness in children, including ROP, are either preventable or treatable.[1] Many advancements have taken place in the management of ROP which have led to decreasing rates of blindness in premature children in developed countries. However, as the ability to save premature infants improves in developing countries, many parts of the world are at risk of seeing history repeat itself and the incidence of blindness from this disease increasing.

ETIOLOGY/PATHOPHYSIOLOGY

The first case reports of ROP were described by Theodore L. Terry in 1942.[2] Affected eyes exhibited a grayish-white, opaque membrane behind the crystalline lens. Neonatal care began to significantly evolve in the 1930s and 1940s. Oxygen administration was recognized for its ability to improve the health of premature infants.[3] Unchecked, empiric use of oxygen became common in the mistaken belief that if a little was good, more was better.

An epidemic of ROP, then called retrolental fibroplasia, followed. Silverman estimated that between 1940 and 1953, as many as 10,000 children (7,000 children in the US) were blinded by the disease.[4]

About 10 years later, Campbell[5] helped to characterize the role of oxygen in the pathogenesis of ROP, reporting in a retrospective study that ROP developed at a higher rate in infants who received higher levels of exogenous oxygen. Randomized studies then confirmed this causal relationship,[6,7] though a 'safe' level of inspired oxygen has never been established. Animal experiments subsequently revealed that high levels of systemic oxygen resulted in permanent obliteration of blood vessels in the developing neonatal retina.[8,9]

Several theories regarding the role of oxygen in promoting the development of ROP were subsequently proposed. Choroidal vessels cannot autoregulate under hyperoxic conditions, while retinal blood vessels can autoregulate. Investigators believe that this dichotomy in response to hyperoxia results in excess oxygen diffusion from the choroid to the retina, prompting constriction of retinal blood vessels to the point of irreversible obliteration.[10,11] Oxygen free radicals have also been theorized to overwhelm antioxidant enzymes and other protective mechanisms in the neonate resulting in damage to stem cells, and thus interrupting the process of normal vessel migration and vasculogenesis.[12] Vasoactive cytokines, such as vascular endothelial growth factor (VEGF), are also believed to be important in the pathogenesis of ROP. High supplemental oxygen in animal models results in suppression of VEGF which is thought to produce excessive pruning of retinal vessels.[13] Researchers have also proposed that later hypoxia results in excessive VEGF expression, neovascularization, and the sequelae of ROP.[13] More recently, deficiency of insulin-like growth factor 1 (IGF-1) has been proposed as an instigator of the disease.[14]

After exogenous oxygen administration was recognized as a significant risk factor for ROP, its use was dramatically curtailed in the neonatal population.[15] The rate of blindness in one survey dropped from 7.9 per 100,000 population to 1.2 per 100,000 population between 1950 and 1965.[16] Concurrent with the decline in the rate of ROP, however, there was a substantial increase in the rate of neonatal mortality and serious morbidity,[15,17] including cerebral palsy.[18] Cross calculated the human cost of oxygen restriction to be the death of 16 infants for every case of blindness prevented.[17] Recognizing this dilemma, the use of oxygen was liberalized, but monitored carefully.[19]

The most significant risk factors for serious ROP are low birth weight and young gestational age at birth.[20–22] Many other risk factors that have been inconsistently linked to ROP severity include hypoxia,[23,24] oxygen administration,[23,25] intraventricular hemorrhage,[22,26] surfactant therapy,[27] hypotension,[28] fungemia,[29–31] sepsis,[26] and anemia.[32,33] The overwhelming impact of both low birth weight and prematurity makes establishing the relative contributions of other risk factors difficult. Infants at greatest risk for ROP, and therefore requiring examination for ROP in the neonatal period, include those with a birth weight less than or equal to 1500 g and/or an estimated gestational age of less than or equal to 30 weeks at birth.

PATHOPHYSIOLOGY

The relationship between premature birth, oxygen exposure, and ROP can be explained at a molecular level, but a full appreciation of the pathogenesis of ROP still requires a basic understanding of ocular embryology and anatomy. Retinal vascular development begins at the optic disc at approximately 16 weeks gestation. It then progresses relatively circumferentially anteriorly and is complete by approximately 40 weeks gestation. Thus, the proportion of immature, avascular retina present at birth is directly related to the degree of prematurity. Exposure to excessive concentrations of oxygen during the neonatal period can lead to vascular injury causing arrest of vascular development, obliteration of newly formed capillaries, and clinically visible ROP. The retina is generally well vascularized in a full-term or near-term infant and ROP cannot occur.

Acute ROP progresses in two main conceptual phases. The retinal blood vessels are capable of autoregulation and can respond to increased oxygen tension after birth by constricting.[10,11] Thus, initial postnatal hyperoxia paradoxically leads to regional ischemia of the developing avascular retina. Hyperoxia of the retina also inhibits the release of the vasoactive cytokines, such as VEGF.[24] Later, worsening retinal ischemia triggers the release of vasoactive cytokines in an effort to re-establish normal retinal perfusion. Dysregulation of these vasoactive cytokines can lead to aberrant vascular development and is believed to be responsible for the development of ROP.[24] In the majority of cases, ROP will involute spontaneously with little or no residual retinal damage. Vision loss and even blindness may occur in a small number of infants as a result of contraction of neovascular tissue on the retinal surface, leading to retinal traction and/or detachment.

IGF-1 appears to be a critical oxygen-independent factor in the pathogenesis of ROP. Recent research has shown that serum levels of IGF-1 in premature infants correlate directly with the clinical severity of ROP.[34–37] IGF-1 acts indirectly as a permissive factor by allowing maximal VEGF stimulation of retinal vessel growth. Lack of IGF-1 in preterm infants prevents normal retinal vascular growth in the early stages of ROP, despite the presence of VEGF.[34] As the neonate matures, rising levels of IGF-1 in the later stages of ROP facilitate VEGF-stimulated pathological neovascularization.

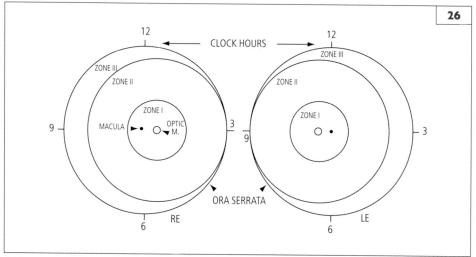

26 Three zones used to classify ROP. (The International Classification of Retinopathy of Prematurity revisited. *Arch Ophthalmol* 2005; **123**(7):991–9. Copyright 2005, American Medical Association. All rights reserved.)

CLINICAL PRESENTATION

ROP can be divided clinically into two phases. In the *acute phase*, the normal process of retinal vascular development is interrupted by the proliferation of abnormal vessels and of fibrous tissue. In the chronic or late proliferation phase of the disease, retinal detachment, macular ectopia, and severe visual loss may occur. ROP is classified according to the International Classification of ROP (ICROP).[12, 38–40] This classification system utilizes retinal landmarks to reduce interexaminer variability and to facilitate communication about disease status among examiners. ROP is classified based on the *zone, stage,* and *extent* of the disease, followed by assessment of the status of the vessels in the posterior pole (known as *plus disease*).

Zone

The zone of ROP refers to the location of disease. Three zones are centered on the optic disc (**26**). The radius of zone I is twice the disk-to-fovea distance in all directions from the optic disk and subtends an angle of 30°. Zone II extends from the edge of zone I peripherally to the nasal ora serrata and continues temporally along the same radius of curvature. Zone III is the residual temporal retina anterior to zone II. In general, the more posterior the ROP, the worse the prognosis. Thus, eyes with zone 1 ROP have the most guarded prognosis.

Stage

The stage of ROP indicates the severity of abnormal vascular changes at the junction of the vascular and avascular retina. The vascularized retina of premature infants without ROP blends almost imperceptibly into the anterior avascularized retina (**27**). When stage 1 ROP develops, the junction between the vascularized and avascularized retina becomes distinct, with the development of a white line (**28**). In stage 1, the clinically visible disease lies within the plane of the retina. In stage 2 ROP, there is elevation of a white ridge above the plane of the retina (**29**). Stage 3 ROP is characterized by the development of extraretinal neovascularization, with fibrovascular tissue extending posteriorly from the ridge into the vitreous (**30**). Isolated tufts of neovascular tissue, referred to as 'popcorn tufts', may lie posterior to the ridge and do not represent stage 3 ROP.

Cicatricial changes in this fibrovascular tissue (stage 3 ROP) may result in partial retinal detachment, referred to as stage 4 ROP. If the partial retinal detachment spares the fovea, the disease is classified as stage 4a ROP. If the partial retinal detachment includes the fovea, it is classified as stage 4b ROP. The visual implications of this distinction are very important, as the fovea contains the photoreceptors responsible for optimal visual acuity. Detachment of the entire retina is termed stage 5 ROP. The staging for an entire eye is reported as the most severe manifestation observed.

Extent

The extent of disease is recorded in 12 sectors or clock hours, each sector subtending an angle of 30°. As the number of clock hours involved increases, the extent of disease is said to be worse and is considered more severe. This is especially true of stage 3 ROP.

Plus disease

The state of the arterioles and venuoles in the posterior aspect of the eye is critically important in determining which eye(s) requires treatment to prevent vision loss from ROP. Normally these vessels exhibit a smooth course toward the ora serrata (the peripheral boundary of the retina) and fall within a typical range of vessel thickness. As the severity of ROP increases, these vessels may become dilated and/or tortuous. Plus disease refers to venous dilation and arterial tortuosity of the vasculature in the posterior pole as defined by a standardized photograph (**31**) demonstrating the minimum amount of vascular dilation and tortuosity required to make a diagnosis of plus disease. These qualifying changes must be present in at least 2 quadrants in the posterior aspect of the eye before the diagnosis of plus disease can be made.

Preplus disease refers to arterial tortuosity and venous engorgement that is outside of normal limits but insufficient to qualify for a diagnosis of plus disease. Progressive vascular disease may also manifest as engorgement of vessels on the iris and may result in pupil rigidity and poor dilation after the administration of dilating drops.

Prior to 2003, ROP that warranted treatment was classified as *threshold* ROP. Threshold ROP, as defined by the Cryo-ROP Study,[41] is characterized by the presence of five or more contiguous or eight cumulative clock hours of extraretinal neovascularization (stage 3 ROP) with plus disease involving zone I or II. *Prethreshold* disease was a term used by early researchers and clinicians to describe a constellation of findings associated with an increased risk of progression to threshold disease.

Both the terms threshold and prethreshold ROP are primarily of historical significance, having been replaced with terms to describe newer treatment parameters. Treatment at threshold was associated with a high rate of unfavorable outcomes. Based on the findings of the Early Treatment of Retinopathy of Prematurity Study (ET-ROP Study),[42] eyes are now considered for treatment when Type I (high-risk prethreshold) ROP is present. Type I ROP is defined as one of the following: (1) zone I ROP, any stage with plus disease; (2) zone I ROP: stage 3, without plus disease; or (3) zone II, stage 2 or 3 with plus disease.

Eyes with Type II ROP (low-risk prethreshold) are considered at increased risk of further progression, and warrant close observation. Eyes with type II ROP often are examined every 2–4 days until the risk of further progression is believed to have declined. Type II ROP is defined as one of the following: (1) zone I, stage 1 or 2 without plus disease, or (2) zone II, stage 3 without plus disease.[43]

Aggressive posterior ROP (or AP-ROP) is a relatively uncommon condition. It is a rapidly progressing and severe form of ROP, formerly

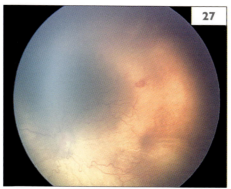

27 Immature retina, without clinically visible ROP. Note the gradual change from vascular to avascular retina.

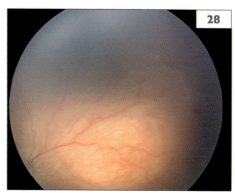

28 Stage I ROP.

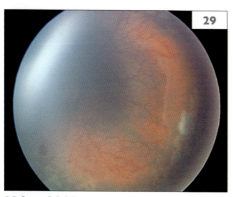

29 Stage 2 ROP.

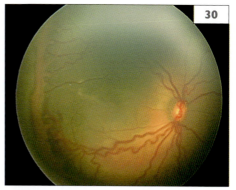

30 Stage 3 ROP.

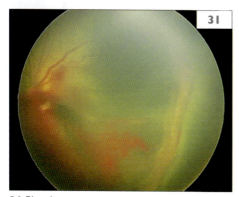

31 Plus disease.

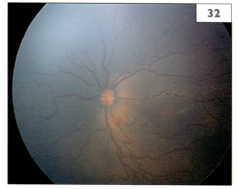

32 Aggressive posterior ROP.

referred to as Rush disease. The hallmarks of the condition are its location in the posterior aspect of the eye (zone I), the presence of plus disease, and ill-defined neovascularization (stage 3 ROP) (**32**). When AP-ROP is present, the posterior pole vessels usually exhibit dilation and tortuosity in all four quadrants. AP-ROP may rapidly progress to stage 5 disease without intervention.

COURSE OF ACUTE PHASE
ROP progression

The timing of retinal disease is more closely linked to postmenstrual age than postnatal age.[41] According to the Cryo-ROP Study,[41] the median postmenstrual ages of onset for stage 1, 2, and 3 disease were 34.3, 35.4, and 36.6 weeks, respectively. Plus disease occurred at a median age of 36.3 weeks. The earliest appearance of prethreshold disease was approximately 26 weeks, of plus disease 31 weeks, and of threshold 31 weeks. Ninety-five percent of all infants who reached threshold did so by 42 weeks postconceptional age. The incidence and severity of ROP were inversely related to birth weight and estimated postmenstrual age.

ROP involution

Acute ROP generally begins to involute at a mean of 38.6 weeks postmenstrual age and 90% of eyes demonstrate onset of involution before 44 weeks postmenstrual age.[44] Flynn and coworkers[45] reported that ROP will last an average of 15 weeks from inception to resolution in eyes that regress.

Whereas involution occurs safely and predictably in the majority of treated and untreated eyes, it can be marked by the development of detrimental vitreoretinal abnormalities resulting in permanent retinal damage, including retinal detachment and blindness. Remnant myofibroblasts in the vitreous may contract for up to 4 months following treatment of ROP,[46] increasing the risk of tractional retinal detachment.[47] Extensive fibrous-appearing organization of the vitreous above the retina and severe vitreous hemorrhage are associated with the development of retinal detachments in eyes treated at threshold.[48] Full involution does not typically occur in most eyes until 2 or more weeks after laser intervention.[48]

DIAGNOSIS

An effective screening program identifies the small number of neonates who require treatment for ROP within a much larger population of at-risk infants[37,48,49] while simultaneously conserving resources and minimizing the number of stressful (and potentially even harmful) examinations required to diagnose vision-threatening ROP.

The screening and treatment guidelines that follow were adapted from a recent consensus statement.[49] The sensitivity of these guidelines in detecting ROP before ROP becomes severe enough to produce a retinal detachment is predicted to be 99% in US institutions.

Infants requiring examination

Infants with a birth weight of less than 1500 g or estimated gestational age (EGA) of 30 weeks or less require examination. Selected infants with a birth weight between 1500 g and 2000 g or EGA of more than 30 weeks who have had an unstable clinical course and who are believed to be at high risk by their neonatologist also should be examined. A single examination by an ophthalmologist skilled in the examination of infants at risk for ROP is only sufficient if the examination unequivocally shows the retina to be fully vascularized in both eyes.

Timing of examinations

Because the onset of serious ROP correlates more closely with postmenstrual age than postnatal age (that is, the youngest infants at birth take the longest time to develop serious ROP), the timing of the first examination should be based on the gestational age at birth. The suggested minimum timing for initial examination is reviewed in *Table 3*. Limited data are available to support these timing guidelines on the most premature babies, such as those born at 23–24 weeks EGA. Follow-up examinations should be scheduled based on examination findings and risks as assessed by the examining ophthalmologist.

MANAGEMENT/TREATMENT

Treatment should be considered for eyes with Type I ROP if the examining ophthalmologist believes treatment is warranted. The decision to withhold treatment despite the presence of Type I ROP is based on clinical judgment after assessing a variety of issues including severity of disease, postmenstrual age, progression of the disease, and other factors. Treatment may also be warranted in situations not prescribed by standard recommendations, and such treatment must be considered on a case-by-case basis.

Cessation of examinations

Cessation of examinations by the ophthalmologist should be based on postmenstrual age

Table 3 Suggested timing of first ROP examination based on estimated gestational age. Note that the guideline for 22 and 23 weeks is considered tentative and not evidence based because of the small number of survivors in these groups

Gestational age at birth (weeks)	Age at initial examination (postmenstrual) (weeks)	Age at initial examination (chronologic) (weeks)
22	31	9
23	31	8
24	31	7
25	31	6
26	31	5
27	31	4
28	32	4
29	33	4
30	34	4
31	35	4
32	36	4

and retinal ophthalmoscopic findings. Findings that suggest examinations can be curtailed include the following: (1) retinal vascularization into zone III without previous zone I or II ROP (in infants with a postmenstrual age of less than 35 weeks, confirmatory examinations are usually warranted since vascularization into zone III is unusual prior to 36 weeks postmenstrual age); (2) full retinal vascularization; (3) postmenstrual age of 45 weeks and no prethreshold disease or worse ROP is present; and (4) regression of ROP, and absence of abnormal vascular tissue that is capable of reactivation and progression. Examinations must continue for at-risk infants even after discharge from the hospital and this should be made clear to the parents of an affected infant, as they often do not follow through with follow-up appointments during the critical examination window.[50] Because timing of examination for ROP may have a significant impact on outcome, it is often optimal for the neonatal unit staff to schedule the first outpatient appointment within the recommended time frame (see below).

Optimally, the responsibility for examination and follow-up of infants at risk of ROP should be defined by the neonatal care unit. Appropriate follow-up care must be available if hospital discharge or transfer is planned while the infant is still at risk for serious ROP. The transferring primary physician generally has the responsibility of communicating eye-care needs to the accepting physician at the time of transfer. If responsibility for arranging follow-up is to be delegated to the parents at the time of discharge, parents should be aware of the fact that there is a critical time window for evaluation and treatment.

Neonatologists and pediatricians caring for a premature infant should be aware of the child's risk for ROP and they should be kept informed by the examining ophthalmologist through appropriate documentation in the medical record. Parents should also be kept informed and optimally should have some understanding of ROP and its potential to impact on their child. Communications methods that have been found to be helpful include prepared written information about ROP, individual examination reports, lectures, bedside communication, and telephone updates. Documentation of such conversations and communication with parents is desirable, when possible, to minimize miscommunication and medicolegal disputes.

Treatment for acute phase disease
Fortunately most neonates who develop ROP undergo spontaneous regression. Intervention to reduce the risk of disease progression is required in advanced cases. Treatment is

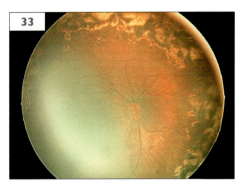

33 Appearance of the retina after diode laser photocoagulation for ROP.

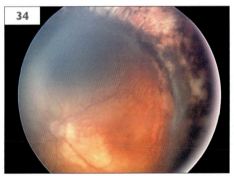

34 Fibrous-appearing organization of the vitreous in ROP.

generally considered for eyes with Type I ROP. Treatment should generally be accomplished within 72 hours of the time that a recommendation for treatment is made to reduce the risk of development of retinal detachment and vision loss. More urgent treatment may be warranted in some situations, such as the presence of aggressive posterior ROP.

Transpupillary laser photocoagulation delivered through an indirect ophthalmoscope is now the most commonly used treatment modality.[51] Diode or argon laser may be used to treat the entire peripheral avascular retina, though argon laser may be associated with an increased incidence of cataracts.[52,53] Photocoagulation destroys the peripheral avascular retina responsible for increased cytokine production, thereby reducing the stimulus for neovascularization and the subsequent risk of retinal detachment (**33**). The optimal setting for treatment depends on several factors including the health of the infant and the preferences of the neonatologist and treating ophthalmologist. Treatment can be accomplished in the intensive care unit or operating room and under sedation, retrobulbar anesthesia, or general anesthesia.[37]

Involution and monitoring of infants after treatment

No official recommendations exist to guide the postoperative management of eyes that have been treated for ROP. Practitioners depend on training and experience to guide postoperative care. In a study on ROP involution following treatment of threshold ROP, Coats and coworkers[20] reported that complete involution occurred in the majority of eyes within 3 weeks of laser treatment and all eyes had fully involuted or developed a retinal detachment by 9 +/− 3 weeks after treatment. Retinal detachments typically were not diagnosed until several weeks after treatment, suggesting the need for close and frequent follow-up after treatment. Eyes most likely to develop a retinal detachment in this study included eyes with zone I disease, marked vitreous organization, and marked vitreous hemorrhage[20,48] (**34**).

Treatment of retinal detachments (stages 4 and 5 ROP)

There are few controlled scientific data available to guide management of retinal detachments. Physicians rely in large part on experience and clinical judgment to gauge the need for surgical intervention in patients who develop or who are considered at high risk for the development of a retinal detachment. Because of the universally poor outcomes associated with stages 4a and 5 retinal detachments,[54] most vitreoretinal surgeons who are experienced in the treatment of late-stage ROP advocate treatment of stage 4a retinal detachments in selected eyes. Anatomical outcomes for treatment of stage 4a retinal detachments are generally good, and surgery at this stage is believed to reduce the risk of progression.[55]

Treatment of retinal detachments is accomplished through the use of a scleral buckle and/or a vitrectomy. A vitrectomy, the most common approach to the treatment of ROP-related retinal detachments, involves surgical removal of the vitreous. The goal of treatment is to release tractional forces on the retina that are emanating in the vitreous. Release of these tractional forces can limit progression of the detachment and can permit re-attachment of the retina. The lens of the eye is not disturbed during the procedure, if possible (lens-sparing vitrectomy). Unfortunately, the detachment profile sometimes requires removal of the crystalline lens of the eye. This results in more complex long-term management issues and a poorer visual prognosis. A scleral buckle procedure involves placement of an encircling silicone band around the globe. As this band is tightened, the force of vitreous tractional elements on the retina is relieved.

When lens-sparing vitrectomy with or without concurrent scleral buckling is preformed for a stage 4a retinal detachment, it has been shown to result in nonprogression of retinal detachments beyond stage 4a in up to 90% of eyes.[55] Visual outcomes can be good with one study reporting a mean visual acuity of 20/58 (range 20/200 to 20/20).[56] Early vitrectomy has recently been reported as an effective means for preventing retinal detachment in aggressive posterior ROP.[57]

Telemedicine
Imaging technologies are evolving rapidly to allow telemedicine to play an increasingly important role in the management of ROP in the future. Telemedicine has the potential to impact on the delivery, quality, and accessibility of ophthalmic care for infants with ROP, especially in communities where ophthalmologists may be unwilling or unable to manage ROP secondary to medicolegal risk (see below). Before image-based screening can be implemented on a large scale, clinical standards, diagnostic accuracy, sensitivity/specificity profiles, and reliability must be established.

PROGNOSIS
Even timely treatment of Type I ROP does not guarantee a favorable outcome. The ETROP study reported an unfavorable structural outcome in 9.0% of eyes treated at high-risk prethreshold compared with 15.6% of eyes managed conventionally.[43] The rate of unfavorable visual outcome in eyes treated at prethreshold in the ETROP study was 19.8%.[43] Infants who have been treated for ROP may be

at a lifelong increased risk of later retinal detachment and require ongoing care.[58]

Comorbidities
An infant treated for ROP can have an excellent anatomical outcome but still have severe visual impairment or even blindness without developing a retinal detachment. The fact that other factors can lead to poor vision in premature infants is underscored by the fact that visual outcomes are less favorable than structural outcomes. These factors include optic atrophy, cortical (cerebral) visual impairment, and subclinical retinal abnormalities.

Infants treated for ROP and infants who developed serious ROP that involuted spontaneously (not requiring treatment) are also at risk for comorbidities, though the risk is significantly lower in treated infants. These comorbidities include, but are not limited to, high myopia (nearsightedness), strabismus (ocular misalignment), contrast sensitivity, and amblyopia.[59,60] Potential comorbidities associated with more severe ROP may include macular dragging producing pseudoexotropia, cataract, and glaucoma.

PREVENTION
ROP was not described until the advent of technologies that permitted the survival of preterm infants with immature retinas. The disease does not occur when the retina is allowed to develop *in utero* under normal physiologic conditions. For this reason, the most effective means of decreasing the incidence of disease is to prevent premature birth itself. Currently, there is no method to absolutely prevent the development and progression of disease in the youngest preterm infants and no means to predict with certainty which infants will fare better than others, though management options are continuously being explored in several clinical and laboratory trials.

Antioxidant therapy
Antioxidant therapy with vitamins E,[61–63] A,[64] and D-penicillamine[65] has been studied based on the theory that reducing oxygen free radical damage may prevent or treat ROP. Each has shown some potential but concerns over side-effects and efficacy have generally limited their use.

Exogenous oxygen curtailment

Control of exogenous oxygen administration to maintain oxygen saturation at a level between 88 and 93% has been shown to minimize the risk of lung injury caused by exposure to excessive oxygen concentrations.[65–68] The incidental finding of a reduced incidence of severe ROP in these studies has led many to recommend oxygen restriction as a means of mitigating the development of severe ROP.[68–70]

Vasoactive cytokines

Localized inhibition of VEGF has been shown to inhibit pathologic retinal neovascularization without adversely affecting pre-existing retinal vessels in rodent models of ROP.[71] Anecdotal use of the VEGF inhibitor bevacizumab has been reported in the treatment of infants with ROP. Though these reports have been generally favorable, widespread, uncontrolled use of these therapies is discouraged until further studies establish both safety and efficacy. The upcoming prospective, multicenter BLOCK-ROP trial will explore the utility of the anti-VEGF drug bevacizumab as local therapy for severe ROP not responsive to laser ablation.

Medicolegal considerations

Medicolegal risk to those who examine and treat ROP is high.[72] It remains a fact that despite significant advances in both the diagnosis and management of severe ROP, infants can and still do suffer severe visual complications and even blindness as a result of ROP. This can occur in spite of an optimal screening program, an experienced examiner, optimal diagnosis and expert treatment. An unfavorable structural outcome can be expected to occur in as many as 9% of eyes treated at high-risk prethreshold, according to the ETROP study.[43]

Parents of premature infants are often unrealistic both in their understanding of their child's medical condition and their expectations regarding outcomes. Parental understanding of ROP and expectations of treatment can be similarly unrealistic. Despite frequent communication with parents about the seriousness of the disease and the risks involved, parents are often surprised when an unfavorable outcome occurs. Surprise over an unfavorable outcome, other medical comorbidities, family dynamics, and the financial stress of caring for a disabled child can be overwhelming. Sympathy elicited by a blind, disabled child may be enough to interest a plaintiff attorney in the pursuit of medicolegal action, even in a properly managed case.

When a medicolegal claim is filed, defendants often include the examining and treating ophthalmologist, the neonatologist, and the hospital. If the infant has been discharged from the hospital, the pediatrician may also be named as a defendant. Misguided and even frankly unethical physicians are sometimes willing to support claims of medical malpractice in these situations, an unfortunate reality that has contributed to the gradual attrition of ophthalmologists willing to remain or become involved in the care of premature infants. Medicolegal risks can be mitigated through training, experience, general adherence to formal ROP screening and treatment guidelines (with documented justification for deviations), and ongoing communication with parents of at-risk infants.

CONCLUSIONS

ROP remains a leading cause of severe visual impairment and blindness in developed countries.[73] Advances in the classification, diagnosis, and treatment of the disease have improved the prognosis for most affected infants. Despite this, approximately 9% of infants who undergo timely treatment for ROP will develop retinal abnormalities associated with an unfavorable outcome and legal blindness. A well-developed screening protocol is crucial in reducing the risk of blindness due to a delayed or omitted examination. Telemedicine may play an increasing role in the management of ROP. Curtailment of exogenous oxygen and therapy to block vasoactive cytokines may result in further advances in the prognosis of ROP.

Amblyopia

Robert W. Arnold, MD, Scott E. Olitsky, MD, and David K. Coats, MD

DEFINITION/OVERVIEW

Amblyopia is derived from Greek and means 'dullness of vision'. Amblyopia is a unilateral or, less commonly, bilateral reduction of best-corrected visual acuity that cannot be attributed solely to the effect of a structural abnormality of the eye or the posterior visual pathways. It is caused by abnormal visual experience early in life. Ophthalmologic examination of the eye typically reveals no organic abnormality. In most cases it is reversible by therapeutic measures.[1]

EPIDEMIOLOGY/ETIOLOGY

The prevalence of amblyopia in the US is estimated to be between 1% and 3%.[2–4] Prevalence rates for amblyopia are higher in developing countries.[5] The National Eye Institute has reported that amblyopia is the most common cause of unilateral visual loss in patients under the age of 70 years in the US.[6] The mean age at presentation of amblyopia varies depending on its cause.[7,8] Patients with strabismus and amblyopia are more likely to present at an early age than are patients with straight eyes. The upper age limit for the development of amblyopia in children who are exposed to an amblyopia-inducing condition (e.g. traumatic cataract) has been reported to be 6–10 years.[9]

Social and psychosocial factors

Detection and treatment of amblyopia are important for a variety of reasons. Affected patients may have reduced vocational and socioeconomic opportunities because normal vision in both eyes is required for many jobs.[10] Individuals with amblyopia are at increased risk for loss of vision and blindness in the nonamblyopic eye.[11,12] The projected lifetime risk of vision loss in the fellow eye has been estimated to be 1.2%.[11] The risk of bilateral visual impairment in patients with amblyopia is greater than twice that of patients without amblyopia.[13] Amblyopia leads to a reduction in binocularity which may lead to the development of strabismus, if not already present.

Psychosocial implications are important to patients who suffer from amblyopia. Significant psychosocial stress related to amblyopia therapy has been reported by amblyopic children and the families of amblyopic children during the treatment period.[14,15] Even adults with a history of amblyopia treatment in childhood continue to have psychosocial difficulties related to the previous amblyopia therapy that can adversely affect self-image, work, education, and friendships.[16]

Amblyopia treatment is cost efficient.[17] The care of children with poor vision secondary to amblyopia may be one of the most economically productive treatments for any vision disorder.

Visual development

During fetal development, differentiation and organization of the visual system are likely guided by intrinsic control mechanisms. At birth, the process is not complete and must continue to develop throughout the first decade of life. Environmental factors and visual experience influence the process in postnatal life. For normal visual development to occur, both eyes must be presented with equally clear and similar images.[18] This constant stimulation is crucial to the development of normal vision. Any factor that interferes with this process can lead to the development of amblyopia.[19] The human visual system is sensitive to the effects of depriving vision only during a limited period of time in childhood. This time period is often called the sensitive or critical period. For humans, this period extends roughly from birth through the end of the first decade of life.[9,20] Vulnerability is greatest during the first few months of life and thereafter gradually decreases.

Classification of amblyopia

Amblyopia is often defined as a difference in visual acuity of two lines or more (Snellen or equivalent) in a child with an otherwise healthy visual system. In reality, amblyopia may be present any time visual acuity is reduced, even if the difference is one line or less. Amblyopia may also occur in association with organic defects of the eye or elsewhere in the visual system (see Organic amblyopia). Amblyopia is most commonly characterized by clinical associations which initiate the problem. Therefore, amblyopia is most often classified based upon the causal mechanism. Familiarity with this classification system is important for clinicians and can be useful in designing and implementing appropriate treatment strategies.

Strabismic amblyopia

Strabismic amblyopia is one of the most common forms of amblyopia. It results from abnormal binocular interaction that occurs when the visual axes of the two eyes are misaligned and the patient develops a preference for one eye. Amblyopia generally does not develop if the patient alternates the use of each eye throughout the day. This abnormal interaction causes the eyes to be presented with different images. Disparate input from the deviating eye stimulates active inhibition of the complex cortical pathways originating in the normal eye. A decrease in the function of these pathways can then lead to the development of amblyopia.

Surgery to correct the strabismus is generally considered ineffective in the treatment of associated strabismic amblyopia. Strabismus surgery is generally deferred until the amblyopia has been maximally treated.[21] This practice allows easier monitoring of amblyopia treatment in preverbal children and helps to encourage parents to comply with the sometimes difficult task of amblyopia therapy. Many strabismus surgeons worry that parents may incorrectly determine that their child's eye problem has been completely treated once the eyes are surgically aligned.

Anisometropic amblyopia

Anisometropia is another frequent cause of amblyopia. Anisometropia refers to the condition in which the need for glasses differs significantly between the two eyes. Anisometropic amblyopia may occur in children with hyperopia (farsightedness), myopia (nearsightedness), or astigmatism (uneven curvature of the cornea).

In contrast to the other types of amblyopia, anisometropic amblyopia may not be detected until the child is old enough to undergo vision screening performed by a pediatrician or school system. The typical child with anisometropic amblyopia lacks obvious external abnormalities of the eyes (e.g. cataracts, strabismus), and visual function appears normal because the child sees well with the fellow eye. It is in these patients that photoscreening may be especially useful in order to detect amblyopia earlier than may otherwise be possible.

Ametropic amblyopia

Severe symmetric refractive error (isoametropia) may cause bilateral amblyopia of mild to moderate degree. Excessive hyperopia is most likely to cause this type of amblyopia. Myopia, even when present at very high levels, rarely causes bilateral amblyopia because the sharply focused images of objects held close to the eyes support normal visual development. Patients with high degrees of hyperopia or astigmatism may show less reduction in their vision and therefore may not be discovered until they undergo some form of screening or testing.

Visual-deprivation amblyopia

Deprivation amblyopia is the least common and most serious form of amblyopia. Visual deprivation is caused by occlusion of the visual axis. Congenital cataracts, ptosis, congenital corneal opacities, and vitreous hemorrhage may lead to deprivation amblyopia. Even temporary obstruction of the visual axis, such as that caused by a hyphema or temporary eyelid edema in a very young child, can produce visual-deprivation amblyopia. Visual-deprivation amblyopia can be unilateral or bilateral. Amblyopia is more likely to occur, be more severe and be more resistant to treatment when the defect promoting its development is unilateral.

Organic amblyopia

Although amblyopia generally occurs in an otherwise normal eye, it can sometimes be superimposed on visual loss directly caused by a structural abnormality of the eye such as optic nerve hypoplasia, coloboma, or a partial cataract.[22] When such a situation ('organic amblyopia') is encountered in a young child it is appropriate to undertake a trial of amblyopia therapy. The attempted treatment can be both diagnostic and therapeutic in doubtful or borderline cases. Improvement in vision confirms that amblyopia was indeed present.

PATHOPHYSIOLOGY

The mechanism and pathogenesis of amblyopia have been topics of intense interest and research. However, the question of the exact location of the disturbance within the visual system responsible for ultimately producing amblyopia still remains unanswered today.

Laboratory research has collected a large volume of information concerning the effects of abnormal visual experience on the immature nervous system through the study of animals placed under various experimental conditions. These studies include the Nobel Prize-winning work of Hubel and Wiesel in the 1960s. Animals, like humans, are vulnerable to the effects of abnormal visual experience only for a limited period of time early in life. The similarities between human amblyopia and the abnormalities induced by differing forms of visual deprivation in animals have allowed conclusions to be drawn concerning the former from data provided by the latter.

Amblyopia is associated with histologic and electrophysiologic abnormalities in the visual pathways. Hubel and Wiesel pioneered methods of studying the effects of changing visual experience in kittens by suturing an eyelid closed.[23] Similar findings have been found in a primate model.[24] Anatomic studies of animals who have had one lid sutured closed indicate that the cortical regions that receive axon terminals from geniculocortical neurons driven by the affected eye contract, while the regions receiving input from the normally experienced eye expand in comparison with normal brains.[25] The lack of cortical responsiveness to a unilaterally deprived eye seems to result not only from loss of synaptic connections, but also from an ongoing process of inhibition that is dependent on input from the normal eye and may be mediated through the neurotransmitter gamma aminobutyric acid (GABA).[26]

CLINICAL PRESENTATION

While it is most often detected, and even defined, by demonstrating a reduction in visual acuity, amblyopia leads to other defects in vision, including changes in contrast sensitivity and abnormalities in the visual field. The full range of abnormalities present in the amblyopic eye is probably not yet fully understood. They may have important clinical applications. Some of these abnormalities may be useful in detecting amblyopia or determining its cause.

Visual acuity

Amblyopic patients are deficient in their ability to *resolve* closely spaced contours and *recognize* the patterns they form. Measurement of visual acuity is therefore the primary manner in which amblyopia is detected. Children old enough to identify letters are usually tested with standard letter optotypes, either projected, wall mounted, or computer generated (**35**). For the less verbal child, testing may be modified to permit the use of manual pointing responses.

Currently, the nonverbal Snellen equivalents most widely used in North America are the tumbling E test and the HOTV test (**36**). For most 3-year-olds and nearly all developmentally normal 4-year-olds, fairly reliable visual acuity measurements can be obtained with either of these tests after a minute or two of instruction (and confirmation of the patient's competence in responding) using large demonstration letters. An advantage of the HOTV test is that there is no need to discriminate left/right mirror image figures, which may be difficult for the young patient.

Various acuity tests have been devised that substitute pictures for letters. These include Allen pictures and Lea symbols (**37**). They have been carefully calibrated and assessed for reliability.[27] Some small children who will not point to identify letters respond well to testing with these figures. Lack of familiarity with the pictured objects or inability to recognize the stylized images may be a problem for some children; testing should begin with a review of the cards up close, and any that are not readily identified should be eliminated (three or four remaining different pictures are sufficient for testing).

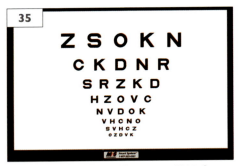

35 Snellen acuity chart. (Courtesy of M & S Technologies, Inc.)

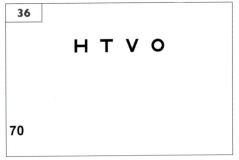

36 HOTV acuity chart. (Courtesy of M & S Technologies, Inc.)

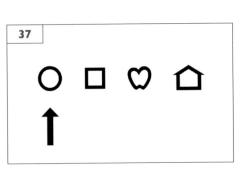

37 Lea symbols. (Courtesy of M & S Technologies, Inc.)

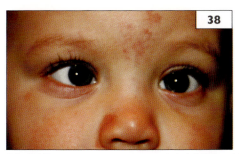
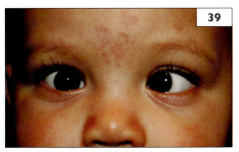

38, 39 Fixation testing in a preverbal child. The child is fixating with the left eye (**38**). Following occlusion of the left eye, the child holds fixation with the right eye (**39**) demonstrating good vision in each eye.

DIAGNOSIS

Amblyopia is optimally treated earlier in life, but can be effectively treated later in life. Screening programs designed to detect visual system anomalies in preschool and elementary school-aged children are commonplace. Screening is most commonly done in the primary care physician's office and/or at school. It is typically done by lay screeners or by nurse screeners, with each achieving similar success in detecting children in need of comprehensive examination.[28]

Parents also play a key role in amblyopia detection. Detection of obvious abnormalities capable of producing amblyopia, such as strabismus and dense cataracts, are typically easily detected by parents prompting formal ophthalmologic evaluation.

Vision assessment techniques vary depending on the age and abilities of the individual child. In preliterate children, techniques that assess visual behavior are utilized, while in older and literate children, psychophysical (quantitative) recognition testing of visual acuity is usually possible.

Visual behavior assessment

Assessment of visual behavior is a key element in the diagnosis of amblyopia in preliterate children. Initial assessment generally includes evaluation of the child's ability to fixate on and follow a visual target, such as the examiner's face or a small toy. A child who exhibits eager fixation and following behavior with one eye but fails to do so with the fellow eye most often has reduced vision in the poorly performing eye. Obvious abnormalities in fixation and following behavior are usually not present unless relatively pronounced visual impairment is present. Inequality of fixation and following behavior between the eyes does not necessarily indicate the presence of amblyopia, but instead may simply indicate the presence of an uncorrected refractive error or other easily remedied problem. It is, however, highly suspicious of amblyopia in a young child.

Fixation preference testing is another commonly used method for identifying amblyopia. The test is easiest to perform in a strabismic patient. The examiner attempts to determine if the child is able to maintain fixation with each eye sequentially. This is most easily accomplished by occluding the fixating eye until the deviating eye fixates on the visual target. The eyes are then observed upon removal of the occluder with several possible responses. Vision can be considered relatively symmetric in each eye if the child maintains fixation with the formerly nonfixating eye (**38, 39**). The formerly nonfixating eye can be considered to have amblyopia (or an amblyopiogenic risk factor) if upon removal of the cover the child immediately returns to fixating with the fellow eye.

Visual acuity assessment

Visual acuity testing should begin as early in life as practical. A child as young as 2 years of age

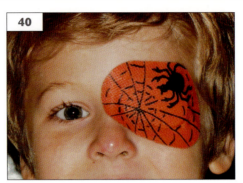

40 Adhesive patch used for occlusion therapy in the treatment of amblyopia.

can occasionally participate in recognition acuity testing while the majority of 3-year-old children can participate in formal visual acuity testing, using optotypes such as Snellen letters, Lea pictures, tumbling E, HOTV, and Allen figures.

A difference in best-corrected visual acuity difference of two lines between fellow eyes (e.g. 6/6 in the left eye and 6/9 in the right eye) is clinically indicative of amblyopia, and is usually associated with the presence of an identifiable amblyopiogenic risk factor such as strabismus, anisometropia, or obstruction of the visual axis.

Younger children often do not achieve a visual acuity of 6/6 during standard clinical testing, due presumably to the young child's inability to fully and optimally participate in the testing process. In the absence of pathology, children younger than 3–4 years old can be considered to have normal vision if their visual acuity is equal and in the range of 6/12 or better.

MANAGEMENT/TREATMENT

The management of patients with amblyopia is less straightforward than the preceding discussions of etiology and diagnosis might imply. In reality children can be difficult to evaluate, and can be inconsistent in their responses during clinical testing. Furthermore, compliance with treatment recommendations is often suboptimal.

The goal of amblyopia treatment is the achievement of the maximum visual acuity and visual function possible for an individual patient. Treatment consists of eliminating any identifiable causes of amblyopia as an initial step.

Elimination of factors obstructing the visual axis, such as cataracts and ptosis, is critical for patients with deprivational amblyopia. Other steps include correction of significant refractive errors, and encouraging use of and development of vision in the amblyopic eye through occlusion therapy and/or penalization.

Optical correction

Correction of significant refractive errors is important to ensure that a clear image is focused onto the fovea of each eye. Without this prerequisite step, other measures are likely to be less successful or even unsuccessful. Anisometropic amblyopia frequently responds to refractive correction alone without the need to institute occlusion or penalization therapy.[29–31] Other treatment measures may be initiated at the same time or only if residual amblyopia remains after correction of refractive error.

Occlusion therapy

Occlusion therapy remains a mainstay of amblyopia. It is preferred by many ophthalmologists because it lacks systemic side-effects, is effective, and is inexpensive. Occlusion is typically accomplished by placement of an adhesive patch directly over the sound eye or use of a patch that fits over the spectacle lens (**40**). Several commercially available patches have been devised that fit over the front of the spectacle lens and contain side shields to produce optimal occlusion. These patches are often better tolerated by spectacle-wearing amblyopes, especially in hot, humid climates.

During the time of occlusion, the sound eye is deprived of form vision, requiring the patient to fixate with the amblyopic eye.

Penalization

Penalization refers to a series of techniques used to diminish the vision of the sound eye temporarily, thereby encouraging use of the amblyopic eye. Penalization can be accomplished through pharmacologic means, through optical blur, or both, and can result in long-term improvement in visual acuity of the amblyopic eye.[32,33]

Pharmologic penalization

Pharmacologic penalization is most commonly accomplished through the instillation of cycloplegic ophthalmic preparations into the sound eye. Atropine 0.5–1% drops are probably most commonly used, but homatropine, scopolamine (hyoscine), and cyclopentolate are preferred by some clinicians. Each of these topical anticholinergic agents results in temporary significant reduction of accommodation. Reduction in ability to accommodate reduces the ability of the sound eye to fixate, thereby providing some incentive to utilize the amblyopic eye.

Optical penalization

Optical penalization involves altering the spectacle or contact lens correction of the sound eye to produce image blur, providing incentive to fixate with the amblyopic eye. Optical penalization may be used alone, or more typically, in combination with pharmacologic penalization. The disadvantage to isolated optical penalization utilizing a fogging lens is that children often avoid the undesired spectacle blur by simply removing or looking over their spectacles in many cases.

Long-term follow-up

Children with amblyopia require ongoing care. In general, younger children should be seen more frequently than older children during the treatment phase of amblyopia. A common follow-up recommendation is that children should be seen at least every 2–4 months during active treatment, though there are no scientific data to support these recommendations. Active treatment for 6–12 months may be required. While most children will achieve resolution of their amblyopia during this period of treatment, some may continue to respond to treatment for a prolonged period of time. Treatment should continue until progress has stalled, and reasonable treatment alternatives have been exhausted. Periodic follow-up thereafter is important because of the potential for amblyopia recurrence.

Nonresponders

The vast majority of children with anisometropic and/or strabismic amblyopia will respond favorably to standard treatment measures. When a child fails to show the expected favorable treatment response, the clinician should inquire about compliance. If compliance with the ongoing treatment regimen is poor or unclear, a change in treatment should be considered and the family counseled about the importance of compliance. Additionally, the clinician should consider reassessment of the child's eyes to ensure that the child's refractive correction is accurate, and that an organic cause of visual impairment is not present.

Older children and teenagers

Classic teaching has been that amblyopia cannot be treated effectively after the first decade of life. Several studies have reported anectodotal experience in the successful treatment of anisometropic amblyopia in older children and teenagers. A recent prospective, randomized study evaluated the effectiveness of treatment of anisometropic and/or strabismic amblyopia in children ages 7 years to <18 years of age.[34] The study concluded that older children often responded favorably to treatment. Those without a history of prior treatment were most likely to respond.

Strabismus disorders

Scott E. Olitsky, MD and Leonard B. Nelson, MD

- **Strabismus**

- **Comitant strabismus**
  Congenital esotropia
  Accommodative esotropia
  Congenital exotropia
  Intermittent exotropia

- **Incomitant strabismus**
  Third cranial nerve palsy
  Fourth nerve palsy
  Sixth nerve palsy

- **Strabismus syndromes**
  Duane's syndrome
  Brown's syndrome
  Monocular elevation deficiency (MED)
  Möbius syndrome

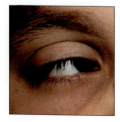
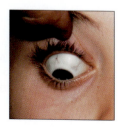
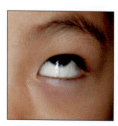
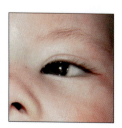

Strabismus

DEFINITION/OVERVIEW

Strabismus denotes a misalignment of the eyes. It is one of the most common eye problems encountered in children, affecting approximately 4% of children younger than 6 years of age. Strabismus can result in vision loss (amblyopia) and can have important and lifelong psychological effects. Early detection and treatment of strabismus are vital to prevent permanent visual impairment. In order to provide the best opportunity for children with strabismus to develop normal binocular vision, alignment of the visual axes must occur at an early stage of visual development. Several terms are used in characterizing the various forms of strabismus and are important in understanding its etiology, treatment, and prognosis.

Orthophoria is the ideal condition of exact ocular balance. It defines that state when the oculomotor apparatus is in perfect equilibrium so that the eyes remain coordinated and perfectly aligned. Even when binocular vision is interrupted, as by occlusion of one eye, truly orthophoric individuals maintain straight eyes. True orthophoria is uncommon, the majority of individuals have a small latent deviation (heterophoria).

Heterophoria is a latent tendency for the eyes to deviate. The latent deviation is normally controlled by fusional mechanisms that provide binocular vision or avoid diplopia (double vision). The eyes deviate only under certain conditions, such as fatigue, illness, stress, or during tests that interfere with maintenance of these normal fusional controls (such as covering one eye). If the amount of heterophoria is large, it may give rise to bothersome symptoms, such as intermittent diplopia, headaches, or asthenopia (eyestrain). Some degree of heterophoria is found in the majority of normal individuals; it is usually asymptomatic.

Heterotropia is a misalignment of the eyes that is constant. It occurs because of an inability of the fusional mechanisms to control the deviation. Tropias can be alternating, involving both eyes, or unilateral. In an alternating tropia, there is no preference for fixation of either eye, and both eyes drift with equal frequency. Because each eye is used periodically, vision in each eye usually develops normally although binocular vision will not. A unilateral tropia is a serious situation because only one eye is constantly misaligned. The undeviated or 'fixating' eye becomes the preferred eye, resulting in loss of vision or amblyopia of the deviated eye.

It is also necessary to describe the type of deviation that is present. The prefixes eso-, exo-, hyper-, and hypo- are added to the terms phoria and tropia to further delineate the type of strabismus. *Esophorias* and *esotropias* are inward or convergent deviations of the eyes, commonly known as crossed eyes. *Exophorias* and *exotropias* are divergent or outward-turning deviations, walleyed being the lay term. *Hyperdeviations* and *hypodeviations* designate upward or downward deviations of an eye. In cases where only one eye is seen to be misaligned, the deviating eye is often part of the description of the misalignment (left esotropia).

Ocular deviations may be constant in all fields of gaze or they may change depending on where the patient is looking. This characteristic of a strabismus describes its '*comitancy*'. A comitant strabismus does not change with movement of the eyes into different gazes whereas an incomitant strabismus does. Detecting the presence of an incomitant strabismus can be extremely important. Many forms of incomitant strabismus may be neurologic in nature and demand urgent evaluation, especially if they are of acute onset. It is customary to divide strabismus disorders into comitant and incomitant forms as will be done in this chapter.

DIAGNOSIS

Many techniques are used to assess ocular alignment and movement of the eyes to aid in evaluating and diagnosing strabismic disorders. In a child with strabismus, as with any ocular disorder, assessment of visual acuity is essential. Decreased vision in one eye requires evaluation for a strabismus or other ocular abnormalities, which may be difficult to discern on a brief screening evaluation. Strabismic deviations of only a few degrees in magnitude, too small to be evident by gross inspection, may lead to amblyopia and devastating vision loss.

Corneal light reflex testing is perhaps the most rapid and easiest performed diagnostic test for strabismus. It is especially useful in children who are uncooperative and in those who have poor ocular fixation. The Hirschberg corneal reflex test is performed by projecting a light source onto the cornea of both eyes simultaneously as a child looks directly at the light. Comparison should then be made of the placement of the corneal light reflex in each eye. In straight eyes, the light reflection appears symmetric and, because of the relationship between the cornea and the macula, slightly nasal to the center of each pupil. When a strabismus is present, the reflected light is asymmetric and appears displaced in one eye. The Krimsky method of corneal reflex testing requires a prism that is placed over one or both eyes to align the light reflections (**41, 42**). The amount of prism needed to align the reflections is used to measure the degree of deviation. Although corneal light reflex testing is a useful screening tool, it may fail to detect a small deviation or an intermittent strabismus.

Cover tests for strabismus allow for more accurate and detailed strabismus measurements but require a child's attention and cooperation, good eye movement, and reasonably good vision in both eyes. If any of these elements are lacking, the results of a cover test may be invalid. Cover tests include the cover–uncover test and the alternate cover test. In the cover–uncover test, a child looks at an object in the distance, 6 m (20 feet) is standard. As the child looks at the distant object, the examiner covers one eye and watches for movement of the uncovered eye. If no movement occurs, there is no apparent misalignment of that eye. After one eye is tested, the same procedure is repeated on the other eye. When performing the alternate cover test, the examiner rapidly covers and uncovers each eye, shifting back and forth from one eye to the other. If the child has an ocular deviation, the eye rapidly moves as the cover is shifted to the other eye. Both the cover–uncover test and the alternate cover test should be performed at both distance and near fixation. The cover–uncover test differentiates manifest deviations (tropias), from latent deviations (phorias).

Strabismus during infancy

Many children will display unstable ocular alignment during the first few months of life and ocular deviations during this period do not necessarily indicate an abnormality. Infants are rarely born with their eyes aligned. During the first months of life, alignment may vary intermittently from esotropia to orthotropia to exotropia. A number of large population studies have confirmed that strabismus is common in early infancy. Because of this, adequate

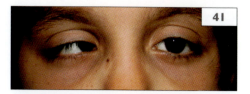

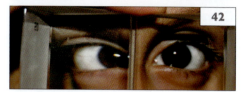

41, 42 Krimsky method of light reflex testing. A prism is placed in front of one (or both) eyes to center the corneal light reflexes.

assessment of alignment usually is not made until the patient is approximately 3 months of age and any angle of strabismus that is present is stable.

Pseudostrabismus

Pseudostrabismus (pseudoesotropia) is one of the most common reasons a pediatric ophthalmologist is asked to evaluate an infant. Pseudoesotropia is characterized by the false appearance of strabismus when the visual axes are actually aligned. This appearance is usually caused by a flat, broad nasal bridge, prominent epicanthal folds, or a narrow interpupillary distance. An observer may perceive less white sclera nasally than would be expected, and the impression is that the eye is turned in toward the nose, especially when the child looks to either side. Parents may comment that the eye almost disappears when their child looks to the side.

Pseudoesotropia can be differentiated from a true strabismus when the corneal light reflex is seen to be centered in both eyes and/or when the cover–uncover test shows no refixation movement. Tightening the epicanthal folds by pinching the bridge of the nose can also be effective in demonstrating that the 'crossing' is not real. Once the diagnosis of pseudoesotropia has been confirmed, parents can be reassured that the child will outgrow the appearance of esotropia. As the child grows, the bridge of the nose becomes more prominent and displaces the epicanthal folds, and the medial sclera becomes proportional to the amount visible on the lateral aspect of the eye.

Comitant strabismus

Esodeviations are the most common type of ocular misalignment in children and represent over 50% of all ocular deviations.

Congenital esotropia

Few children who are diagnosed with congenital esotropia are actually born with crossed eyes. Most pediatric ophthalmologists consider infants with confirmed onset of esotropia earlier than 6 months of age as having congenital esotropia. Some pediatric ophthalmologists prefer the term infantile esotropia to differentiate those children whose eyes were not crossed at birth.

ETIOLOGY

The cause of congenital esotropia is unknown. Theories include both a primary defect in sensory development of the brain that leads to the abnormal alignment as well as a primary 'motor' theory in which the ocular mis-alignment is the primary abnormality which then leads to a secondary disruption of binocular vision. It is likely that both causes exist and may also be equally responsible for the development of the disorder in many children.

CLINICAL PRESENTATION

The characteristic angle of congenital esotropia is large and constant (**43**). Because of the large deviation, cross-fixation is frequently encountered. This is a condition in which the child looks to the right with the left eye and to the left with the right eye. With cross-fixation, there is no need for the eye to turn away from the nose (abduction) as the adducting eye is used in side gaze. Cross-fixation may therefore simulate a 6th nerve palsy. Abduction can be demonstrated by the doll's head maneuver or by patching one eye for a short time. Children with congenital esotropia tend to have refractive errors similar to those of normal children of the same age. This contrasts with the characteristic high level of farsightedness associated with accommodative esotropia. Amblyopia is common in children with congenital esotropia.

DIFFERENTIAL DIAGNOSIS

During the first year of life, a number of conditions can simulate congenital esotropia (*Table 4*). Because the management of these conditions may differ from the treatment of congenital esotropia, it is important to recognize these other possibilities. In general, a relatively small angle deviation should raise doubt when contemplating the diagnosis of congenital esotropia. The majority of these other disorders can be ruled out following a thorough ophthalmologic evaluation. For this reason, all infants presenting with esotropia require a full evaluation, including a dilated funduscopic examination.

Table 4 Differential diagnosis of congenital esotropia

Pseudoesotropia
Duane's retraction syndrome
Möbius syndrome
Congenital sixth nerve palsy
Early-onset accommodative esotropia
Sensory esotropia
Esotropia in the neurologically impaired

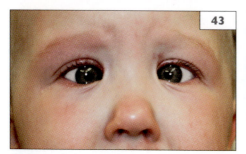

43 Congenital esotropia.

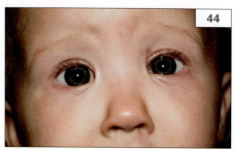

44 Three days following surgery for congenital esotropia.

DIAGNOSIS

The diagnosis is generally made when an infant presents prior to 6 months of age with a large, constant esotropia, full abduction, a normal level of hyperopia, and no underlying ophthalmic disorder that could lead to vision loss and a secondary strabismus. It is not infrequent to encounter a child who meets some but not all of these criteria. Some children may present with all the findings of congenital esotropia but with a higher than average level of farsightedness. In order to rule out the possibility that the farsightedness is the cause of the strabismus (accommodative esotropia), a trial of glasses may be necessary. If the glasses do not significantly change the deviation, the diagnosis of congenital esotropia can then be made. In children, or even adults, who present later in life, the typical history of early crossing in association with the other expected findings can also be used to confirm this diagnosis.

MANAGEMENT/TREATMENT

The treatment for congenital esotropia consists of strabismus surgery (**44**). The primary goal of treatment in congenital esotropia is to eliminate or reduce the deviation as much as possible. Ideally, this results in normal sight in each eye, in straight-looking eyes, and in the development of binocular vision. Surgery is performed after any associated amblyopia, if present, is treated. It is important to treat amblyopia prior to surgery. It is much easier to follow the progress of amblyopia in a preverbal child while their eyes are crossed. In addition, parental compliance with amblyopia treatment tends to be much lower once the eyes are straightened and appear 'normal'.

PROGNOSIS

It is important that parents realize that early successful surgical alignment is only the beginning of the treatment process for children with congenital esotropia. Many children with a history of congenital esotropia may redevelop strabismus or amblyopia and therefore they need to be monitored closely during the visually immature period of life. Early treatment is more likely to lead to the development of binocular vision, which helps to maintain long-term ocular alignment. Even with successful surgical alignment, it is common for vertical deviations to develop in children with a history of congenital esotropia. These generally develop months or years after the initial surgery has been performed. The two most common forms of vertical deviation to develop are inferior oblique muscle overaction (IOOA) and dissociated vertical deviation (DVD). In IOOA, the overactive inferior oblique muscle produces an upshoot of the eye closest to the nose when the patient looks to the side. In DVD, one eye drifts up slowly with no movement of the other eye. Surgery may be necessary to treat either or both of these conditions. In addition, a significant number of children may develop a recurrent esotropia where glasses will help to eliminate the crossing (accommodative esotropia) even if they did not prior to surgery.

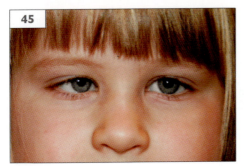
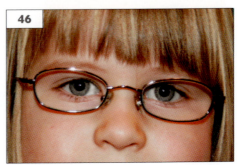

45, 46 Accommodative esotropia. Glasses eliminate the need to accommodate and therefore the esotropia.

Accommodative esotropia

Accommodative esotropia is defined as a 'convergent deviation of the eyes associated with activation of the accommodative (focusing) reflex'.

ETIOLOGY

The mechanism of accommodative esotropia involves uncorrected hyperopia, accommodation, and accommodative convergence. The image entering a hyperopic (farsighted) eye is blurred. If the amount of hyperopia is not significant, the blurred image can be sharpened by accommodating (focusing of the lens of the eye). Accommodation is closely linked with convergence (eyes turning inward). If a child's hyperopic refractive error is large, esotropia may develop.

CLINICAL PRESENTATION

Accommodative esotropia usually occurs in a child who is between 2 and 3 years of age and who has a history of acquired intermittent or constant crossing. Occasionally, children under 1 year of age may present with all the clinical features of accommodative esotropia. They may also present with a history suggestive of congenital esotropia but have a higher than expected level of farsightedness. Amblyopia occurs in a large percentage of patients.

MANAGEMENT/TREATMENT

To treat accommodative esotropia, the full hyperopic (farsighted) correction is initially prescribed. These glasses eliminate a child's need to accommodate and therefore correct the esotropia (**45, 46**). Although many parents are initially concerned that their child will not want to wear glasses, the benefits of binocular vision and the decrease in the focusing effort required to see clearly provide a strong stimulus to wear glasses, and they are generally accepted well. The full hyperopic correction sometimes straightens the eyes at distance fixation but leaves a residual deviation at near fixation; this may be observed or treated with bifocal lenses, antiaccommodative drops, or surgery.

PROGNOSIS

Most children maintain straight eyes once initially treated. Because hyperopia generally decreases with age, many patients outgrow the need to wear glasses to maintain alignment. In some patients, a residual esodeviation persists even when wearing their glasses. This condition commonly occurs when there is a delay between the onset of accommodative esotropia and treatment. In others, the esotropia may initially be eliminated with glasses but crossing redevelops. The crossing that is no longer correctable with glasses is the deteriorated or nonaccommodative portion. Surgery for this portion of the crossing may be indicated to restore binocular vision.

It is important to tell parents of children with accommodative esotropia that the esodeviation may appear to increase without glasses after the initial correction is worn. Parents frequently state that before wearing glasses, their child had a small esodeviation, whereas after removal of the glasses the esodeviation becomes quite large. Parents often blame the increased esodeviation on the glasses. This apparent increase is due to a child using the appropriate amount of accommodative effort after the glasses have been worn.

Congenital exotropia

Congenital exotropia behaves in a very similar fashion to congenital esotropia. It typically occurs early in life and presents with a large, constant out-turning. Amblyopia is common. Treatment for congenital exotropia requires strabismus surgery. As with congenital esotropia, early surgery gives the best chance of developing binocular vision although vertical strabismus (IOOA and DVD) frequently occurs later in life. Congenital exotropia may be associated with neurologic disease or abnormalities of the bony orbit, as in Crouzon syndrome.

Intermittent exotropia

Intermittent exotropia is the most common exodeviation in childhood.

CLINICAL PRESENTATION

The age of onset of intermittent exotropia varies but is often between age 6 months and 4 years. It is characterized by outward drifting of one eye, which usually occurs when a child is fixating at distance (**47**). The deviation is generally more frequent with fatigue or illness. Exposure to bright light may cause reflex closure of the exotropic eye. Because the deviation generally begins with distance fixation and is only seen when the child is tired, it is often not seen when examined by a primary medical doctor at close distance or during a well child visit. A history reported by the parents of an out-turned eye which occurs mostly when tired or sick is so typical that this history alone is highly suggestive for the disorder, and consultation with an ophthalmologist may be advisable. With time, the deviation usually becomes manifest more frequently.

DIAGNOSIS

The diagnosis of intermittent exotropia is made based upon the history and findings at the time of the motility examination. While the exam findings may help to determine the level of control that is present to maintain proper alignment, the history from the family may be crucial in deciding how often the deviation is present. This may be especially helpful when determining when treatment should be suggested.

MANAGEMENT/TREATMENT

While there are some forms of medical treatment that may be used by some ophthalmologists, most pediatric ophthalmologists agree that strabismus surgery is needed in the overwhelming majority of patients with intermittent exotropia and that medical treatments serve only to delay surgery in most patients.

The decision to perform eye muscle surgery is based on the magnitude and frequency of the deviation. If the deviation is small and infrequent, it is reasonable to observe the child. If the exotropia is large and increasing in frequency, surgery is indicated to maintain normal binocular vision.

PROGNOSIS

Because the eyes initially can be kept straight most of the time, visual acuity tends to be good in both eyes and binocular vision is initially normal during early stages of the disease. Left untreated, patients with intermittent exotropia show a typical progression: the deviation becomes more frequent until it becomes constant. Strabismus surgery has a high success rate although some patients may redevelop an exotropia later in life.

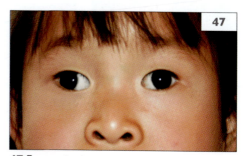

47 Exotropia.

Incomitant strabismus

Third cranial nerve palsy

ETIOLOGY

In children, 3rd nerve palsies are usually congenital. The congenital form is often associated with a developmental anomaly or birth trauma. Acquired 3rd nerve palsies in children can be an ominous sign and may indicate a neurologic abnormality such as an intracranial neoplasm or an aneurysm. Other less serious causes include an inflammatory or infectious lesion, head trauma, postviral syndromes, and migraines.

CLINICAL PRESENTATION

A 3rd nerve palsy, whether congenital or acquired, usually results in an exotropia and a hypotropia, (outward and downward) deviation of the affected eye, as well as complete or partial ptosis of the upper lid. This characteristic strabismus results from the action of the normal, unopposed muscles, the lateral rectus muscle and the superior oblique muscle. If the internal branch of the 3rd nerve is involved, pupillary dilation may be noted as well. Eye movements are usually limited nasally, in elevation and in depression (**48–53**). In congenital and traumatic cases of 3rd nerve palsy a misdirection of regenerating nerve fibers may develop, referred to as aberrant regeneration. This results in anomalous and paradoxical eyelid, eye, and pupil movement such as elevation of the eyelid, constriction of the pupil, or depression of the globe on attempted medial gaze.

DIAGNOSIS

Diagnosis is based upon the characteristic exotropia and hypotropia with associated limitation in adduction and vertical movements of the eye. Pupillary involvement is an especially important sign as it may indicate an expanding intracranial aneurysm and need for emergent neurologic evaluation and treatment.

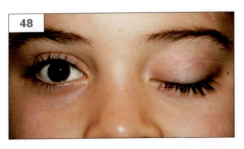

48–53 Third cranial nerve palsy. Complete ptosis (**48**); duction deficits (**49–53**).

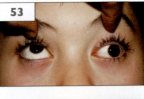

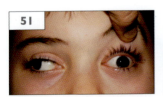

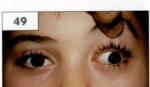

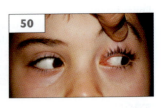

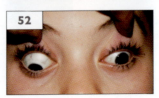

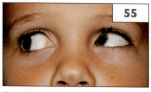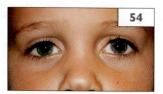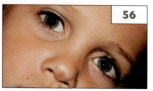

54–56 Left fourth cranial nerve palsy demonstrating left hypertropia which increases in right gaze and in left head tilt.

MANAGEMENT/TREATMENT

Initial ophthalmic treatment for patients with acquired 3rd nerve palsy involves relief of diplopia. If there is complete 3rd nerve palsy, the associated complete ptosis will cover the pupil and prevent diplopia. However, in partial 3rd nerve palsy, the lid may not cover the pupillary space, so that diplopia may remain a problem. Occlusion therapy is then the best solution to the diplopia. In children young enough to develop amblyopia, the patch should be alternated so that the affected eye will continue to develop normal vision.

Surgery to correct acquired 3rd nerve palsy should be postponed for several months after the onset of the condition when possible. If the ptosis is complete and the eyelid cannot open, early ptosis surgery may be needed in younger children in order to prevent the development of amblyopia.

PROGNOSIS

Many patients with acquired 3rd nerve palsies will show improvement with time. Those patients with congenital palsies may be given limited binocular vision with early treatment. Multiple procedures are often required to achieve alignment in straight-ahead gaze.

Fourth nerve palsy

ETIOLOGY

A fourth nerve palsy can be congenital or acquired. Because the 4th nerve has a long intracranial course, it is susceptible to damage resulting from head trauma. In children, however, 4th nerve palsies are more frequently congenital than traumatic.

CLINICAL PRESENTATION

A palsied 4th nerve results in weakness in the superior oblique muscle, which causes an upward deviation of the eye, a hypertropia. Because the antagonist muscle, the inferior oblique, is relatively unopposed, the affected eye demonstrates an upshoot when looking toward the nose. Children typically present with a head tilt to the shoulder opposite the affected eye, their chin down and their face turned away from the affected side. This head position places the eye away from the area of greatest action of the affected muscle and therefore minimizes the deviation and the associated double vision. Long-standing head tilts may lead to facial asymmetry. Because the abnormal head posture maintains the child's ocular alignment, amblyopia is uncommon. As no abnormality exists in the neck muscles, attempts to correct the head tilt by exercises and neck muscle surgeries are ineffective. Recognition of a superior oblique paresis can be difficult because deviation of the head and the eye may be minimal.

DIAGNOSIS

The pattern of strabismus seen in a patient with a 4th nerve palsy is diagnostic. The deviation increases when looking to the unaffected side and when the head it tilted to the same side (54–56). The 'three step test' allows for the diagnosis to be made in the vast majority of cases. Sometimes there can be a question as to whether the deviation is of new onset or just newly discovered. The presence of facial asymmetry and/or a long-standing head posture seen in old photographs can often help to answer this question.

MANAGEMENT/TREATMENT

Eye muscle surgery is indicated in order to improve the ocular alignment and eliminate the abnormal head posture. In cases of traumatic palsy, treatment is delayed until there is lack of spontaneous resolution, which will occur in a majority of cases.

PROGNOSIS

Surgery for both congenital and traumatic 4th nerve palsies carries an excellent prognosis for improvement of both the associated torticollis and improving the field of single binocular vision.

Sixth nerve palsy

ETIOLOGY

Acquired 6th nerve palsies in childhood can be an ominous sign because the 6th nerve is susceptible to increased intracranial pressure associated with hydrocephalus and intracranial tumors. Other causes of 6th nerve defects in children include trauma, vascular malformations, meningitis, and Gradenigo syndrome. A benign 6th nerve palsy, which is painless and acquired, can be noted in infants and older children. This is frequently preceded by a febrile illness or upper respiratory tract infection and may be recurrent. Complete resolution of the palsy is usual. Although not uncommon, other causes of acute 6th nerve palsy should be eliminated before this diagnosis is made.

CLINICAL PRESENTATION

A 6th nerve palsy produces markedly crossed eyes with limited ability to move the afflicted eye laterally (**57–59**). Children frequently may present with their head turned toward the palsied muscle, a position that helps preserve binocular vision. The esotropia is largest when the eye is moved toward the affected muscle.

DIFFERENTIAL DIAGNOSIS

Congenital 6th nerve palsies are rare. Decreased lateral gaze in infants is often associated with other disorders, such as congenital esotropia or Duane's retraction syndrome. In neonates, a transient 6th nerve paresis can occur; it usually clears spontaneously by 6 weeks. Increased intracranial pressure associated with labor and delivery may be the contributing factor.

MANAGEMENT/TREATMENT

As with other forms of traumatic cranial nerve palsies, surgical treatment is delayed until there is no sign of spontaneous improvement. Occlusion can be used for relief of diplopia. If the deviation does not improve with time, strabismus surgery may be warranted. If there is some function of the lateral rectus muscle, standard strabismus surgery may be used. If there continues to be complete absence of lateral rectus function, a transposition procedure may be needed in which the inferior and superior rectus muscles are moved next to the lateral rectus muscle to generate outward tension on the eye.

PROGNOSIS

Most cases of 6th nerve palsy will resolve with time. For those that do not, surgery is effective in eliminating the deviation in straight-ahead gaze but often will not improve the lateral movement of the eye.

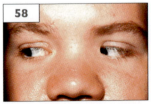
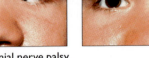
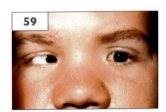

57–59 Sixth cranial nerve palsy.

Strabismus syndromes

Special types of strabismus have unusual clinical features. Most of these disorders are caused by structural anomalies of the extraocular muscles, adjacent tissues, or neurologic development. Most strabismus syndromes produce incomitant misalignments.

Duane's syndrome

Duane's syndrome is a congenital motility disorder that is characterized by limited ocular movement and retraction of the globe on adduction. There are several forms of Duane's syndrome based upon the specific limitation of movement that is seen.

ETIOLOGY

The cause of Duane's syndrome is thought to be an absence of the 6th nerve nucleus and anomalous innervation of the lateral rectus muscle. This results in cocontraction of the medial and lateral rectus muscles on attempted adduction of the affected eye, which leads to the observed retraction of the globe.

CLINICAL PRESENTATION

Within the spectrum of Duane's syndrome, patients may exhibit impairment of abduction, impairment of adduction, or a limitation of both abduction and adduction (**60–62**). An upshoot or downshoot of the involved eye on adduction occurs in some cases. They may have esotropia, exotropia, or relatively straight eyes. The majority of patients with Duane's syndrome exhibit a compensatory head posture to maintain single vision. Amblyopia is uncommon. Duane's syndrome usually occurs sporadically. It is sometimes inherited as an autosomal dominant trait. It usually occurs as an isolated condition but may occur in association with various other ocular and systemic anomalies.

DIFFERENTIAL DIAGNOSIS

The diagnosis of Duane's syndrome may be difficult to make in a young child where the limitation of movement of the eye may be difficult to see. Patients with esotropia that is noted shortly after birth may have Duane's syndrome. In contrast to those patients with congenital esotropia, the deviation in Duane's syndrome is usually relatively small. Patients with congenital esotropia have full ocular rotations. The most important disorder with which Duane's syndrome can be confused is 6th nerve palsy. The need to distinguish between these entities is vital in order to eliminate an unnecessary neurologic work-up in a patient with Duane's syndrome, or not to miss the need for one in a patient with a 6th nerve palsy. Patients with Duane's syndrome have a relatively small crossing of their eyes given their large abduction deficit. The presence of globe retraction can also be helpful.

MANAGEMENT/TREATMENT

Surgery is indicated to treat a large compensatory face turn, a noticeable upshoot or downshoot, or significant globe retraction. While surgery to improve alignment or to reduce a noticeable face turn can be helpful, surgery cannot significantly improve the movement of the eye.

PROGNOSIS

Most patients with Duane's syndrome do not require surgery and remain stable for life. They adjust to the lack of movement of their eye by moving their head to look to the affected side.

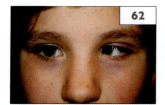 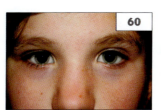 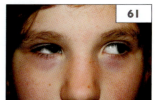

60–62 Duane's syndrome right eye. Eyelid fissure narrowing with adduction.

Brown's syndrome

ETIOLOGY

Most cases of Brown's syndrome are congenital, but acquired Brown's syndrome may follow trauma to the orbit involving the region of the trochlea or after sinus surgery. It may also occur with inflammatory processes, particularly sinusitis and juvenile rheumatoid arthritis. Some cases have been attributed to structural abnormalities such as a tight superior oblique tendon, congenital shortening or thickening of the superior oblique tendon sheath, or connective tissue trabeculae between the superior oblique tendon and the trochlea.

CLINICAL PRESENTATION

In Brown's syndrome, elevation of the eye in the adducted position is restricted (**63, 64**). An associated downward deviation of the affected eye in adduction may also occur. A compensatory head posture may be present to move the eye away from the adducted position. Parents often notice the 'abnormal' movement of the other eye; that it elevates higher than the actual affected eye. This apparent 'over-elevation' is a result of normal movement compared to the limited elevation of the involved side.

DIAGNOSIS

Although the clinical characteristics of Brown's syndrome usually allow a diagnosis to be made, a definitive diagnosis requires a positive forced duction test. In children, this is often done at the time of surgery. Forceps are placed on the eye and an attempt is made to manually rotate the globe toward the nose while it is being elevated. An inability to move the globe into this position confirms the diagnosis of Brown's syndrome.

MANAGEMENT/TREATMENT

Surgical intervention may be warranted for cases that involve a compensatory head posture, a large downshoot in adduction, or a vertical strabismus in straight-ahead gaze. Surgery consists of weakening the involved superior oblique. Treatment is not indicated for the lack of elevation in adduction.

PROGNOSIS

Most patients with Brown's syndrome do not require surgery. While surgery is often successful in eliminating a torticollis or significant ocular deviation, it does carry the risk of producing an iatrogenic 4th nerve palsy.

Monocular elevation deficiency (MED)

ETIOLOGY

Monocular elevation deficiency (MED), also called double elevator palsy, describes a monocular elevation deficit in both abduction and adduction. When an affected child fixates with the nonparetic eye, the paretic eye is low and the ipsilateral upper eyelid may appear ptotic. Fixation with the paretic eye causes a hypertropia of the nonparetic eye and a disappearance of the ptosis (**65–67**). MED may represent a paresis of both elevators, the superior rectus and inferior oblique muscles, or a possible restriction to elevation from a fibrotic inferior rectus muscle (a limited form of a more generalized fibrosis syndrome).

CLINICAL PRESENTATION

Patients may present because of the pseudoptosis and the vertical misalignment may not be noted. A compensatory chin up head posture may be present to allow for binocular vision.

DIFFERENTIAL DIAGNOSIS

MED may mimic Brown's syndrome. Both produce a limitation of elevation in adduction. Severe cases of Brown's syndrome may display some degree of limitation in abduction as well. Attempted movement of the eye at the time of surgery (forced duction testing) is useful to differentiate these disorders. It is also important to distinguish the type of MED (restrictive versus paralytic) as the treatments are different.

MANAGEMENT/TREATMENT

Treatment for MED is indicated when a deviation exists in straight-ahead gaze or when a compensatory head posture exists. Treatment consists of weakening of the inferior rectus muscle if its restriction is the cause of the deviation, and transposition eye muscle surgery for the paretic form of the disease. Because the apparent ptosis is actually secondary to the strabismus, correction of the hypotropia treats the pseudoptosis.

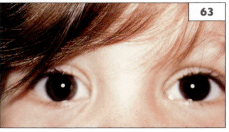 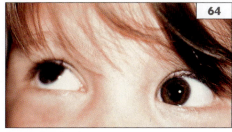

63, 64 Brown's syndrome. (Courtesy of Ken K. Nischal FRCOphth.)

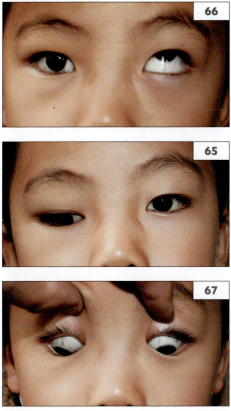

65–67 Monocular elevation deficiency.

Möbius syndrome

ETIOLOGY

The cause of Möbius syndrome is unknown. Whether the primary defect is maldevelopment of cranial nerve nuclei, hypoplasia of the muscles, or a combination of central and peripheral factors is unclear. Some familial cases have been reported.

CLINICAL PRESENTATION

The distinctive features of Möbius syndrome are congenital facial paresis and abduction weakness. The facial palsy is commonly bilateral, frequently asymmetric, and often incomplete, tending to spare the lower face and platysma. The abduction defect may be unilateral or bilateral. Esotropia is common although some children will have relative straight eyes (**68**). Associated developmental defects may include ptosis, palatal and lingual palsy, hearing loss, pectoral and lingual muscle defects, micrognathia, syndactyly, supernumerary digits, or the absence of hands, feet, fingers, or toes.

DIFFERENTIAL DIAGNOSIS

Because of the early onset, Möbius syndrome may present as a congenital esotropia. The abduction deficit(s) may lead to a diagnosis of 6th nerve palsy. However, the presence of facial palsy and swallowing difficulties generally makes this diagnosis distinguishable from other forms of strabismus.

MANAGEMENT/TREATMENT

Surgical correction of the esotropia is indicated and any attendant amblyopia should be treated. As with other cases of 6th nerve palsy, abduction may not improve following successful alignment surgery.

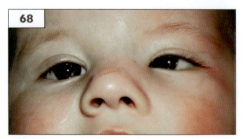

68 Möbius syndrome.

Conjunctiva

Steven J. Lichtenstein, MD, FAAP

- **Introduction**

- **Conjunctivitis**

- **Bacterial conjunctivitis**

- **Viral conjunctivitis**

- **Herpes conjunctivitis**

- **Giant papillary conjunctivitis**

- **Allergic conjunctivitis**

- **Vernal keratoconjunctivitis**

- **Phlyctenular keratoconjunctivitis (phlyctenulosis)**

- **Ophthalmia neonatorum**

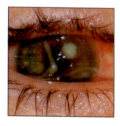
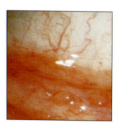
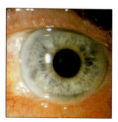
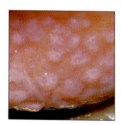

Introduction

While problems with the cornea can cause permanent visual loss, and a leukocoria can indicate the possible presence of a cataract or retinoblastoma, which can be visually devastating or even life threatening, the conjunctiva often causes relatively little concern. However, the conjunctiva is one of the most important structures that helps to maintain the health and wellbeing of the eye. Without this extremely thin covering of the anterior portion of the globe, the eye would be exposed to an extremely harsh environment. Although most cases of routine conjunctivitis will resolve spontaneously over 10–14 days, with or without treatment, the physician should be alert to the case which can potentially cause serious and permanent vision problems. These serious conditions, although rare, that are thought of as 'only pink eye' can cause a lifetime of vision problems in the patient. This chapter will look at the anatomy, physiology, pathophysiology, and treatment of the conjunctiva and conjunctival disorders to help the primary care provider in maintaining the health of the child's eye.

The conjunctiva is a thin, translucent mucous membrane that is vascularized and serves as both a barrier and as a reservoir of immunologic components to protect the eye (**69**). The only portion of the anterior segment of the eye that is not covered by the conjunctiva is the cornea. The conjunctiva has two anatomical components: the tarsal conjunctiva and the bulbar conjunctiva. The tarsal conjunctiva starts on the lids at the mucocutaneous junction, referred to by ophthalmologists as the 'gray line'. It is firmly attached to the inside portion of the eyelid, creating the mucosal surface of the lid. The bulbar conjunctiva starts approximately 1 mm from the limbus, the area where the sclera and cornea meet, and is loosely attached to the globe, except at the limbus where it is tightly attached to the episclera. The tarsal and bulbar conjunctivae then meet in the superior, temporal, and inferior portions of the globe, forming a sac called the fornix of the eye. The superior fornix extends up approximately 25 mm from the open eyelid margin, while the inferior fornix extends down approximately 9–10 mm from the eyelid margin.[1] The tarsal and bulbar conjunctivae join laterally to create the lateral boundary of the fornix, but medially, the conjunctiva ends at the caruncle, which contains skin as well as conjunctival components. Tenon's capsule, also known as the fascia bulbi, is a thin tissue which covers the globe from the optic nerve to the limbus, separating it from the orbital fat. The bulbar conjunctiva sits on Tenon's capsule, and is fused with this tissue at the limbus at the episclera.

The conjunctiva is composed of non-keratinized, stratified columnar epithelium which sits on top of the substantia propria, a highly vascularized connective tissue. These tissues then meet at the limbus and the columnar epithelium then transitions to stratified squamous epithelium and joins the corneal epithelium. The conjunctiva is highly populated with cells that produce the aqueous, mucin, and outer lipid layers of the tear film. The conjunctival goblet cells produce the mucopolysaccharides that form the protective mucous layer of the tear film. These cells also produce immunoglobulin A (IgA), which forms the immunologic barrier. Goblet cells are found in greater quantities in the young, and decrease as we age, accounting for the increased occurrence of dry eyes in the elderly. They are distributed throughout the conjunctiva, but with a great preponderance in the inferonasal portion of the conjunctiva. The aqueous portion of the tear film is produced by the lacrimal glands and accessory lacrimal glands. The ducts of these glands open onto the surface of the conjunctiva, and along with keeping the eye moist and comfortable, bring a vast array of immunologic factors which protect the eye from foreign substances.

The conjunctival fornices prevent a contact lens from slipping off of the cornea and becoming dislocated behind the eye of the wearer. If a contact lens remains on the globe, it will be located in either the superior or inferior fornix. The substantia propria contains abundant mast cells, plasma cells and neutrophils, which, although possibly linked to allergy and anaphylaxis, also play a significant role in immunologic protection, as well as wound healing.[2]

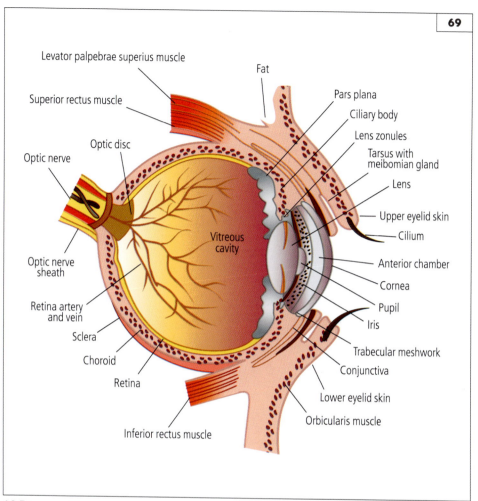

69 Diagram of the eye.

Conjunctivitis

Conjunctivitis literally means an inflammation of the conjunctiva. When this membrane becomes inflamed, it is commonly referred to as 'pink eye' or 'red eye'.[3] The etiology of the inflammatory process is complicated (**70**). The inflammation can result from both an infectious and noninfectious etiology and proper diagnosis of the etiology is imperative in order to deliver effective treatment.[4–7] Outbreaks of conjunctivitis are seasonal in nature; they occur most frequently when children are in close contact with each other in the winter, and tend to decrease during warm weather, when close contact decreases. This is evident in the number of prescriptions written for ocular antibiotics. However, conjunctivitis does occur year round. The etiology of the inflammation also somewhat follows the age of the patient, with a bacterial etiology occurring most frequently in younger, preschool age children, and a viral etiology occurring most frequently in older children and adults.[8] However, there have been reported outbreaks of bacterial conjunctivitis occurring in older children as well as adults.[9,10] *Table 5* presents the various etiologies of conjunctivitis seen in the pediatric population.

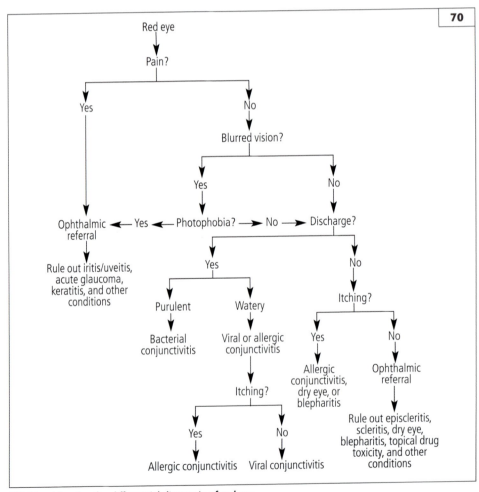

70 Algorithm for the differential diagnosis of red eye.

Determining the etiology of conjunctivitis is not always easy. Cultures are rarely, if ever, obtained, and a significant number of cases are diagnosed by telephone triage. The most important information to elicit from either telephone triage or the office visit is an accurate history of the child's signs and symptoms (*Table 6*).

Table 5 Types of conjunctivitis

Infectious	Bacterial, Viral
Noninfectious	Allergic (environmental pollutants, seasonal & perennial)
	Dry eye
	Trauma (including subconjunctival hemorrhage)
	Foreign body
	Toxic or chemical
	Thermal injuries
	Neoplasm
	Factitious
	Idiopathic
Other causes	Uveitis
	Acute angle closure glaucoma
	Episcleritis/scleritis
	Keratitis (infectious/noninfectious)
	Corneal ulcer (infectious/noninfectious)

Bacterial conjunctivitis

DEFINITION/OVERVIEW

Acute conjunctivitis is the most common ocular infection in childhood, usually affecting children less than 6 years of age. The belief that most causes of conjunctivitis in children are viral in etiology is not supported by the literature. The literature, from the early 1980s through 2007, shows that the most common form of acute conjunctivitis in the pediatric population is bacterial in nature.[4,11–14] If the child is under 1 year of age, the presence of a congenital dacryostenosis causing a purulent discharge must be excluded from the diagnosis of acute bacterial conjunctivitis. Bacterial conjunctivitis can occur in three forms: acute, hyperacute, and chronic.

ETIOLOGY

The eye has a number of different defense mechanisms that help to protect it from a bacterial infection. These include the presence of normal, nonpathogenic colonies of bacteria on the conjunctiva – which help prevent the establishment of invading pathologic organisms, the presence of immunologic agents secreted in the normal tear film, and physical shearing forces of the natural blink. These all provide a defense mechanism for the eye. When any of these protective mechanisms are compromised, an acute bacterial infection can result. The organisms that have been shown in all of the published papers from 1981 through

Table 6 Signs and symptoms of bacterial conjunctivitis

Acute
- Begins unilaterally
- Tearing
- Lid crusting in morning

- Purulent or mucopurulent discharge
- Eyelid edema
- Moderate diffuse hyperemia

Hyperacute
- Pain and tenderness of the globe
- Intense diffuse hyperemia
- Papillae

- Copious purulent discharge
- Occasional preauricular lymphadenopathy
- Conjunctival edema and chemosis

Chronic
- Lid crusting
- Foreign body sensation

- Mucoid discharge
- Conjunctival injection

2007 are *Staphylococcus aureus, Streptococcus pneumoniae, Hemophilus influenzae,* and *Moraxella catarrhalis*.[3,11–16]

CLINICAL PRESENTATION

The signs and symptoms of bacterial conjunctivitis are listed in *Table 6*. The history might reveal that the child has been rubbing their eyes and showing ocular irritation over the past 12–24 hours. The patient will usually present with conjunctival injection of the bulbar and tarsal conjunctival vessels (**71**). The conjunctival injection might also involve the episcleral vessels. There might be mild discomfort or irritation, but frank pain is atypical and should lead the primary care provider away from the diagnosis of routine bacterial conjunctivitis and towards the differential diagnosis of a more serious etiology for the red eye. There might also be a mild amount of photophobia present, but any significant degree of photophobia is not consistent with the diagnosis of acute bacterial conjunctivitis. Special mention should be made of conjunctivitis in a contact lens wearer. Concerns about *Pseudomonas aeruginosa* should be at the forefront of the differential diagnosis of conjunctivitis in this population (**72**). A contact lens wearer with signs of conjunctivitis and pain or decreased vision should be referred to an ophthalmologist promptly.

The hallmark of acute bacterial conjunctivitis is the presence of purulent or mucopurulent discharge from the eye with matting of the lashes. The matting will usually be seen after the child awakens in the morning, or after an extended nap. Visual acuity is not altered except possibly briefly with the purulent discharge obscuring the vision. This should clear with blinking. If the child is seen in the office, attempts to obtain a visual acuity measurement should be made, especially in the older child who can cooperate. Lymphadenopathy is usually not present except possibly during the late stages of the disease when the symptoms are spontaneously starting to clear without treatment in 7–10 days. The presence of lymphadenopathy with either preauricular or submandibular involvement should lead the primary care provider towards the diagnosis of a viral etiology for the conjunctivitis. Both membranous as well as pseudomembranous conjunctivitis can be seen (**73**). The difference between membranous and pseudomembranous conjunctivitis is the way the membrane peels off of the conjunctiva. In pseudomembranous conjunctivitis, the membrane is easily removed and causes no bleeding, where in membranous conjunctivitis, peeling of the membrane causes bleeding and discomfort, and is much more difficult to accomplish. Membranous conjunctivitis can be caused by bacterial conjunctivitis with an etiology of β-hemolytic streptococci, pneumococci, *Corynebacterium diptheriae*, and *Neisseria gonorrhoeae*. Pseudomembranous conjunctivitis can be seen in all

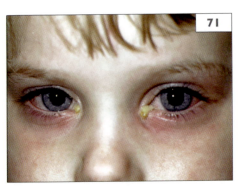

71 Bacterial conjunctivitis. (Courtesy of Rudy J. Wagner, MD.)

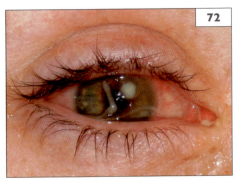

72 *Pseudomonas* corneal ulcer secondary to contact lens wear. (Courtesy of Robert D. Gross, MD, MPH.)

of the causes of membranous conjunctivitis as well as ocular cicatricial pemphigoid, superior limbic keratoconjunctivitis, and chlamydial conjunctivitis in newborns. Viral conjunctivitis with an etiology of adenovirus, herpes simplex virus and ocular vaccinia, as well as ligneous conjunctivitis, Stevens–Johnson syndrome, and chemical and thermal burns can all cause membrane formation.

Although bacterial conjunctivitis is very often a bilateral disease, with one eye usually showing more involvement than the fellow eye, it can also occur as a unilateral condition. It can be seen in the pediatric population associated with another acute infection, acute otitis media (AOM) in what is known as the conjunctivitis–otitis media syndrome.[14–16] Conjunctivitis–otitis media syndrome can be seen in as high as 35% of children who have conjunctivitis, and is indicative of a bacterial etiology.

The natural history of bacterial conjunctivitis will lead to the return of the normal bacterial flora and eradication of the offending organism. However, if there is a large pathologic organism load and disruption of any of the natural defense mechanisms of the cornea (i.e. breakdown of the intact corneal epithelium from continual rubbing secondary to irritation), a corneal infection (keratitis) or corneal ulcer formation can occur. A corneal ulcer has the potential to interfere with normal vision by causing a corneal scar to form following healing of the ulcer. The healing ulcer causes disruption of the regular alignment of the corneal fibrils, and thus opacification of the clear cornea. If this scar is in the visual axis, permanent visual damage can occur.

MANAGEMENT/TREATMENT

Table 7 (overleaf) summarizes the modalities available for treatment of bacterial conjunctivitis in 2008, compiled from the package inserts of the various antibiotics. This information will continually change as newer antibiotics are added to the pharmaceutical armamentarium, and bacteria continue to develop resistance to chemotherapeutic agents. The use of the algorithm in Figure **70**, especially if telephone triage is used, can help the physician in choosing the most appropriate treatment regimen for the child's inflamed eye.

A contact lens wearer who shows signs of a bacterial conjunctivitis should be evaluated and may require cultures prior to the initiation of antibiotic therapy. If treatment is started without obtaining cultures, and any patient does not respond to treatment of a significant purulent conjunctivitis, the primary care provider should consult an ophthalmologist, especially if the patient is a contact lens wearer. At this point, cultures and Gram stain of the conjunctiva are often obtained prior to any change in therapy, to ascertain the etiology of the infective organism to prevent the possibility of visually devastating sequelae (**74**).

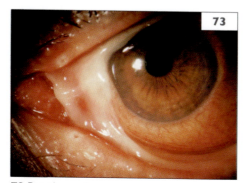

73 Pseudomembrane.

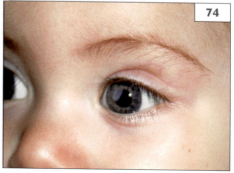

74 *Pseudomonas* corneal ulcer 6 months postinfection.

Table 7 Antimicrobial agents for bacterial conjunctivitis in topical preparations

Antimicrobial agent	Dosage	Comments
Sulfonamides Sulfisoxazole (4% solution)	q.2–3 h × 7–10 days	Bacteriostatic rather than bactericidal, no longer effective against Gram-positive organisms, highly irritating, may cause severe hypersensitivity reactions
Sulfacetamide sodium (1–30% solutions, 10% ointment)	q.2 h – q.i.d.	
Aminoglycosides Gentamicin (0.3% solution)	q.i.d.	Weak activity against Gram-positive pathogens, particularly *Streptococcus* sp.
Tobramycin (0.3% solution)		May cause hyperemia or keratopathy
Bacitracin (500 U/g ointment)	q.h.s. to q.i.d.	Effective only against Gram-positive organisms
Macrolides Erythromycin (0.5% ointment)	q.h.s. to q.i.d.	*Staphylococci* sp. have become resistant to erythromycin
Azithromycin (1% solution)	b.i.d. × 2 days then q.d. × 5 days	
Chloramphenicol (1% ointment, 5% solution)	q.2 h to q.i.d.	Broad spectrum of activity. No longer used in the US due to its association with aplastic anemia
Polymyxin B/trimethoprim sulfate (solution 10,000 U; 1 mg/ml)	q.3 h × 7–10 days Not to exceed 6×/day	Effective against *H. influenzae* and *S. pneumoniae*. Not reliably bactericidal, cure of infection may take more than 1 week. Few hypersensitivity reactions
Antibiotic/steroid combinations	Should be used by ophthalmologist or optometrist only	Can exacerbate ocular viral infections, may induce glaucoma or cataracts with prolonged use. Should only be used under the supervision of an ophthalmologist
Fluoroquinolones **second-generation** Ciprofloxacin (0.3% solution or ointment)	q.2 h × 2 days, up to 8 times/day, then q.i.d. × 5 days (class labeling)	Highly effective against a broad spectrum of Gram-negative and Gram-positive ocular pathogens. However, resistance has emerged in *S. pneumoniae* against both second- and third- generation agents
Ofloxacin (0.3% solution)	Same as above (class labeling)	
Third-generation Levofloxacin (0.5% solution)	Same as above (class labeling)	Highly effective against a broad spectrum of Gram-negative and Gram-positive ocular pathogens
Levofloxacin (1.5% solution)	Not indicated for the treatment of bacterial conjunctivitis	Indicated only for the treatment of bacterial corneal ulcers, not conjunctivitis
Fourth-generation Gatifloxacin (0.3% solution)	Same as above (class labeling)	Highly effective against a broad spectrum of Gram-negative and Gram-positive ocular pathogens
Moxifloxacin (0.5% solution)	t.i.d. × 7 days (the only fluoroquinolone not to be given class labeling by the F.D.A.)	All of the fluoroquinolones with indications for the treatment of bacterial conjunctivitis have benzalkonium chloride (BAK – alkyldimethylbenzyl-ammonium chloride) as a preservative except moxifloxacin (Vigamox®) which is preservative-free

(All dosages from *Physician's Desk Reference*, 62nd edn, 2008. Thomson, Montvale.)

Rationale for the treatment of bacterial conjunctivitis

The use of antibiotics, in any circumstance, systemically or topically, must be well thought out, and antibiotics should not be used in a haphazard or 'shotgun' approach. Unless the etiology of the disease process, or its sequelae, is bacterial in nature, the use of antibiotics is inappropriate and should be avoided. To treat everything 'with a pill or drop' will accelerate the emergence of 'super bugs' such as methicillin-resistant *Staphylococcus aureus* (MRSA), both hospital and community acquired (HA-MRSA, CA-MRSA). The treatment of bacterial conjunctivitis should include the following goals:

- A rapid rate of bacterial kill to minimize the spread of the contagion.
- A high concentration of the antibiotic in the target tissue to exceed the minimum inhibitory concentration (MIC) for the suspected pathogens.
- A broad range of coverage to include all of the known bacterial etiologies of the disease, including staphylococci, streptococci, *Haemophilus influenzae*, and *Moraxella catarrhalis*.
- A low incidence of bacterial resistance.
- A low level of ocular toxicity.
- A drop that is comfortable and well tolerated by the pediatric population.
- A convenient dosing schedule to enhance parental compliance.

If any of these points are not met, the treatment of the disease could prove to be worse than this self-limiting disease itself. In addition, treating suspected bacterial conjunctivitis with an antibiotic that meets all of these criteria facilitates rapid identification of a masquerade syndrome; a disease may present as a 'routine' case of conjunctivitis, but is actually a process that can cause significant damage to the eye, or even blindness. With the use of an antibiotic that is bacteriocidal and shows minimal resistance to the most common bacteria causing conjunctivitis in the pediatric population, these masquerade syndromes can be rapidly identified, and appropriate therapy can be initiated.

With increasing bacterial resistance, the most logical approach to the choice of an appropriate antibiotic would be to limit the use of newer antibiotics, and use an older antibiotic until failure of treatment is seen. This is commonly called the 'Big Gun' theory, and is very relevant to systemic disease. However, in topical treatment of bacterial conjunctivitis, the use of the 'Correct Gun' is much more appropriate and will help to identify a masquerade syndrome much more rapidly. A virtual 'safety net' can be achieved by prescribing a bacteriocidal antibiotic which can rapidly eradicate the organism.[17] The newer generation fluoroquinolones fit this profile extremely well because of their rapid action on the bacteria.[18] The appropriate way to treat bacterial conjunctivitis is therefore to make the diagnosis, select the appropriate antibiotic, treat for a short period of time, and then discontinue the use of the antibiotic; this will not lead to increasing resistance of the bacteria.

Resistance

One of the most frightening things seen in medicine is the emergence of bacteria that have mutated to become resistant to antimicrobial agents. The prolonged use of antibiotics, along with tapering dosage regimens, is the most likely cause of increasing resistance. There are definite correlations between the inappropriate use of antibiotics and patient noncompliance with the emergence of resistant organisms.[19] The use of antibiotics in animal feed to help bring livestock to market has also played a role in the development of antibiotic resistance in humans.[20] Bacteria have shown a definite increase in resistance to the fluoroquinolones. Although this group shows excellent Gram-negative coverage, Gram-positive organisms are developing increasing resistance to the second- and third-generation fluoroquinolones, especially *S. pneumoniae*.[21] A retrospective study of isolates recovered from bacterial conjunctivitis and keratitis was conducted during the 12-year period from 1990 to 2001 to determine the resistance of methicillin-sensitive *S. aureus* (MSSA) to ciprofloxacin and levofloxacin.[22] There was a definite pattern of increasing resistance, which was statistically significant. In a 15-year study in Sao Paulo, Brazil, from 1985 to 2000, of 4585 conjunctival cultures examined, there was a marked decrease of *in vitro* activity of gentamycin and tobramycin against *S. pneumoniae* and *S. aureus*.[23] Recent findings show that approximately half of the *S. epidermidis* isolates from the normal human conjunctiva had one or more mutations of topoisomerase II and topoisomerase IV, which is strongly associated with reduced susceptibility to fluoroquinolones.[24]

Viral conjunctivitis

DEFINITION/OVERVIEW
A common misperception of conjunctivitis is that it is routinely secondary to viral and not bacterial infection. Even the most current version of the AAP *Red Book* lists viral conjunctivitis as the most common form of the disease in children.[8] However, the literature does not support this assertion. Nevertheless, viral conjunctivitis is common and practitioners should be particularly attuned to its signs and symptoms since it should not be treated with antibiotics.

ETIOLOGY
Children with viral conjunctivitis are contagious for at least 7 days from the first appearance of their symptoms. Although the spread of the disease is thought to be caused mainly by direct contact with the virus by contaminated fingers to the eye, the virus may also be spread by coughing and sneezing of airborne particles. For this reason, the most important strategy to halt the spread of the virus is good hygiene and washing hands. The child should be isolated to prevent spread of the contagion. Adenovirus is the most common etiology of viral conjunctivitis, and as discussed previously, is seen more commonly in the fall and winter months.

CLINICAL PRESENTATION
Table 8 presents the signs and symptoms of viral conjunctivitis. There is an acute onset of unilateral symptoms that can rapidly spread to being bilateral through cross contamination of the fellow eye. A watery or serous discharge is present, along with the conjunctival injection (**75**). A hemorrhagic component may be seen in some cases (**76**). The presence of acute preauricular and/or submandibular lymphadenopathy may help to confirm the diagnosis. The child may be febrile and may have a pharyngitis associated with the conjunctivitis. Follicles of the conjunctiva can be seen if the lower lid is pulled down slightly (**77**). Acute follicular conjunctivitis is usually associated with a viral etiology (epidemic keratoconjunctivitis, herpes zoster keratoconjunctivitis, infectious mononucleosis, Epstein–Barr virus infection) or chlamydial infections (inclusion conjunctivitis), while chronic follicular changes can be seen in chronic chlamydial infection (trachoma, lymphogranuloma venereum) or as a toxic or reactive inflammatory response to topical medications and molluscum contagiosum. The follicles appear as gray-white, round to oval elevations which measure 0.5–1.5 mm in diameter and can be seen in the inferior and superior tarsal conjunctivae, and less often, on bulbar or limbal conjunctiva.

Table 8 Signs and symptoms of viral conjunctivitis

Adenoviral
- Water discharge
- Hyperemia
- Petechial hemorrhages
  Punctate keratitis
- Frequent preauricular lymphadenopathy
- Serous, mucoid, or mucopurulent discharge
- Pharyngitis

Herpetic
- Usually unilateral
- Vesicular eruptions on eyelids
- Diffuse hyperemia
- Follicles
- Serous–mucoid discharge
- Occasional preauricular lymphadenopathy
- Dendritic epithelial keratitis of conjunctiva
  or cornea

MANAGEMENT/TREATMENT

Supportive care and isolation of the child to decrease the spread of the contagion is the only treatment indicated for routine viral conjunctivitis. Because the necessity of isolation requires children to miss school, after-school, and daycare, parents often request a 'drop' to get their child back into their daily routine. Most schools or daycare will only allow a child back if they are 'on a drop', but this is not even standardized from community to community.[25] Nevertheless, the use of an antibiotic drop is inappropriate when the etiology is presumed to be viral in nature. The use of an antibiotic has no effect on the infection, other than to eradicate the normal bacterial flora of the conjunctiva. Moreover, the child is no less contagious, and may actually spread the virus quicker because good hygiene and hand washing may be less rigorous if the caregiver thinks that the antibiotic is having an effect on the disease process.

Most cases of viral conjunctivitis are self-limiting and overtreatment should be avoided. Corneal subepithelial infiltrates may be seen in some cases of epidemic keratoconjunctivitis (**78**).

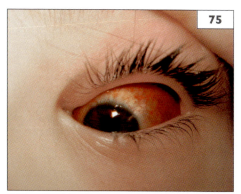

75 Viral conjunctivitis. (Courtesy of Robert D. Gross, MD, MPH.)

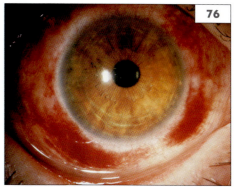

76 Hemorrhagic conjunctivitis. (Courtesy of Casey Eye Institute, Oregon Health Sciences University.)

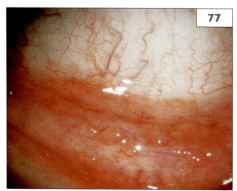

77 Conjunctival follicles. (Courtesy of Casey Eye Institute, Oregon Health Sciences University.)

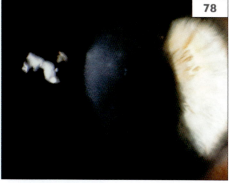

78 Adenoviral conjunctivitis, corneal infiltrates. (Courtesy of Casey Eye Institute, Oregon Health Sciences University.)

Herpes conjunctivitis

Viral conjunctivitis caused by the herpes simplex (HSV) or herpes zoster (HZV) viruses can cause serious and permanent damage to the eye and vision. Herpes zoster infections are not as common as herpes simplex in the pediatric patient. These infections can show periocular as well as ocular involvement, and are most often unilateral in nature. Herpes simplex infections can also be recurrent, causing repeated bouts of conjunctivitis, keratitis, and periorbital disease.

ETIOLOGY

Most cases of secondary conjunctivitis are caused by HSV-1 and are associated with recurrent orolabial infection (cold sores). HSV-2 is associated with genital infection and is the more common cause of neonatal eye infections.

CLINICAL PRESENTATION

Patients can exhibit a serous discharge, bulbar and tarsal conjunctival injection, photophobia, epiphora, lid edema, and vesicular eruptions of the lids. There may also be dendritic ulcerations of the cornea which can leave permanent scarring and visual acuity damage. The dendrites will stain with fluorescein and be visible with a Wood's light or cobalt blue light (**79**). They will also stain with Rose Bengal, which stains devitalized cells of the cornea, giving the classic dendrite appearance. A Wood's light is not necessary to observe the staining with Rose Bengal. If herpetic involvement is suspected in a child with conjunctivitis, a referral to an ophthalmologist is warranted.[26] The use by a primary care provider of any ophthalmic drop containing a steroid is contraindicated and it should only be prescribed by an ophthalmologist because of the possibility of herpetic involvement. The use of a steroid in a child with herpes can cause permanent and possibly devastating complications, including acute corneal perforation.

MANAGEMENT/TREATMENT

Treatment of viral conjunctival disease may shorten its duration but does not seem to otherwise alter the course of disease. Treatment is indicated when the cornea is involved. Oral acyclovir (aciclovir) has been shown to be effective for treatment of herpetic epithelial keratitis and for reducing the rate of recurrence when used prophylactically. Topical antiviral medications carry a risk of corneal toxicity and their use should be reserved for patients under the care of an ophthalmologist.

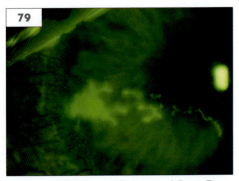

79 Corneal dendrites. (Courtesy of Casey Eye Institute, Oregon Health Sciences University.)

Giant papillary conjunctivitis

ETIOLOGY

GPC is a noninfectious condition that occurs when there is a chronic foreign body irritation of the eye. In the past, it was most frequently seen in children and young adults with an ocular prosthesis and in patients with exposed sutures or scleral buckles after retinal detachment surgery. GPC is also associated with patients who have undergone glaucoma filtering procedures with the formation of a conjunctival bleb, or elevation of the conjunctiva near or at the limbus, to allow the aqueous humor to escape the anterior chamber, therefore maintaining a controlled intraocular pressure.[39] However, as the use of cosmetic contact lenses finds its way into younger and younger children, GPC is now commonly being seen with the use, and misuse, of contact lenses in both children and adults. Rigid, gas-permeable lenses as well as soft contact lenses have both been associated with GPC, although the incidence of GPC with the use of rigid gas-permeable lenses is less than with soft contact lens use.

The symptoms of GPC are low grade as the condition starts to evolve. There may be a mild amount of itching, or mild contact lens discomfort. However, since many of the patients are extremely motivated to continue their contact lens wear, the symptoms will worsen with increasing itching, blurring of vision, mucoid production, and then finally contact lens intolerance. Involvement of the cornea is rare, but with continued use of soft contact lenses, even in the presence of increasing conjunctival irritation, pannus formation can occur.

CLINICAL PRESENTATION

The symptoms of GPC can begin months or even years after the patient starts to wear his or her contact lenses. There is no sex or racial predilection, but the symptoms of GPC seem to be more aggressive in children who wear contact lenses. Papillae are seen on the superior tarsal conjunctiva and can measure up to 1 mm in diameter (**80**). The same type of papillae are seen in VKC, but the giant papillae in VKC are usually larger than in GPC, and the permanent ocular changes seen in VKC are not seen in GPC. However, pannus formation can be seen in children from chronic misuse of their contact lenses. Itching on initial insertion of the contact lenses is an early symptom of GPC. If not treated properly, progression to complete contact lens intolerance may occur.

MANAGEMENT/TREATMENT

The only definitive treatment for patients who are experiencing signs and symptoms of GPC is removal of the foreign material from contact with the eye. This means removing exposed scleral buckles, altering an ocular prosthesis to create less conjunctival irritation, or discontinuation of the use of contact lenses until the symptoms resolve. Since, as previously mentioned, the motivation of these patients to continue their cosmetic contact lens wear is usually high, complete discontinuation may be very difficult to accomplish. In these cases, improving the patient's compliance with hygiene in handling their lenses, decreasing the time that the contact lenses are inserted, the use of disposable lenses, or a different lens material should be employed. Since the primary care provider does not have expertise in this area, the importance of compliance should be stressed, and the patient should be referred back to the eye care professional providing the contact lenses.

PROGNOSIS

The symptoms of most patients can be controlled with topical medications. In those cases that cannot, removal of the offending agent is generally curative.

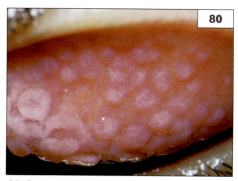

80 Giant papillary conjunctivitis. (Courtesy of Casey Eye Institute, Oregon Health Sciences University.)

Allergic conjunctivitis

DEFINITION/OVERVIEW

Allergic conjunctivitis can be divided into five common forms, two acute (seasonal allergic conjunctivitis [SAC] and perennial allergic conjunctivitis [PAC]), and three chronic (vernal keratoconjunctivitis [VKC], atopic keratoconjunctivitis [AKC], and giant papillary conjunctivitis [GPC]) (*Table 9*).[27] AKC is usually seen in late adolescents and adults, so will not be discussed here.

'If it doesn't itch, it's probably not allergy' is probably the best way to start thinking about allergy as the etiology of an inflamed eye.

ETIOLOGY

Allergic conjunctivitis is usually associated with type 1 hypersensitivity reactions. The main component of ocular allergy is the mast cell along with IgE. When an allergen comes in contact with the conjunctiva of a previously sensitized patient, the mast cell, which is filled with granules of histamine, will degranulate, spilling the contents into the surrounding tissue. The release of histamine causes a cascading release of chemical mediators, which causes vasodilatation, increased vascular permeability, and increased mucoid production. The main mediators in mast cell degranulation are histamine, tryptase, kininogenase, and eosinophil chemotactic factor of anaphylaxis (ECF-A). If the allergic reaction has a long protracted course, a late-phase response can occur. The main mediators of this late-phase response includes leukotriene B4, leukotriene C4, D4, prostaglandins D2, and platelet activation factor.[28]

Seasonal conjunctivitis is the most common form of ocular allergic disease.[26] The ocular manifestations occur either seasonally (SAC) or perennially (PAC). Although the symptoms, including rhinitis and congestion, can be treated quickly by primary care providers, the ocular complaints may not be elucidated during the examination. The symptomatic patient is usually miserable and treatment of their systemic symptoms as well as their ocular symptoms is beneficial. SAC is associated with release of pollens in the early spring from grasses and trees, or in the late summer and early fall secondary to ragweed. PAC can occur at any time throughout the year. This is usually associated with allergens such as pet dander and dust mites. Once an individual is exposed to a sensitizing agent, the symptoms of the allergic response occur quickly. Although PAC sufferers have symptoms year round, they will usually experience seasonal exacerbations.[29,30]

Table 9 Signs and symptoms of allergic conjunctivitis

Seasonal
- Bilateral
- Itching
- Tearing
- Conjunctival injection
- Chemosis
- Ropey or stringy mucoid discharge

Vernal
- Severe itching
- Ropey mucoid discharge
- Blurred vision
- Trantas' dots
- Giant papillae

Giant papillary
- Itching
- Contact lens intolerance
- Mild hyperemia
- Giant papillae
- Mucoid discharge

CLINICAL PRESENTATION

Although acute allergic conjunctivitis is usually seen bilaterally, it is not uncommon for a patient to complain of unilateral symptoms, even when bilateral signs are present. Besides the itching, patients will often complain of a stringy or ropey mucoid discharge, lid edema, chemosis (edema of the conjunctiva), and red, hyperemic conjunctiva (**81**).[31] Patients will often show other signs of atopy, with allergic rhinitis being extremely common. Patients with atopic disease will sometimes not have a primary complaint of itching eyes, but instead other symptoms of allergic reactions including wheezing, rhinoconjunctivitis, and eczema.[32]

MANAGEMENT/TREATMENT

The treatment of acute allergic conjunctivitis centers around symptomatic relief. By reducing the allergic response to the allergen and reducing the inflammatory response of the eye and periorbital region, the patient will be much more comfortable and less symptomatic.[33] The most important goal is to reduce the amount of allergic load to the patient. If the child is suffering from PAC, then eliminating the allergen will be the most beneficial approach. Eliminating pet dander or laundry detergent, or reducing contact with dust mites can show significant relief of the patient's symptoms. If the allergic response is caused by seasonal allergens, this is not an easy task. SAC will also benefit from any reduction in the allergen load, including keeping windows closed and using an air filtration system in the house. When the child is outside exposed to various pollens and other allergens, these allergens will collect in his or her hair, which can be transferred to the pillow at night, putting a significant allergen load in direct contact with the ocular adnexa. By simply washing the child's hair before they go to bed, the allergen load will not be transferred to the pillow and thus the eyes. Cool or cold compresses are also beneficial for symptomatic relief. The use of topical ophthalmic drops can also help to lower the allergic response, and the patient's symptoms. These medications are divided into five categories: antihistamines, mast cell stabilizers, antihistamine/mast cell stabilizer combinations, corticosteroids, and nonsteroidal anti-inflammatory drugs (NSAIDs).

PROGNOSIS

The treatment of SAC is often frustrating for both the physician and patient. Recurrences are common and complete resolution of symptoms without the use, and risk, of steroids is not always possible. However, many patients can be helped significantly. Patients will show a definite increase in the quality of life when their symptoms are controlled.[34] Patients with chronic disease can show permanent changes and potential visual impairment.

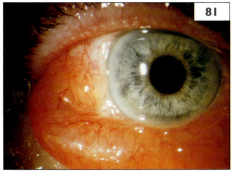

81 Conjunctival chemosis. (Courtesy of Casey Eye Institute, Oregon Health Sciences University.)

Vernal keratoconjunctivitis

ETIOLOGY

VKC is caused by the exuberant reaction of the body's immune system towards an allergen. VKC is thought to be mainly a type I hypersensitivity reaction, with eosinophils, as well as mast cells the most involved cells. There has also been some speculation that a type IV hypersensitivity reaction may also play a role in this condition, with mononuclear cells, fibroblasts, and newly secreted collagen seen.[35]

CLINICAL PRESENTATION

VKC is a chronic form of allergic conjunctivitis. It is bilateral and will usually be seen affecting the superior and limbal conjunctivae. There is a definite predilection for VKC affecting males more than females,[36] and it is seen in warmer climates more often than cooler climates. It usually presents before age 10 years, and will often resolve following puberty. There is also a history of eczema or asthma in 75% of patients.[37] Although this is a chronic condition, seasonal exacerbations are often seen. The symptoms that are reported are similar to those seen in acute allergic conjunctivitis but are usually more severe and chronic. The primary complaints are severe itching, and a thick, ropey discharge. The patient will usually have a history of allergies and atopy. Along with conjunctival injection, small whitish dots on the cornea at the superior limbus will often be visible with a direct ophthalmoscope. These dots, Trantas or Horner–Trantas dots, are pathognomonic for VKC (**82**). The superior tarsal conjunctiva will often show large 'cobblestone-like' papillae (**83**). In severe and chronic cases of VKC, sterile corneal ulcers, known as corneal shield (Togby's) ulcers, may be present (**84**). They are usually seen at the superior limbus, and can be painful, serious vision-threatening lesions. These ulcers need to be aggressively managed if they do not show rapid re-epithelialization.[38] Other symptoms seen in VKC are foreign body sensation, epiphora or excess tearing, photophobia, and ocular burning and stinging (*Table 10*).

MANAGEMENT/TREATMENT

Treatment is centered on reducing the patient's symptoms, controlling the hypersensitivity reaction, and keeping the ocular structures well lubricated to prevent the serious vision-threatening sequelae that can be seen with VKC. The initiation of therapy as early as possible to prevent these sequelae is highly recommended once the diagnosis of VKC is made. The use of cool or cold compresses, artificial tears, as well as bland ophthalmic ointments can help reduce the early symptoms. Systemic as well as topical antihistamines, along with mast cell stabilizers can keep the symptoms under control, but play a less prominent role during an acute exacerbation. The use of NSAIDs as well as topical steroidal anti-inflammatory drops will usually be required during an acute exacerbation.

In patients that have corneal shield ulcers, aggressive therapy is indicated. Since these ulcers are painful, the use of a cycloplegic drop is indicated and will reduce the ciliary spasm and

---

Table 10 Signs and symptoms of vernal keratoconjunctivitis

Signs	Symptoms
• Bilateral	• Red injected conjunctiva
• Conjunctival injection	• Severe ocular itching
• Giant cobblestone-like papillae seen on the superior tarsal conjunctiva (usually larger than those seen in giant papillary conjunctivitis)	• Epiphora (tearing)
	• Mucoid discharge
• Superior limbal conjunctivitis	• Ocular burning
• Trantas' or Horner–Trantas dots	• Photophobia
• Corneal shield (Togby's) ulcers	

pain that the child may experience. If the ulcer does not rapidly re-epithelialize, the use of topical antibiotics is also indicated. A physical barrier with a low water content hydrogel lens can be used to stop the cobblestone-like giant papillae from re-abrading the corneal epithelium. If a patient is showing these significant symptoms during an acute exacerbation, consultation with an ophthalmologist is highly recommended.

PROGNOSIS

VKC is often a chronic and recurring problem. Mild cases can be effectively managed and patients can be made comfortable. More severe cases place the patient at significant risk for vision loss, usually as a result of the disease process itself. However, the overly aggressive use of topical corticosteroids to treat the disease may also cause problems.

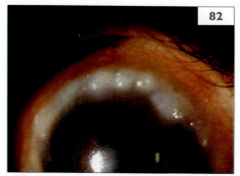

82 Horner–Trantas dots. (Courtesy of Casey Eye Institute, Oregon Health Sciences University.)

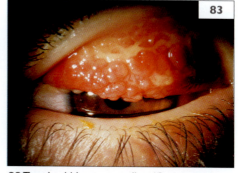

83 Tarsal cobblestone papillae. (Courtesy of Casey Eye Institute, Oregon Health Sciences University.)

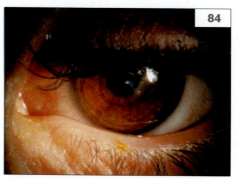

84 Shield ulcer. (Courtesy of Casey Eye Institute, Oregon Health Sciences University.)

Phlyctenular keratoconjunctivitis (phlyctenulosis)

ETIOLOGY

Phlyctenular keratoconjunctivitis represents an inflammatory process secondary to an allergic hypersensitivity response of the conjunctiva and cornea. Phlyctenular keratoconjunctivitis results from a hypersensitivity reaction to bacterial antigens, primarily *Staphylococcus aureus*, but has also been associated with *Mycobacterium tuberculosis, Chlamydia* sp., *Candida albicans*, and some parasites (*Ascaris lumbricoides, Ancylostoma duodenale*). There has also been an association of phlyctenular keratoconjunctivitis in patients with rosacea, Behçet's disease, and human immunodeficiency virus (HIV). It is more common in females especially in the first two decades of life.

The exact mechanism by which the elevated, hard, yellowish-white nodules (phlyctenules) are produced is unclear. Since their presence is associated with foreign antigens, it is believed to represent a delayed allergic hypersensitivity reaction.[40] The presence of accompanying lid disease, with a staphlococcal blepharitis, is a frequent finding in children with phlyctenular keratoconjunctivitis.

CLINICAL PRESENTATION

The classic signs of phlyctenular keratoconjunctivitis are conjunctival injection with the presence of phlyctenules, usually at the limbus. The phlyctenules can also be found on the conjunctiva away from the limbus, as well as on the clear cornea. The patients will typically present with a chronically inflamed red eye, lasting longer than the natural history of viral or bacterial conjunctivitis of 10–14 days, with most of the conjunctival injection surrounding the phlyctenule. The patient may also have failed to improve with the use of a topical antibiotic. Their symptoms may include epiphora, ocular irritation, and a muco-purulent, and/or ropey discharge. The phlyctenules can measure 1–3 mm, and can be bilateral. When there are corneal phlyctenules present, the symptoms tend to be more severe.

MANAGEMENT/TREATMENT

The treatment of phlyctenular keratoconjunctivitis must be aimed at eliminating the antigen that is causing the eye to exhibit the delayed hypersensitivity reaction. The use of good lid hygiene is imperative if blepharitis is present. Lid scrubs two to three times a day, along with the use of a topical antibiotic ointment, will help to get rid of the offending organism and the hypersensitivity reaction. In mild cases, this along with the use of lubricating drops may alleviate the problem completely. In moderate to severe cases of phlyctenular keratoconjunctivitis, especially with significant corneal involvement, the use of a topical steroid, or a topical steroid/antibiotic combination, may be necessary. Because these lesions are sensitive to treatment with a topical steroid, the child can show rapid improvement in signs and symptoms. However, the patient may show exacerbation of signs if the antigen is still present, and the steroids are tapered too quickly. Because the use of topical steroids in these patients may be associated with significant sequelae, management of the treatment should be directed by an ophthalmologist. If there is a significant blepharitis present, the addition of doxycycline to the treatment regime can be considered, but is contraindicated in children younger than 8 years due to the side-effects on the teeth and bones. In cases of phlyctenular keratoconjunctivitis that do not show a significant blepharitis or otherwise appear atypical, a complete workup of the patient, including a purified protein derivative (PPD), chest X-ray, HIV titer, and HLA typing should be performed.

PROGNOSIS

Phlyctenular keratoconjunctivitis can often be controlled and symptoms improved with local treatment. In more severe cases, vision can be reduced secondary to corneal scarring.

Ophthalmia neonatorum

ETIOLOGY

Ophthalmia neonatorum represents a distinct form of conjunctivitis seen during the first 4 weeks postpartum. If conjunctivitis is suspected during this time period, consultation with an ophthalmologist, neonatologist, and infectious disease specialist is highly recommended.

The most common etiologies of ophthalmia neonatorum are chemical conjunctivitis (hyperemia and mucoid discharge during the first 24 hours postpartum) caused by silver nitrate or erythromycin prophylaxis, herpes simplex, *Neisseria gonorrhoeae* and *N. meningitidis*, and *Chlamydia trachomatis* (**85**).[26] The four latter etiologies are all potentially vision- and eye-threatening and will require aggressive treatment. These organisms must be part of the clinician's differential diagnosis for the newborn early on after delivery, especially if the mother has experienced a spontaneous rupture of membranes, and delivery has been intentionally delayed by the obstetrician. With access of these organisms to the unborn child through the cervix and into the uterus, without the protection of an intact amniotic sac, a newborn infant can exhibit the signs and symptoms of an infection earlier than would be expected.

CLINICAL PRESENTATION

The onset of the conjunctivitis may occur in the first few days of life but may be delayed for up to 1 month (*Table 11*). Infants may present with mild conjunctival hyperemia and discharge or with marked conjunctival swelling and copious discharge. Some cases may lead to rapid corneal ulceration and perforation of the eye. Systemic infection can cause sepsis and meningitis.

DIAGNOSIS

Chemical conjunctivitis is a mild irritation and redness of the conjunctiva occurring in the first 24 hours after instillation of silver nitrate prophylaxis of ophthalmia neonatorum. These symptoms can suggest the onset of

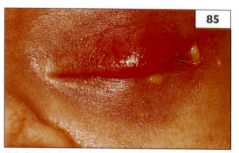

85 Ophthalmia neonatorum caused by chlamydia. (From Vernon S, *Differential Diagnosis in Ophthalmology*, Manson Publishing.)

Table 11 Time line of ophthalmia neonatorum

First 24 hours postpartum	Toxic (chemical conjunctivitis) secondary to instillation of ocular prophylaxis
Postpartum Day 2–5	*Neisseria gonorrhoeae* *N. meningitidis*
Postpartum Day 5–8	*Haemophilus* sp. *Streptococcus pneumoniae* *Staphylococcus aureus,* *Pseudomonas aeruginosa* (rare)
Postpartum Day 5–14	*Chlamydia trachomatis* (serotype D–K)
Postpartum Day 6–14	Herpes simplex virus

conjunctivitis in the newborn, but the condition will improve spontaneously by the second day.

During the first 4 weeks postpartum, cultures and Gram stains of ocular discharge are important before initiating any treatment. The physician must remember that he or she has a minimum of three patients who must be investigated: the newborn baby, the mother, and all of the mother's sexual partners. Unless a suspicion of a severe etiology of an ocular infection is maintained during the ophthalmia neonatorum period, significant and devastating ocular and visual sequelae can occur.

MANAGEMENT/TREATMENT

Treatment is based on the causative organism. Treatment of gonococcal ophthalmia neonatorum includes systemic ceftriaxone. Neonatal chlamydial disease should also be treated systemically due to the risk of pneumonia. The treatment of choice is oral erythromycin, 50 mg/kg per day in four divided doses for 14 days. Topical treatment is not effective.

Prophylaxis for gonorrheal ophthalmia neonatorum with 2% silver nitrate was first introduced by Crede in 1880. It significantly reduced the incidence of gonorrheal conjunctivitis and is still used in many places today. In other areas it has been replaced by erythromycin and tetracycline ointments, which are effective against both *Gonococcus* and trachoma inclusion conjunctivitis agent (TRIC). Povidone–iodine drops have been shown effective and less toxic when compared to erythromycin or silver nitrate ointment, and may be particularly useful in developing countries due to the low cost.

Cornea

Brandon D. Ayres, MD

- **Introduction**

- **Congenital corneal opacity**
Embryology
Peters anomaly
Sclerocornea
Congenital dermoid
Birth trauma
Congenital hereditary endothelial
    dystrophy
Congenital hereditary stromal
    dystrophy
Posterior polymorphous membrane
    dystrophy

- **Metabolic diseases**
Mucopolysaccharidosis
Hurler's syndrome (MPS I-H)
Scheie's syndrome (MPS I-S)
Hunter's syndrome (MPS II)
Morquio's syndrome (MPS IV
    A and B)

Maroteaux–Lamy syndrome (MPS VI
    A and B)
Sly's syndrome (MPS VII)
Idiopathic mucopolysaccharidoses
Mucolipidosis
Sialidosis (ML I)
I-Cell disease (ML II)
Pseudo-Hurler dystrophy (ML III)
ML IV

- **Miscellaneous metabolic diseases**
Fabry's disease
Cystinosis
Tyrosinemia

- **Infectious diseases**
Herpes simplex virus (HSV)
Congenital syphilis
Rubella

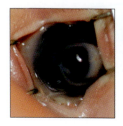 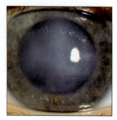 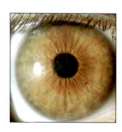 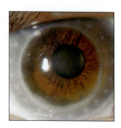

Introduction

The treatment of corneal conditions in children can prove to be challenging. Not only are children at risk for infectious and inflammatory corneal conditions, but they can also have congenital conditions affecting the cornea and anterior segment. Recognizing these conditions is of the utmost importance because treatment can prevent corneal scarring and permanent visual loss. This chapter will be divided into several major subdivisions of congenital corneal opacification, developmental abnormalities, metabolic disease, and infectious etiologies.

Congenital corneal opacity

Embryology

To fully understand the origins of many of the congenital opacities of the cornea it is important to understand the embryogenesis of the anterior segment (meaning the cornea, anterior chamber, iris, and lens). The development of the cornea is triggered by the formation of the lens vesicle at about the sixth week of gestation.[1] At this point the primitive corneal epithelium is resting on a thin acellular basement membrane, adjacent to which is the lens basement membrane and primitive lens vesicle. With separation of the lens vesicle, neural crest-derived mesenchymal cells migrate behind the epithelium forming the corneal endothelium. A second migration of neural crest cells occurs posterior to the forming endothelium, which is destined to form the iris. At the same time cells migrate between the epithelium and endothelium forming the keratocytes of the corneal stroma. By 3 months the endothelium thins to a single cell layer resting on its basal lamina, which is later called Descemet's membrane.[1] One of the more important concepts in the development of the cornea is that it is dependent on proper development of the lens.

Peters anomaly

ETIOLOGY

Peters anomaly was first desribed in 1906 by Peters[2] and is the most common cause of congenital corneal opacity, accounting for approximately 40% of cases.[3] It is an anomaly due to inadequate migration and differentiation of the neural crest cells in forming the anterior segment of the eye and is best classified as a neurocrestopathy.[4,5]

The exact etiology of Peters anomaly is not fully understood. The majority of cases are sporadic and in these cases teratogens such as prenatal rubella infection have been implicated.[6] In cases where there is a family history of Peters anomaly, mutations in the genes FOXC1, PAX6, PITX2, FOXE3, and CYP1B1 have been implicated.[7] Both autosomal dominant and recessive patterns of inheritance have been described.[8] Most likely the findings in Peters anomaly are multifactorial in nature, arising from both genetic and environmental factors.

CLINICAL PRESENTATION

In Peters anomaly there is an area of corneal opacification with associated defects in the corneal stroma, Descemet's membrane, and endothelium.[9,10] In the majority of cases both eyes are involved.[11] The opacity in the cornea may be quite subtle or encompass the entire cornea (**86**). It is also very common to see

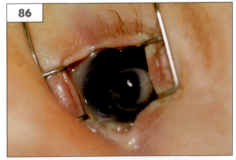

86 8-week-old healthy boy born with anterior segment dysgenesis. Note the irregular cornea with scar tissue. The iris and lens are atrophic.

strands of iris tissue adherent to the margins of the corneal opacity. The lens may be clear or cataractous, and may be adherent to the posterior surface of the cornea. Many physicians will use the status of the lens to classify the anomaly into type I (no lens involvement) and type II (lens involvement).[12]

Peters anomaly can be associated with other ocular and nonocular findings. Glaucoma is a common finding in these patients. The proposed mechanism for the development of the glaucoma is inadequate formation of the pathway for aqueous drainage.[13] Small eyes and retinal conditions have also been reported in association with Peters anomaly. Some of the nonocular conditions reported include developmental delay, congenital heart disease, external ear anormalies, central nervous system (CNS) abnormalities, genitourinary abnormalities, hearing loss, cleft lip and palate, and spinal defects. As most of the associated defects affect midline structures, the recommendation is to screen patients for heart and pituitary defects.[14]

MANAGEMENT/TREATMENT AND PROGNOSIS

Many children with Peters anomaly will require surgery to maintain vision. This is often corneal transplantation and glaucoma surgery to help keep the intraocular pressure under control. Major ophthalmic surgery in young children is quite challenging due to the severity of the disease.

Children with Peters anomaly require frequent follow-up. Often these examinations need to be performed under anesthesia. These frequent trips to the operating room can create both an emotional and financial burden for many families. Studies have shown the transplant survival rate to be between 40 and 60% at 3 years, and perhaps 50% of those children will achieve a final vision of 20/200 or better.[15,16]

Sclerocornea

ETIOLOGY

Sclerocornea is a second congenital condition where the junction between the cornea and the adjacent sclera becomes indistinct. Sclerocornea tends to be a sporadic condition; however, as in most cases of anterior segment dysgenesis, both autosomal dominant and recessive patterns have been reported.[17] In 1993 the MIDAS syndrome was introduced.[18] This syndrome consists of microphthalmia, dermal aplasia, and sclerocornea and is due to deletion at Xp22.3. Typically in this syndrome there are skin defects that involve the upper body including the scalp, face, and neck. Nonocular findings include congenital heart defects, short stature, hypospadias, developmental delay, absence of the corpus callosum, nail dystrophy, and hydrocephalus.[19] Though MIDAS syndrome has a defined area of chromosomal deletion, the exact genetic locus has not been identified.

CLINICAL PRESENTATION

The condition is nonprogressive and tends to be bilateral though often asymmetric.[20] The opacification of the cornea may be peripheral or include the entire cornea, with fine blood vessels continuous with the surrounding conjunctiva. Sclerocornea can be seen as an isolated peripheral corneal opacity or it may be associated with other ocular and systemic abnormalities.[10,21]

MANAGEMENT/TREATMENT AND PROGNOSIS

As in Peters anomaly, many children will need corneal surgery for visual restoration. The destruction of the normal anatomy of the peripheral cornea reduces the success rate in corneal transplantation in sclerocornea. Preoperative ultrasound of the anterior segment (ultrasound biomicroscopy) to look for associated damage to the iris and angle has been helpful in surgical planning.[22]

Congenital dermoid

ETIOLOGY

Congenital dermoid tumors are limbal growths most commonly found in the inferonasal quadrant at the corneal limbus (**87**). They are typically composed of epidermal appendages but also may contain bone, cartilage, teeth, and even brain tissue. In the majority of patients corneal dermoids are an isolated finding. Systemic findings such as eyelid abnormalities and Goldenhar syndrome (**88**) have been reported with corneal dermoids.[23,24] Any patient diagnosed with a dermoid tumor of the cornea should be closely examined for other associated eye, ear, and vertebral abnormalities. Though dermoids are generally thought to be spontaneous in nature, some familial transmission has been documented, where defects to Xq24-qter have been implicated.[25] In other forms of dermoid tumors mutations to the gene PITX2 have been detected.[26]

CLINICAL PRESENTATION

The lesions appear clinically as smooth elevated masses most commonly crossing the corneal limbus in the inferonasal quadrant. Dermoid tumors rarely involve intraocular structures.[24] Dermoids tend to be unilateral but bilateral cases have been reported.[27]

MANAGEMENT/TREATMENT AND PROGNOSIS

The treatment of corneal dermoids is based upon the threat to normal visual development and the concerns of the parents and the patient. Corneal dermoids may induce a unilateral astigmatism which can lead to amblyopia. Removal of the dermoid may be indicated as part of amblyopia treatment or to prevent its development. In some cases, the dermoid can be quite noticeable and becomes a social concern. Surgery can be performed in such cases. Surgery may consist of a partial keratectomy (removal of the anterior portion of the cornea) or a full thickness corneal graft, depending upon how deep the dermoid penetrates the cornea.

Birth trauma

ETIOLOGY

Severe corneal edema and opacity can result from birth trauma. The proposed mechanism of action in these cases is the blade of the forceps compresses the eye causing a rise in intraocular pressure and distention of the eye. These forces cause tears in Descemet's membrane allowing swelling of the cornea.[28] The injured and swollen cornea will often heal without surgical intervention but leaves vertical scars on Descemet's membrane visible with a slit-lamp.

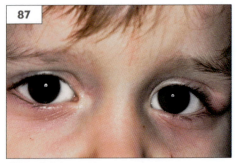

87 Limbal dermoid.

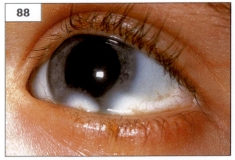

88 Limbal dermoids seen in a child with Goldenhar syndrome. (From Strobel S *et al. Paediatrics and Child Health – The Great Ormond Street Colour Handbook*, Manson Publishing.)

DIAGNOSIS

Diagnosis is made in a child with a history of birth trauma and findings consistent with that trauma. Other causes for corneal clouding need to be eliminated. As with any infant with corneal opacity, suspected birth trauma needs to be evaluated by an ophthalmologist.

MANAGEMENT/TREATMENT AND PROGNOSIS

In those patients who develop large levels of astigmatism, a contact lens can be used to create a more uniform corneal curvature. Even in these very young patients contact lens fitting can be performed and used to prevent permanent visual loss.[29] Even if the cornea remains clear, high astigmatism leading to amblyopia can be seen.[30,31] Birth trauma can lead to problems later in life. Late endothelial decompensation has been reported in patients with birth trauma after cataract surgery leading to corneal edema.[32]

Congenital hereditary endothelial dystrophy

ETIOLOGY

The congenital hereditary endothelial dystrophies (CHED) come in two forms, autosomal dominant (AD) and autosomal recessive (AR).[33] The search for the genetic locus for CHED (both AD and AR) has led to chromosome 20.[34,35] Studies using homozygosity mapping have shown that the genetic loci for the AD and AR forms of CHED are both on chromosome 20, but are distinct. These same studies have led to isolation of the gene SLC4A11 on chromosome 20p in association with the AR form of CHED.[36,37] With this new genetic information, testing and counseling may be beneficial to families in which a parent is affected and for sporadic cases of CHED.

CLINICAL PRESENTATION

In both AD and AR forms there are irregular endothelial cells and loss of cells. Descemet's membrane shows fibrillar deposits in the posterior nonbanded zone. These changes allow hydropic swelling of the corneal stroma and epithelium, leading to increased thickness and a ground glass opacification.[38] The AR form of CHED tends to present at birth with corneal opacification and nystagmus. The infants do not seem to have pain or light sensitivity. In contrast, the AD form of CHED presents at about 2 years of life with corneal swelling, light sensitivity and pain, but lacks the nystagmus.[39] CHED tends to be isolated to the cornea and it is rare for it to be associated with other ocular or systemic conditions.

MANAGEMENT/TREATMENT AND PROGNOSIS

Unfortunately there is no medical treatment for endothelial diseases in children and adults alike. Children with either form of CHED have a poor visual prognosis if untreated and the majority of children will need corneal transplantation (89).[38] Although the prognosis is still guarded, children with CHED seem to have a better prognosis then those with other causes of corneal opacity.[40] The higher success may be related to the relative lack of associated damage to other structures of the eye.

Patients with a later onset of CHED (AD) seem to have a better prognosis than those presenting earlier in life.[41] Early intervention is recommended to reduce the chances for amblyopia and permanently reduced vision.

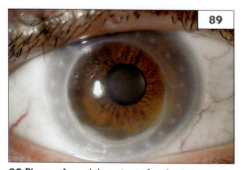

89 Photo of an adult patient after having a transplant as a child for congenital hereditary endothelial dystrophy. Note the clear central corneal transplant and the cloudy peripheral cornea.

Congenital hereditary stromal dystrophy

ETIOLOGY

Congenital hereditary stromal dystrophy (CHSD) is a very rare AD corneal dystrophy. Most of the genetic evidence points to the gene for decorin on chromosome 12.[42] CHSD has not been linked to other associated ocular or systemic conditions.

CLINICAL PRESENTATION

Children with CHSD are born with bilateral corneal opacities. The opacity tends to be worse in the center of the cornea with gradual clearing in the peripheral cornea. Corneal thickness is normal in these patients, indicating irregular arrangement of collagen fibers as the cause of the opacity rather than swelling of the corneal stroma.[43]

MANAGEMENT/TREATMENT AND PROGNOSIS

Treatment for CHSD is similar to CHED. If the opacity is felt to be visually disabling corneal transplantation can be performed. Prognosis is largely based upon corneal graft survival and amblyopia treatment when needed.

Posterior polymorphous membrane dystrophy

ETIOLOGY

Posterior polymorphous membrane dystrophy (PPMD) is inherited in an autosomal dominant pattern. Multiple genetic loci on different chromosomes have been implicated in PPMD. Chromosomes 20p, 20q, 1p, and 10p have all been linked in different families with PPMD.[44–46]

CLINICAL PRESENTATION

Early opacification of the cornea has been reported with PPMD, but this is not the norm.[47] Most patients with PPMD have a band-like opacity in Descemet's membrane, often described as a 'snail track'. The iris can be quite irregular in PPMD with adhesion to the peripheral cornea. With more severe PPMD, glaucoma and corneal opacity are more common (**90**).[48]

The histopathologic findings in PPMD include areas of irregular corneal endothelial cells that look more like epithelial cells. These cells will grow across the cornea and onto the iris blocking fluid drainage from the eye (causing glaucoma). Irregularities in Descemet's membrane have also been noted.[49]

MANAGEMENT/TREATMENT AND PROGNOSIS

Generally speaking PPMD has a mild course and many patients may not know they are affected. PPMD is not typically associated with other systemic findings. Ocular findings may include irregular pupils, glaucoma, and corneal opacity. Transplant is rarely indicated for PPMD; however, if the opacity is severe enough it may become necessary. One major difference between PPMD and the other corneal dystrophies is that the corneal swelling *may* spontaneously improve, negating the need for transplantation.

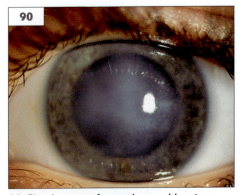

90

90 Cloudy cornea from a 4-year-old patient with posterior polymorphous membrane dystrophy (PPMD).

Metabolic diseases

Metabolic diseases, also known as inborn errors of metabolism, are known to cause corneal opacity. The majority of metabolic diseases are inherited in an AR fashion and are due to dysfunctional lysosomal enzymes (lysosomal storage disease). The poorly or nonfunctioning enzymes allow the collection of metabolic debris in the end organ where that enzyme is being used and often includes the cornea. It is important to understand that the patient with a metabolic disease due to an inborn error of metabolism may be born with a clear cornea and develop clouding over time. The two main classes of inborn errors of metabolism include errors of carbohydrate metabolism (mucopolysaccharidosis) and lipid metabolism (mucolipidosis).

Mucopolysaccharidosis

ETIOLOGY

Not every mucopolysaccharidosis (MPS) causes corneal clouding. The most commonly associated MPS that have corneal findings include MPS I-H (Hurler's syndrome), MPS I-S (Scheie's syndrome), MPS II (Hunter's syndrome), MPS IV A and B (Morquio's syndrome), and MPS VI A and B (Maroteaux–Lamy syndrome). Glycosaminoglycans (GAGs) are very important in maintaining the structure of the cornea. Keratin sulfate and chondroitin sulfate serve as the backbone for the extracellular matrix of the cornea keeping a constant interfibrillar distance.[50] If the distance is altered the clarity of the cornea is reduced. Heparin sulfate and other GAGs are also expressed in the epithelial layer of the cornea and likely play a role in corneal wound healing.[51] With the disruption in GAG metabolism, lysosomal storage products collect, causing a loss of clarity in the cornea as well as symptoms associated with deposition in other target organs.

DIAGNOSIS

Diagnosis is based upon the clinical manifestations of the disease along with laboratory confirmation of the genetic/enzymatic defect involved.

MANAGEMENT/TREATMENT AND PROGNOSIS

The current treatment for many of the mucopolysaccharidoses is bone marrow transplantation to replace hematopoietic stem cells. With early treatment many of the signs of the storage diseases can be minimized including corneal clouding.[52] Enzyme replacement is also an option for these patients; however, the ocular findings may not regress and may continue to worsen.[53] Gene replacement therapy shows promise in treating MPS. Most studies are currently in animal models, but with time this may become a treatment option in humans.[54]

The prognosis for retention of good vision is based upon the clarity of the central cornea and the involvement of other structures of the eye such as the retina or optic nerve. The overall prognosis for these patients is dependent on involvement of other vital organ systems that may occur in each individual disorder.

Hurler's syndrome (MPS I-H)

The ocular findings in Hurler's syndrome include clouding of the cornea, optic nerve swelling, glaucoma, and retinal degeneration (**91–93**). Associated findings include short stature, joint stiffness, gargoyle-like faces, cardiac abnormalities, and progressive mental retardation.

Hurler's syndrome is an AR inborn error of metabolism due to a deficiency in α-iduronidase. The enzyme deficiency leads to accumulation of dermatan and heparin sulfate. Unfortunately children with Hurler's syndrome have a short life expectancy (8–9 years average) even with proper diagnosis and treatment.[55]

Scheie's syndrome (MPS I-S)

Scheie's syndrome is basically a less severe form of Hurler's syndrome. Patients with Scheie's syndrome also have the corneal clouding, joint stiffness, coarse facies, and cardiac manifestations. Mental retardation is not present. Scheie's syndrome is also inherited in an AR fashion. It is caused by a deficiency in α-iduronidase. Hurlers's syndrome and Sheie's syndrome both represent different ends of the spectrum for a similar disease. Patients can present with variable features including heart, skeletal, neurodevelopmental, and ocular findings.

The clouding of the cornea in Scheie's syndrome is slower and may only be in the periphery of the cornea.[56] Corneal transplantation is not likely to be needed. Patients with Scheie's syndrome live to adulthood with normal life expectancy.[57]

Hunter's syndrome (MPS II)

The clinical picture of Hunter's syndrome is similar to that seen in Hurler's and Scheie's syndromes and mental retardation may or may not be present. Congenital clouding of the cornea is not typical in Hunter's syndrome. Rarely, corneal clouding can present later in life. This may be due to swelling of the corneal keratocytes with dermatan and heparan sulfate.[58]

Hunter's syndrome is the only X-linked recessive MPS. Hunter's syndrome is due to a deficiency in iduronosulfate sulfatase.

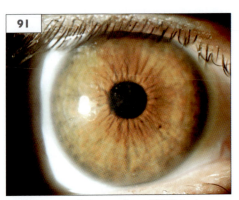

91 Mild corneal changes from PPMD in the mother of the patient in **92**.

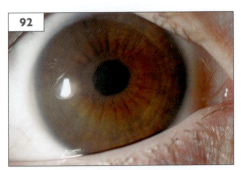

92 Cornea from a pediatric patient with Hurler's syndrome. Note the diffuse haze in the cornea.

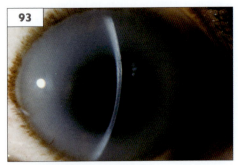

93 Hurler's syndrome.

Morquio's syndrome (MPS IV A and B)

Morquio's syndrome is an AR deficiency of N-acetylgalactosamine-6-sulfate sulfatase. This deficiency leads to the accumulation of keratin sulfate. Corneal clouding can occur with Morquio's syndrome but this is often later in life. Accumulation of membrane-bound inclusion bodies can also be found in the conjunctiva and retina.[59] Severe odontoid hypoplasia is common in this syndrome, leading to cervical dislocation. Spondylo-epiphyseal abnormalities and aortic regurgitation are also hallmarks of this syndrome. Patients with Morquio's syndrome are of normal intelligence.

Maroteaux–Lamy syndrome (MPS VI A and B)

Corneal opacification in Maroteaux–Lamy syndrome is a very common finding. The primary enzyme deficiency is arylsulfatase B and it is inherited in an AR manner. The lack of arylsulfatase B leads to the accumulation of dermatan sulfate. As with many of the other lysosomal storage diseases, skeletal abnormalities are common as is hepato-splenomegaly. Coarse facies (mild), joint stiffness, and heart disease are also common. Corneal opacities and clouding are very common in Maroteaux–Lamy syndrome at a very young age.[60] If the corneal opacification is severe corneal transplantation is necessary. Glaucoma has also been reported in cases of Maroteaux–Lamy syndrome.[61]

Sly's syndrome (MPS VII)

Sly's syndrome is a rare AR syndrome due to a defect in the enzyme β-glucuronidase. The enzyme deficiency leads to the accumulation of dermatan sulfate. Patients with Sly's syndrome have been reported to have corneal opacification. Hepatosplenomegaly, skeletal deformity, and mental retardation have also been reported.[62]

Idiopathic mucopolysaccharidoses

Congenital corneal opacification due to mucopolysaccharide accumulation in the cornea has been reported in the absence of any systemic inborn error of metabolism.[63] This is a very rare cause of congenital corneal opacity and must be a diagnosis of exclusion.

Mucolipidosis

The mucolipidoses (MLs) are a group of storage diseases that have clinical features of both lipidoses and mucopolysaccharidoses.[64] Unlike in the mucopolysaccharidoses, the urinary excretion of GAGs is normal. There are four (I–IV) types of ML and all of them can have corneal clouding. The congenital corneal findings are most common in ML type IV, where it is a hallmark of the disease, and in type II (I-cell disease).

Sialidosis (ML I)

ML I is caused by a deficiency in neuraminidase leading to an accumulation of sialyloligo-saccharides. This disease exists in two major forms: infantile (I) and congenital (II) form. Patients will often show hepatosplenomegaly, mental retardation, skeletal abnormalities, and a cherry red spot on the retina.[65] Corneal clouding is seen, but is relatively uncommon.[66]

I-Cell disease (ML II)

The enzymatic defect in ML II is in N-acetyl-glucosaminyl-phosphotransferase. Affected children with this condition typically have a short life expectancy. Clinical features include gingival hyperplasia, hepatomegaly, delayed motor development, coarse facial features, hirsutism, low-set ears, and corneal clouding. Almost half of infants with I-Cell disease will have some level of congenital clouding of the cornea.[67]

Pseudo-Hurler dystrophy (ML III)

ML III is often considered a less severe form of ML II. The same N-acetyl-glucosaminyl-phosphotransferase enzyme is deficient, but may have more residual activity. Patients will show joint stiffness, short stature, and gingival hyperplasia.[64] Though almost all patients with ML-III will eventually show corneal clouding, it may not be present at birth.[68]

ML IV

ML IV is a condition classically seen in the Ashkenazi Jewish population. The exact enzymatic defect for ML IV is still uncertain. This disease is primarily one with ocular findings including corneal opacities, retinal degeneration, optic neuropathy, ocular misalignment, and psychomotor retardation.[69] Patients with ML IV may also have decreased proton secretion in parietal cells leading to iron deficiency anemia and achlorhydria.[70]

The treatment options for the MLs are limited. The corneal changes seen in ML IV are known to cause significant ocular pain and tearing as well as reduced vision.[71] The pathology in the cornea with ML IV seems to be primarily limited to the corneal epithelium. Transplantation of limbal tissue and conjunctiva has been reported to help improve the corneal epithelial abnormalities from which these patients suffer.[72]

Miscellaneous metabolic diseases

Fabry's disease

ETIOLOGY

Fabry's disease is an X-linked recessive disorder resulting from a deficiency in the α-galactosidase enzyme.[73] The accumulation of glycolipid leads to the observed systemic and ocular findings.

CLINICAL PRESENTATION

Ocular findings in Fabry's disease include cataract formation, retinal vascular tortuosity, and swirls seen in the corneal epithelium called verticillata. The corneal changes are the most commonly seen ophthalmic finding and may be seen by 6 months of age.[74] Systemic findings include angiokeratomas, cardiac conduction defects, mitral valve prolapse, renal dysfunction, and painful peripheral neuropathy.[75]

MANAGEMENT/TREATMENT AND PROGNOSIS

Treatment of Fabry's disease currently focuses on supportive treatment for painful episodes or end-organ failure and enzyme replacement therapy. Early treatment with enzyme replacement has shown promise with reduced end-organ damage and reduced pain.[75]

Cystinosis

ETIOLOGY

Cystinosis is caused by a deficiency of a membrane-bound transport protein allowing transport of cystine out of lysosomes. The accumulation of cystine in the lysosome allows crystals to form and deposit in several different organs including the kidneys, bone marrow, pancreas, muscle, brain, and eye.[76] Cystinosis is a rare AR disorder that can be divided into non-nephropathic (mild) and nephropathic (severe) forms. Nephropathic cystinosis further divides into infantile and intermediate types.[77] Infantile nephropathic cystinosis is the form that has early corneal findings. Needle-like crystals first form in the peripheral cornea and over time migrate centrally.[78] The deposits in the cornea may not reduce vision but will cause light sensitivity and pain.

MANAGEMENT/TREATMENT AND PROGNOSIS

Treatment of the corneal erosions due to cystine crystals was once purely supportive with frequent lubricant drops and ointments. Bandage contact lenses can be used to reduce both the frequency and pain of epithelial erosions. Over the past several years topical cysteamine drops have been used to reduce the corneal signs and symptoms of cystinosis.[79] Treatment with oral cysteamine can minimize many of the systemic findings in cystinosis, but does not reduce crystal formation in the cornea.[80]

Tyrosinemia

ETIOLOGY

Oculocutaneous tyrosinemia (tyrosinemia type II or Richner–Hanhart syndrome) is an AR disorder, caused by a deficiency of hepatic tyrosine aminotransferase.

CLINICAL PRESENTATION

Affected patients suffer from mental retardation, a hyperkeratotic rash on the palms and soles of their feet, and dendritic corneal lesions. The ocular findings can often present before the cutaneous.[81] The lesions seen on the cornea look very much like the lesions seen in herpetic keratitis, and may stain with fluorescein stain. What differentiates these lesions from those seen in HSV is bilateral involvement, lack of response to antiviral therapy, and normal corneal sensation. The corneal changes often present in the first year of life and are associated with a significant amount of pain, light sensitivity, and tearing.[81]

Diagnosis of tyrosinemia II is confirmed by finding elevated levels of plasma or urine tyrosine levels. Any infant diagnosed with bilateral herpetic keratitis should be screened for tyrosinemia.

MANAGEMENT/TREATMENT AND PROGNOSIS

Treatment of tyrosinemia II is through dietary restriction of tyrosine and phenylalanine. With early detection and dietary changes, both systemic and corneal signs can be improved.[82]

Infectious diseases

Corneal infections which lead to scarring and opacity can be caused by both bacterial and viral mediators. These are not seen very commonly but need to be kept in the differential diagnosis of a corneal opacity. In some patients sensation is reduced in the cornea due to either infectious keratitis or other congenital causes such as familial dysautonomia or Goldenhar–Gorlin–Goltz syndrome.[83] The following section reviews the most common causes of keratitis in the pediatric population.

Herpes simplex virus (HSV)

ETIOLOGY

One of the most common corneal infections seen in the adult population is due to the herpes simplex virus, type I. The pediatric patients most affected by this are the neonates. In the neonate herpetic infection is relatively uncommon with estimates as low as 1 in 20,000 to as high as 1 in 3000.[84] An estimated 20% of neonates will manifest ocular infection in the form of periocular dermatitis, dendritic or stromal keratitis, or chorioretinitis.

Approximately 35% of neonatal HSV infection is from HSV I, the remainder is from HSV II.[85] Transmission can be transplacental, exposure during delivery, or exposure shortly after birth.[86]

MANAGEMENT/TREATMENT AND PROGNOSIS

Treatment for neonatal HSV relies on prompt diagnosis. Timely diagnosis is critical due to the relatively high incidence of encephalitis due to HSV, which can lead to death or permanent neurologic sequelae. Many expecting mothers are asymptomatic at the time of delivery but can still transmit the virus. Even C-section delivery does not guarantee nontransmission. The use of intravenous antiviral medication has reduced morbidity and mortality from HSV, but even with early diagnosis and proper treatment an excellent outcome is not guaranteed.[87]

Congenital syphilis

ETIOLOGY

Congenital syphilis occurs in fetuses infected after 16 weeks of gestation. Before that time, transmission to the fetus can occur but does not lead to damage to the developing eye. Almost all children born to mothers with primary syphilis acquired after the fourth month of pregnancy will develop congenital syphilis.

CLINICAL PRESENTATION

Congenital syphilis will often lead to bilateral corneal scarring in association with intraocular inflammation. In the majority of patients corneal scarring is not seen at birth, but presents after the age of 2 years. The keratitis typically presents as peripheral inflammation in the cornea that progresses centrally. The corneal changes tend to be a later ocular sequela of congenital syphilis and signs of retinal damage are already present by the time the keratitis is noted. Corneal scarring associated with hearing loss and notched teeth due to congenital syphilis is commonly known as Hutchinson's triad. Other common nonocular stigmata of congenital syphilis include frontal bossing of the forehead, saddle nose defect,[88] and skin wrinkling radiating from the mouth.[89]

MANAGEMENT/TREATMENT AND PROGNOSIS

Any patient with suspected ocular changes from congenital syphilis needs to be treated by an eye care specialist. Many authorities feel that patients with ocular findings need to be treated as neurosyphilis patients. Early treatment can prevent corneal scarring. Corneal scarring may require transplantation.

Rubella

ETIOLOGY

Ocular involvement in congenital rubella is caused by maternal infection with rubella in the first trimester with transplacental transmission to the fetus. Infection in the later stages of pregnancy does not result in serious ophthalmic sequelae.

Congenital infection with rubella can cause extensive damage to the eye. Cataract formation, congenital glaucoma, corneal opacity, and microphthalmia have all been reported from congenital infection with rubella.[90,91]

MANAGEMENT/TREATMENT AND PROGNOSIS

In most developed countries vaccination has helped to eradicate congenital rubella. If necessary, surgery to reduce the pressure of glaucoma or to remove a congenital cataract can be done. With persistent corneal edema corneal transplantation is necessary for normal visual development. The best way to reduce visual loss due to infectious diseases such as rubella is to continue with aggressive vaccination programs, which have reduced the incidence of vaccine-preventable disease in the US to an all-time low.[92]

Lens disorders

Richard P. Golden, MD

- **Introduction**

- **Structural lens abnormalities**
  Aphakia
  Spherophakia (microspherophakia)
  Coloboma
  Subluxation (ectopia lentis)
  Lenticonus
  Persistant fetal vasculature

- **Cataracts**
  Nuclear cataracts
  Lamellar cataracts
  Anterior polar cataracts
  Posterior polar cataracts
  Sutural cataracts
  Anterior subcapsular cataracts
  Posterior subcapsular cataracts
  Cerulean (blue-dot) cataracts
  Complete cataracts

- **Etiology of cataracts**
  Genetic and metabolic diseases
  Trauma
  Medication and toxicity
  Maternal infection

- **Diagnosis of cataracts**

- **Management/treatment of cataracts**
  Visual significance
  Surgery
  Aphakia
  Pseudophakia
  Amblyopia

- **Cataract prognosis**

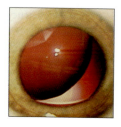
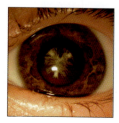
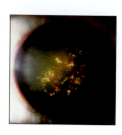
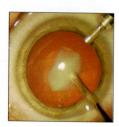

Cataracts

Congenital and infantile cataracts may be classified by their morphology, etiology, presence of specific metabolic disorders, and by associated ocular and systemic anomalies. When bilateral, approximately one-third of these cataracts occur as an inherited trait, one-third are associated with specific diseases or syndromes, and one-third are idiopathic.[4]

Nuclear cataracts

Nuclear cataracts may be unilateral (**99, 100**), but often are seen bilaterally and are associated with an autosomal dominant (AD) inheritance pattern. The location in the embryonal or fetal nucleus suggests a congenital onset, but acquired cases are also seen. They are usually dense and highly visually significant. They may be diagnosed at or shortly after birth due to an abnormal or absent red reflex and leukocoria.

Lamellar cataracts

These opacities are whitish and occupy a layer between the nucleus and cortex. The nucleus and more peripheral cortex are generally clear. The visual significance can vary widely and may be progressive (**101–104**). Lamellar cataracts are occasionally unilateral, but are more often bilateral. The location suggests that these opacities are usually acquired and may be a result of an intrauterine insult.

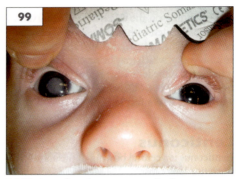

99 Unilateral nuclear cataract of unknown etiology in a 6-week-old infant with hypoplastic left heart syndrome.

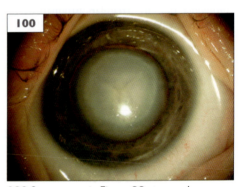

100 Same eye as in Figure **99** seen under operating microscope. Note the clear lens peripheral to the opacity.

Anterior polar cataracts

Anterior polar cataracts are small, white, central opacities. They derive from abnormal separation of the lens vesicle during embryogenesis. These opacities may be transmitted in an AD pattern, but over 90% are sporadic.[5] They are typically 1–2 mm in size and are not progressive, although progression has been described.[6] Approximately one-third are bilateral (**105–107**). They are not often highly visually significant, but may be associated with amblyopia due to variable degrees of anisometropia. Surgical intervention is not frequently necessary.

Posterior polar cataracts

Similar to their anterior equivalents, posterior polar cataracts are small, white, central opacities. They are often seen in association with aniridia. They may be highly visually significant, even when relatively small. Posterior lenticonus may also lead to central posterior opacities that may be similar in appearance. However, the opacities associated with posterior lenticonus may be rapidly progressive, unlike true posterior polar cataracts.

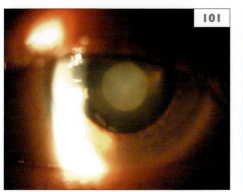 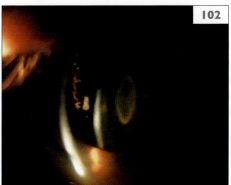

101, 102 Visually significant lamellar cataract in a 5-year-old. Vision was 20/80 prior to surgery.

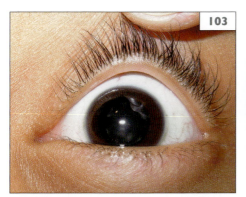 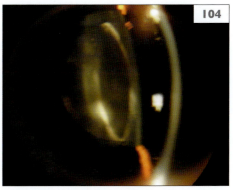

103, 104 Minimally visually significant lamellar cataract in a 9-year-old. Vision was 20/30.

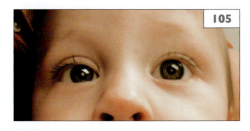 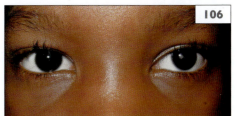

105 Asymmetric bilateral anterior polar cataracts in a 3-year-old. Vision was 20/50 in the right and 20/40 in the left.

106, 107 Unilateral anterior polar cataract in a 7-year-old.

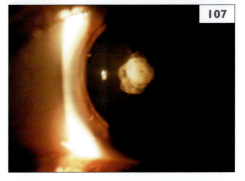

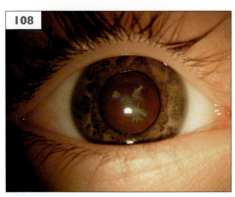 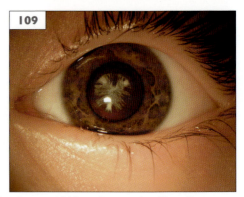

108, 109 Asymmetric bilateral sutural cataracts in a 3-year-old. Note the associated lamellar opacities, worse in the left eye.

Sutural cataracts

These congenital opacities involve the nuclear Y-sutures. They may be unilateral or bilateral (**108, 109**). When bilateral, sutural cataracts are often associated with an AD inheritance pattern. Autosomal recessive (AR) and X-linked recessive patterns have also been described.[7] They can be progressive and the visual significance may vary widely (**110**).

Anterior subcapsular cataracts

Anterior subcapsular opacities occur immediately beneath the anterior lens capsule. They are usually acquired and most commonly associated with abnormalities of the anterior capsule anatomy (anterior lenticonus seen with Alport syndrome) or with trauma (**111**). They may also be idiopathic. The visual significance is generally not severe, but may be variable.

Posterior subcapsular cataracts

Posterior subcapsular opacities are most often idiopathic, but may be associated with trauma (**112, 113**), chronic corticosteroid use, uveitis, or Down's syndrome.[5] They may also develop in conjunction with posterior polar cataracts seen with posterior lenticonus. They are located immediately anterior to the posterior lens capsule and are generally highly visually significant.

Cerulean (blue-dot) cataracts

These are multiple, small, bluish-white opacities seen diffusely throughout the peripheral lens cortex and are almost always bilateral (**114**). Inheritance pattern is usually AD.[8] They may also be idiopathic or seen in association with Down's syndrome. They may be slowly progressive, but are generally only minimally visually significant.

Complete cataracts

The entire lens is opacified and the red reflex is obscured. Complete cataracts may be present at birth or may progress from other subtotal opacities. Trauma is another common etiology. They may be unilateral or bilateral and produce severe visual impairment (**115**).

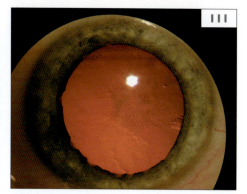

110 Mild sutural cataract seen at the slit-lamp. The opacity was asymptomatic in this 12-year-old.

111 Anterior subcapsular cataract due to trauma from a paintball gun. Note the wrinkling of the anterior capsule from fibrosis and peripheral cortical vacuoles.

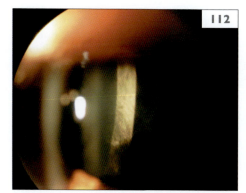

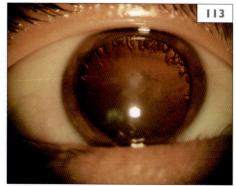

112, 113 Posterior subcapsular cataracts associated with a history of blunt trauma. Note the multiple peripheral cortical vacuoles (**113**).

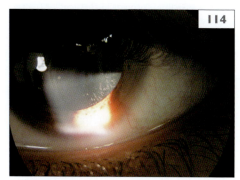

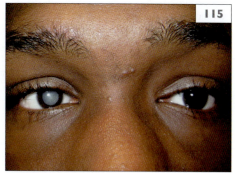

114 Cerulean cataract in a 10-year-old. Similar opacities were seen in the contralateral eye as well as in the mother.

115 Unilateral complete cataract in a 16-year-old from unknown etiology.

Etiology of cataracts

Genetic and metabolic diseases

DOWN'S SYNDROME

Down's syndrome may be associated with cataract formation at any age, but it typically presents within the first year of life. The opacities may vary in location and appearance. Other ocular abnormalities associated with Down's syndrome include epicanthal folds, refractive errors, iris abnormalities (Brushfield spots), strabismus, nasolacrimal duct obstruction, retinal abnormalities, amblyopia, and nystagmus.[9]

GALACTOSEMIA

This is an autosomal recessive disorder caused by a deficiency of one of three enzymes (galactokinase, galactose-1-phosphate uridyl transferase, or uridine diphosphate galactose epimerase). It frequently leads to bilateral cataracts, which may begin with a classic 'oil-droplet' appearance. It may be at least partially reversible with the elimination of galactose from the diet. If left untreated, it may progress to complete opacification of the lens.[10]

LOWE SYNDROME

Lowe syndrome (oculocerebrorenal) is an X-linked recessive disease characterized by cataracts, mental retardation, and renal aminoaciduria. Lens opacities occur in nearly 100% of affected males and may be associated with posterior lenticonus (**116**).[11] Development of glaucoma is also common. Female carriers may have mild peripheral lens opacities as well.[12] Diagnosis is confirmed by identifying amino acids in the urine. Life expectancy is significantly reduced with death often in the second decade.

ALPORT SYNDROME

This is an X-linked dominant disorder characterized by anterior lenticonus, deafness, and interstitial nephritis.[13] Anterior lenticonus is frequently associated with anterior subcapsular cataract formation (**117**). Rarely, the lens capsule may spontaneously rupture, leading to complete cataract.[14]

DIABETES

Diabetes-related cataracts may occasionally be found in children. These cataracts typically appear as diffuse subcapsular or snowflake-like opacities.

HYPOGLYCEMIA

This is often seen in low birth-weight infants. Cataracts are usually bilateral and lamellar, but may cause complete opacity.[5]

MYOTONIC DYSTROPHY

Myotonic dystrophy is an AD muscular dystrophy characterized by progressive muscle wasting. The classic bilateral lens opacities appear as polychromatic, iridescent 'Christmas-tree' cataracts (**118**). Additional ocular features include ptosis, extraocular muscle paresis, microphthalmos, and retinal pigmentary degeneration. Nervous system involvement and cardiac abnormalities are also typical.[15] Hypoparathyroidism occasionally leads to cataract formation in children. The opacities are related to hypocalcemia and consist of multicolored flecks (similar to the 'Christmas-tree' cataract seen in myotonic dystrophy).

FABRY'S SYNDROME

This is a rare X-linked recessive disease caused by a defect in the activity of the alpha-galactosidase A enzyme. It leads to abnormal glycosphingolipid storage, which then accumulates in the eyes, central and peripheral nervous systems, cardiac muscle, kidneys, and vascular tissue. Early signs of the disease include pain and burning in the extremities as well as reddish-purple punctate skin lesions (angiokeratoma corporis diffusum). Affected males generally die in their 3rd–4th decades from cardiovascular disease and renal failure. Lens opacities are common and have a characteristic appearance. They appear as posterior spokelike cataracts, which are pathognomonic for the condition. Anterior subcapsular cataracts may also be seen. Other ocular features of this disease include classic corneal subepithelial whorl-like opacities and vascular abnormalities of the conjunctiva and retina.[16]

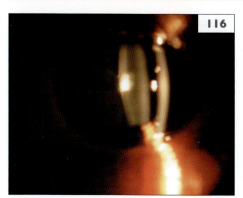

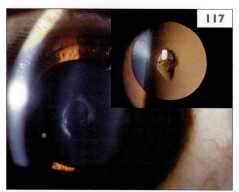

116 Slit-lamp view of a posterior polar cataract associated with posterior lenticonus in a 10-year-old.

117 Anterior lenticonus associated with Alport syndrome seen by direct slit-lamp examination and retroillumination (inset). (Courtesy of M. Edward Wilson, Jr., MD.)

REFSUM SYNDROME

This is a disorder of phytanic acid metabolism that results from defects in phytanoyl-CoA hydroxylase. Ocular associations include pupil abnormalities, retinitis pigmentosa, nystagmus, and cataract.[17] Nonocular associations include deafness, anosmia, cerebellar ataxia, and peripheral polyneuropathy. Treatment consists of restriction of dietary phytanic acid.

WILSON'S DISEASE

This is a rare, AR disorder characterized by abnormal copper metabolism. Copper accumulates in various organs, including the liver, central nervous system, and eye. The classic ocular findings include a Kayser–Fleischer ring (a greenish-brown accumulation in the peripheral cornea) and a yellowish, petaloid, anterior subcapsular opacity termed a 'sunflower' cataract.[18]

CONRADI SYNDROME

This is an X-linked dominant form of chondrodysplasia punctata characterized by asymmetric limb shortening, skin abnormalities, and sparse hair. Cataracts are an occasional feature of this disorder.[19]

MANNOSIDOSIS

This is a rare AR lysosomal storage disease due to a deficiency in alpha- or beta-mannosidase (type 1 and 2 respectively), which leads to defective lipoprotein degradation. An assay for

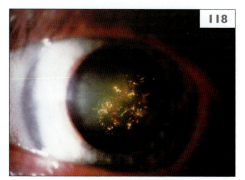

118 Classic 'Christmas-tree' cataract seen in myotonic dystrophy. (Reproduced, with permission, from Johns KJ, *Basic and Clinical Science Course: Cataract and Lens, Section 11*, American Academy of Ophthalmology, 2001–2002.)

the specific enzyme is diagnostic. Posterior spokelike or scattered punctate lens opacities are characteristic and generally form within the first year of life.[20] Type 1 disease is most severe, generally resulting in progressive mental and motor retardation, leading to death in the first decade of life.

ANTERIOR SEGMENT DYSGENESIS SYNDROMES

These are a heterogeneous group of disorders characterized by variable degrees of abnormalities in development of the anterior segment structures. These conditions include Axenfeld–Reiger syndrome (**119, 120**), Peters anomaly, iridocorneal endothelial (ICE) syndrome, and Alagille's syndrome. Glaucoma is a common complicating factor in these disorders and cataracts may also be seen.[21]

ANIRIDIA

Aniridia is an AD or sporadic condition most notably characterized by nearly complete absence of the iris. A rudimentary iris is almost always present, however. Multiple ocular abnormalities are generally found in association with aniridia including glaucoma, cataract, foveal and optic nerve hypoplasia, nystagmus, and progressive corneal opacification. Lens subluxation may also develop. The sporadic form has been associated with Wilm's tumor in approximately one-third of cases.[22,23] It may also be associated with genitourinary abnormalities and mental retardation (WAGR association). Individuals with sporadic aniridia should be followed with serial abdominal ultrasounds to look for Wilm's tumor, which is generally diagnosed by age 5 years.[24]

HALLERMANN–STREIFF SYNDROME

This is an extremely rare condition without any known inheritance pattern. It is thought to occur as a result of new sporadic mutations. Affected individuals exhibit short stature, extremely thin skin, severe dental abnormalities, and an unusual 'birdlike' facies. Cataracts are present in over 90% of cases.[25]

Trauma

Trauma is the most common cause of acquired cataracts in children. Both penetrating and nonpenetrating trauma can lead to cataract formation (**121–124**). Significant damage to other ocular structures is often seen. Occasionally, even seemingly mild trauma may lead to cataract formation. If the lens capsule remains intact, anterior subcapsular, posterior subcapsular, and cortical opacities are most common, but complete cataract may also be seen. If the lens capsule is ruptured, either by direct penetration, or by severe nonpenetrating injuries, complete cataract may form rapidly. In the case of penetrating trauma, computed tomography (CT) scan is useful to assess for retained intraocular foreign bodies. In nonpenetrating trauma, B-scan ultrasound is used to assess for retinal detachments and other posterior segment abnormalities. Once the lens capsule has been breached, early removal of the lens is indicated to help limit intraocular inflammation. Individuals with traumatic cataracts should be monitored for the development of glaucoma, which may arise secondary to damage of other anterior segment structures.

Medication and toxicity

Various medications (topical and systemic) have been implicated in the formation of cataracts. The most common medication-induced cataracts are secondary to corticosteroids (**125**). The incidence is dose and duration dependent. Typical opacities associated with this class of medication appear as posterior subcapsular cataracts, but it may lead to complete opacification as well. Other medications

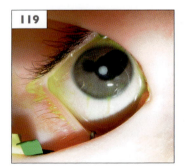
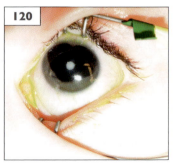

119, 120 Bilateral anterior polar cataracts in a 1-year-old associated with Axenfeld–Reiger syndrome. Note the severe iris hypoplasia in these microphthalmic eyes.

121–124 Traumatic cataracts. Cataracts secondary to blunt trauma from a golf club (**121**), a paintball gun injury with associated anterior capsule rupture and iris synechia (**122**), nonpenetrating BB gun injury with associated iris defect and posterior capsule rupture (**123**), and penetrating injury from a tree branch involving the anterior capsule (**124**) (note the four sutures in the cornea from the corneal laceration repair).

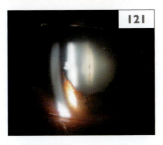

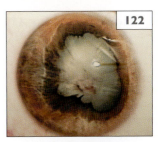

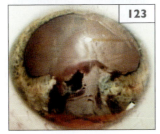

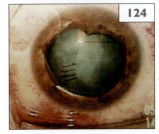

125 Posterior subcapsular cataract associated with chronic prednisone use in a 13-year-old with systemic juvenile rheumatoid arthritis.

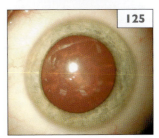

implicated in cataract formation include amiodarone, phenothiazines, chloroquine, busulfan, and the topical anticholinesterase and miotic drugs used to treat chronic open-angle glaucoma.[26]

Toxic chemicals which come in contact with the eye and cause corneal burns may lead to cataract formation. Exposure to radiation or chronic cigarette smoke is also a risk factor for the development of lens opacities. Iron (siderosis), gold (chrysiasis), silver (argyriasis), and copper (chalcosis) may cause cataracts.

Maternal infection

Intrauterine infections may result in cataracts. These opacities are most often bilateral, but may be unilateral. The majority of these infection-related cataracts are caused by toxoplasmosis, rubella, cytomegalovirus, herpes simplex, and syphilis (TORCHS). Varicella, measles, mumps, and human immuno-deficiency virus (HIV) have also been implicated in some cases.[5] Rubella is the most common and most classic etiology of intrauterine infection causing congenital cataracts. Congenital rubella is also associated with a high incidence of sensorineural hearing loss, heart defects, and mental retardation. Other ocular findings may include retinopathy, strabismus, microphthalmos, optic atrophy, keratitis, and glaucoma.[27] Live virus particles may remain dormant in the lens and severe inflammation may ensue when the cataract is removed. Congenital rubella syndrome is now extremely rare in the US since the introduction of the vaccine, but the incidence is much higher in unvaccinated populations.

Diagnosis of cataracts

A critical first step in the optimal management of pediatric cataracts is early recognition of the problem. Diagnosis is often first made by family members or primary care physicians who notice a white or partially white pupil in one or both eyes (leukocoria). Careful examination of the red reflex of both eyes using a direct ophthalmoscope (Bruckner test) can usually detect even the most minor of lens opacities. Asymmetry of the red reflex in a child of any age should raise concern for cataract or other ocular abnormalities and warrants prompt referral to an ophthalmologist. Strabismus (usually in unilateral cases) or nystagmus (usually in bilateral cases) may also be the presenting sign of childhood cataracts. The onset of nystagmus is generally considered a poor prognostic sign for achieving good visual outcomes.[28]

Careful evaluation of the medical and family history of patients with childhood cataracts, along with evaluation of the opacity and other associated ocular and systemic abnormalities, can often lead the clinician to elicit the etiology. If other dysmorphic features are present, consultation with a geneticist should be considered. When the etiology cannot be determined, further laboratory testing may be indicated. In the case of unilateral cataracts, TORCHS titers (IgM) and Venereal disease Research Laboratory (VDRL) for syphilis is all that is generally necessary. If bilateral, urine should be tested for reducing substances (after milk-feeding). Additional optional testing includes calcium and phosphorus levels, red cell galactokinase level, and urine for amino acids.[4,5]

Management/treatment of cataracts

Visual significance

Determination of the visual significance of a particular lens opacity is an important step to help guide treatment. In neonates, this evaluation can at times be especially challenging. Streak retinoscopy and view of the ocular fundus using a direct ophthalmoscope can give the ophthalmologist a good sense of the visual significance. Careful examination of the particular characteristics and morphology of the

cataract is also important. In general, opacities in the visual axis >3 mm can be assumed to be significant. Posterior opacities and confluent opacities (without intervening clear zones) also tend to be more visually significant. If surgical intervention is deemed necessary in a neonate, timing of such intervention is critical to help maximize visual outcomes. When possible, this should take place before 6 weeks of age in unilateral cases and 8 weeks if bilateral.[29,30] Surgery should occur even earlier when possible. Such early intervention can lead to good visual acuities and binocular function.[31]

In older preverbal children, careful assessment of fixation preference and other visual behaviors can be a reliable indicator of visual deficits. The use of special tests, such as pattern visually evoked potentials and the preferential looking test (Teller acuity cards), may be effective tools to help determine levels of reduced vision and are especially useful in determining interocular differences in vision.

In verbal children, acuity can be accurately assessed using various optotypes (Allen figures, tumbling E chart, HOTV matching, or Snellen letters). There still remains the challenge, however, of determining at what level of visual deficit is surgery indicated. Most would agree that cataracts causing a reduction in visual acuity beyond 20/70 require surgery.[5] Some feel that vision of 20/50 or less is a more appropriate cutoff for surgical intervention.[32]

Opacities that are not visually significant can usually be carefully observed over time to monitor for signs of progression or development of amblyopia. Anisometropia (difference in refractive error) is common and should be corrected optically with glasses or contacts. In some cases, amblyopia from anisometropia may be more significant than the cataract itself. Aggressive treatment of the anisometropic amblyopia is indicated prior to considering cataract surgery in these instances. Opacities that are only mildly visually significant can often be managed conservatively. If unilateral or asymmetric, patching the better eye, in addition to optical correction, can be effective at preventing or treating amblyopia.

Surgery

Surgical management of pediatric cataracts differs significantly from that of senile cataracts. Senile cataracts generally have a hard nucleus that requires phacoemulsification (ultrasonic removal) or an extracapsular (manual expression) technique to remove. Pediatric cataracts, in contrast, are much softer and can be removed by aspiration either with vitrectomy instrumentation (allowing aspiration and cutting of any fibrotic lens material) or with aspiration instrumentation only. The surgical technique may involve a posterior approach (from behind the lens) through the pars plana, or an anterior approach (in front of the lens) through the limbus or clear cornea. The anterior approach has become the preferred method of most pediatric ophthalmologists.[5,33]

The central portion of the anterior capsule is first removed and the lens material is then aspirated. If an intraocular lens (IOL) is to be inserted, it is then placed in the capsular bag (**126–133**). Currently, foldable acrylic IOLs are preferred by most surgeons, but rigid polymethylmethacrylate (PMMA) lenses are also used. Foldable silicone IOLs are rarely used in the pediatric population.[34]

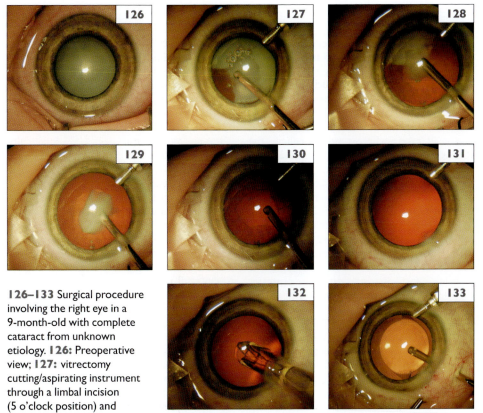

126–133 Surgical procedure involving the right eye in a 9-month-old with complete cataract from unknown etiology. **126:** Preoperative view; **127:** vitrectomy cutting/aspirating instrument through a limbal incision (5 o'clock position) and irrigating cannula (2 o'clock position); **128, 129:** progressive aspiration of lens material; **130:** remaining lens cortex adherent to lens capsule; **131:** lens cortex completely removed. Note the visible anterior capsulorrhexis opening; **132:** injection of foldable one-piece acrylic IOL into capsular bag; **133:** posterior capsulotomy with anterior vitrectomy performed through pars plana incision. Note the IOL is well centered in the capsular bag.

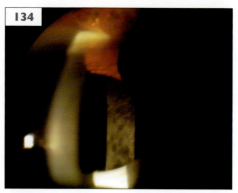

134 Posterior capsule opacification seen 1 year postoperatively in a 10-year-old. Vision was 20/30. Note the anterior capsule opacification seen inferiorly (not in the visual axis).

The long-term safety of placing an IOL has become increasingly well established. However, the earliest age at which to begin implanting IOLs has not. The decision of whether to place an IOL is controversial in children under 2 years of age, and especially in the first few months of life. Some surgeons advocate IOL placement in nearly all cases, whereas others believe the youngest patients should initially be left aphakic and treated with contact lenses or aphakic spectacles. The primary concerns for IOL placement in infants are increased postoperative inflammation, increased risk of needing one or more reoperations, and difficulty in calculating the ideal IOL power to implant due to the dramatic lens power changes that occur over the first year of life.

If left intact, opacification of the posterior capsule after lensectomy occurs in nearly all pediatric patients (**134**). The decision whether to remove the central posterior capsule and perform anterior vitrectomy at the same time as the initial cataract surgery is also age dependent and somewhat controversial. Experts currently recommend performing primary posterior capsulotomy with anterior vitrectomy in most patients under 5 years of age and consider this an optional step in older patients. A secondary posterior capsulotomy may be performed with the use of a slit-lamp mounted YAG laser if the patient is able to cooperate with the procedure. However, up to one-third will close

spontaneously if performed in children under 6 years, forming a secondary membrane.[33] A traditional surgical posterior capsulotomy with anterior vitrectomy may also be performed if the opacification is too dense or if the patient is uncooperative with the YAG laser procedure.

Aphakia

Aphakic eyes are generally extremely hyperopic and require optical correction. In most cases, infantile aphakia is best treated with contact lenses. They should be placed as soon as possible postoperatively and almost always within the first week. The lens power should overcorrect infants by +1.00 to +3.00 diopters to create clear near vision. Once the natural lens of an eye is removed, accommodation is lost. Therefore, bifocal spectacles are used over the contacts after the age of 2–4 years. Bilateral aphakic spectacles can also be used in contact lens intolerant children or as a backup to contacts (**135**). Unilateral aphakia should not be managed with spectacles unless there is no binocular fusion potential. This is because the magnification caused by unilateral aphakic spectacles creates unequal retinal image sizes and disrupts binocular fusion. In these cases, extensive patching of the sound eye is often necessary to promote proper visual development in the aphakic eye.

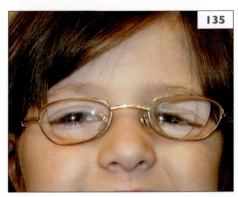

135 Aphakic spectacles on a 5-year-old who underwent bilateral lensectomies for autosomal dominant lens subluxation.

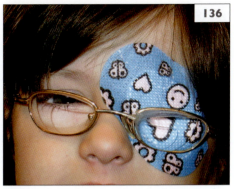

136 Patching of the better seeing left eye in the same patient from Figure 135.

Pseudophakia

Even when an IOL is placed (either at the time of initial surgery, or secondarily), additional optical correction is usually required. This is because postoperatively there is generally residual hyperopia with or without astigmatism. Eyes are frequently deliberately left with a variable amount of hyperopia due to the anticipated myopic shift which occurs as the eye continues to grow throughout development. Several reports have been published establishing the ideal amount of residual hyperopia to target, based on the specific age at which the IOL is placed.[35–37] Depending on the age and level of cooperation of the child, the additional optical correction may be achieved by the use of either spectacles or contact lenses. If tolerated, spectacles are the ideal choice since they allow for the use of bifocals, which are necessary for attaining both near and distance optical correction. Some experts recommend aiming for emmetropia in the case of unilateral cataracts even in very young children.[5] This recommendation is based on the premise that the success rate of amblyopia treatment is higher in an emmetropic eye than in one that requires additional optical correction early on. Multifocal IOLs have been used on a limited basis in an attempt to eliminate the need for lifelong bifocal spectacle dependence. Additional studies are necessary to establish better their role in the pediatric population.

Amblyopia

Once proper optical correction has been achieved, patching constitutes the mainstay of amblyopia treatment. In unilateral (or bilateral asymmetric) congenital cataracts, the degree of amblyopia is highly dependent on the severity of lens opacity and the age at which the lens is removed. Patching regimens may vary with both age and level of amblyopia (136). Recommendations may be as little as 1–2 hours per day or as much as 50% or more of the waking hours. Visual development continues throughout childhood until approximately age 8–9 years and the risk of amblyopia continues through that age as well.[5,38] It is not uncommon to maintain some level of patching until children reach this age in order to achieve and maintain maximal visual potential. In the case of acquired cataracts, amblyopia may not be as severe, but is dependent on the duration and degree of opacity. In the case of equal bilateral amblyopia, appropriate optical correction may be all that is required. If visual acuity is equal, patching is generally not recommended unless strabismus is present, in which case strabismus surgery is often required.

Cataract prognosis

The visual prognosis for pediatric cataracts is worse than that of adult cataracts. Vision may be limited by amblyopia as well as other associated abnormalities of the eye. In the case of congenital cataracts, the most critical factor affecting visual prognosis is the age at which the lens is removed.

Unilateral congenital cataracts have a worse prognosis than bilateral ones. Assuming proper visual rehabilitation, mean visual acuity was found to be 20/60 if operated prior to 2 months of age. Final visual acuity is generally poor if operated after this timeframe. In addition, these children nearly all develop strabismus and lack binocular fusion. Even when operated early, the potential for binocular function is often limited.

Bilateral congenital cataracts tend to have a better visual prognosis, but in the case of dense opacities, early intervention is equally as critical for achieving good visual outcomes. Similar to unilateral cataracts, visual results are best if surgery and subsequent optical correction take place prior to 2 months of age. These patients generally achieve 20/50 or better vision most of the time. Sensory nystagmus may develop if early intervention is not undertaken. Once this occurs, visual potential is often limited and outcomes are usually 20/100 or worse.[28]

Glaucoma

Daniel T. Weaver, MD

- **Introduction**

- **Diagnosis of pediatric glaucoma**
  Ocular examination

- **Differential diagnosis of pediatric glaucoma**

- **Primary infantile glaucoma**

- **Juvenile open-angle glaucoma**

- **Primary pediatric glaucoma associated with systemic disease**
  Lowe's syndrome
  Sturge–Weber syndrome
  Neurofibromatosis

- **Pediatric glaucoma associated with ocular anomalies**
  Axenfeld–Rieger syndrome
  Aniridia
  Peters anomaly

- **Secondary childhood glaucoma**
  Trauma
  Neoplasia
  Uveitis (iritis)
  Glaucoma following pediatric cataract surgery
  Other causes of secondary glaucoma in children

- **Treatment of pediatric glaucoma**
  Drug treatment
  Surgical management

- **Summary**

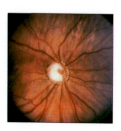
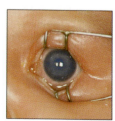
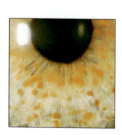
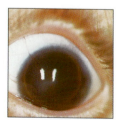

Introduction

Glaucoma in infants and children is rarely encountered by the pediatrician in routine office practice. However, the pediatrician and primary care provider are often the first physicians to encounter the child with the early presenting signs of this vision-threatening process. Recent genetic, pharmacologic, and surgical advances in the management of this complex disease have improved the prognosis for affected patients. Therefore, familiarity with the clinical features of this disease is important in determining the need for timely intervention and treatment for affected children.

Diagnosis of pediatric glaucoma

In the typical adult patient, glaucoma presents as an occult disease process, potentially affecting vision with little or no warning if left untreated. In contrast, glaucoma presenting in the pediatric population often presents with specific signs, symptoms, and clues readily apparent to the nonophthalmic specialist, in many cases requiring no special diagnostic examination equipment aside from what is routinely available.

It is useful to divide the childhood glaucomas into those of primary and secondary origin. Primary glaucoma is caused by a defect in the aqueous outflow mechanism of the developing eye and is often of genetic origin. Multiple associations with systemic and ocular abnormalities are noted in *Table 12*. Secondary glaucoma results from systemic disease, injury, drugs, or otherwise unrelated ocular disease. The causes of secondary glaucoma are numerous and will not all be considered in detail in this chapter.

The elevation of intraocular pressure (IOP) is axiomatic in making the diagnosis of glaucoma in children, but the manifestions of elevated IOP vary greatly depending on the age at presentation and upon the rapidity of pressure rise (*Table 13*). Infants and very young children often present to the pediatrician because the caregivers have noted that something is wrong

---

Table 12 Primary and secondary childhood glaucomas

I. Primary glaucomas
- A. Congenital open-angle glaucoma (PCG)
  1. Newborn congenital glaucoma (iridotrabeculodysgenesis)
  2. Infantile glaucoma (trabeculodysgenesis)
  3. Late recognized
- B. Autosomal dominant juvenile glaucoma
- C. Primary angle-closure glaucoma
- D. Associated with systemic abnormalities
  1. Sturge–Weber syndrome
  2. Neurofibromatosis type 1 (NF-1)
  3. Stickler syndrome
  4. Oculocerebrorenal (Lowe's) syndrome
  5. Rieger syndrome (Axenfeld–Rieger syndrome)
  6. SHORT syndrome
  7. Hepatocerebrorenal syndrome
  8. Marfan syndrome
  9. Rubinstein–Taybi syndrome
  10. Infantile glaucoma with mental retardation and paralysis

II. Secondary glaucomas
- A. Traumatic glaucoma
  1. Acute glaucoma
     a. Angle concussion
     b. Hyphema
     c. Ghost cell glaucoma
  2. Late-onset glaucoma with angle recession
  3. Arteriovenous fistula
- B. Secondary to intraocular neoplasm
  1. Retinoblastoma
  2. Juvenile xanthogranuloma
  3. Leukemia
  4. Melanoma
  5. Melanocytoma
  6. Iris rhabdomyosarcoma
  7. Aggressive nevi of the iris
- C. Secondary to uveitis
  1. Open-angle glaucoma
  2. Angle-blockage glaucoma
     a. Synechial angle closure

Table 12 Primary and secondary childhood glaucomas (*continued*)

I. Primary glaucomas

    11. Oculodentodigital dysplasia
    12. Open-angle glaucoma associated with microcornea and absence of frontal sinuses
    13. Mucopolysaccharidosis
    14. Trisomy 13
    15. Caudal regression syndrome
    16. Trisomy 21 (Down syndrome)
    17. *Cutis marmorata telangiectasia congenita*
    18. Warburg syndrome
    19. Kniest syndrome (skeletal dysplasia)
    20. Michel syndrome
    21. Nonprogressive hemiatrophy
    22. PHACE syndrome
    23. Sotos syndrome
    24. Linear scleroderma
    25. GAPO syndrome
    26. Roberts pseudothalidomide syndrome
    27. Wolf–Hirschhorn (4p) syndrome
    28. Rabinow syndrome
    29. Nail-patella syndrome
    30. Proteus syndrome
    31. Fetal hydantoin syndrome
    32. Cranio-cerebello-cardiac (3C) syndrome
    33. Brachmann–de Lange syndrome

E. Associated with ocular abnormalities

    1. Primary
    2. Aniridia
        a. Congenital glaucoma
        b. Acquired glaucoma
    3. Congenital ocular melanosis
    4. Sclerocornea
    5. Congenital iris ectropion syndrome
    6. Peters anomaly
    7. Iridotrabeculodysgenesis (iris hypoplasia)
    8. Posterior polymorphous dystrophy
    9. Idiopathic or familial elevated episcleral venous pressure
    10. Anterior corneal staphyloma
    11. Congenital microcornea with myopia
    12. Congenital hereditary endothelial dystrophy
    13. Iridocorneal endothelial syndrome (ICE)

II. Secondary glaucomas

    b. Iris bombe with pupillary block
    c. Trabecular endothelialization

D. Lens-induced glaucoma

    1. Subluxation-dislocation and pupillary block
        a. Marfan syndrome
        b. Homocystinuria
        c. Weill–Marchesani syndrome
    2. Spherophakia and pupillary block
    3. Phacolytic glaucoma

E. Following surgery for congenital cataract

    1. Lens tissue trabecular obstruction
    2. Pupillary block
    3. Chronic open-angle glaucoma associated with angle abnormalities

F. Steroid-induced glaucoma

G. Secondary to rubeosis

    1. Retinoblastoma
    2. Coats disease
    3. Medulloepithelioma
    4. Familial exudative vitreoretinopathy
    5. Chronic retinal detachment

H. Secondary angle-closure glaucoma

    1. Retinopathy of prematurity
    2. Microphthalmos
    3. Nanophthalmos
    4. Retinoblastoma
    5. Persistent fetal vasculature
    6. Congenital pupillary iris-lens membrane
    7. Topiramate
    8. Central retinal vein occlusion
    9. Ciliary body cysts

I. Malignant glaucoma

J. Glaucoma associated with increased venous pressure

    1. Cavernous or dural-venous fistula
    2. Orbital disease

K. Secondary to maternal rubella

L. Secondary to intraocular infection

    1. Acute recurrent toxoplasmosis
    2. Acute herpetic iritis
    3. Endogenous endophthalmitis

Table 13 Signs and symptoms of pediatric glaucoma

Epiphora (tearing)	Corneal clouding with loss of iris detail
Photophobia (light sensitivity)	Corneal enlargement
Blepharospasm/pain	Decreased vision/rapid myopic shift (older children)

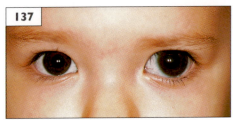

137 This patient with unilateral congenital glaucoma was referred by her mother's obstetrician because the left eye 'didn't look right'. Note left corneal enlargement with mild clouding. Tearing and photophobia were prominent symptoms. IOP was controlled following two goniotomies but cupping persists with poor vision in the left eye despite patching and spectacles. Right eye remains normal.

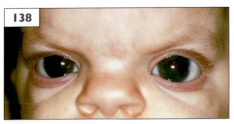

138 Severe bilateral corneal enlargement in congenital glaucoma. Corneas measured 15 mm right eye and 16 mm left eye at 10 months of age when referred for treatment (normal adult cornea measures 12 mm). Multiple surgeries have been required including diode laser treatment. Patient is now on topical and systemic glaucoma medication with borderline control 11 years later. Refraction is −9.50 + 1.00 × 180 right eye and −12.00 left eye.

with the eyes. Corneal clouding and ocular enlargement are hard signs not to be overlooked by the primary care provider, but the classic triad of epiphora, photophobia, and blepharospasm is often present in early childhood (**137**). These changes occur due to progressive corneal enlargement leading eventually to breaks in Descemet's membrane and can be progressive over months to even years if left untreated. In contradistinction to glaucoma in the adult patient, progressive corneal enlargement can occur during the first 2 years of life up to 18 mm in extreme cases (**138**) creating severe myopia (nearsightedness), optic disc cupping, and even ocular rupture resulting from minor trauma.

Optic disc cupping (**139**) can be seen with the direct ophthalmoscope in the office setting. It can be reversible if the glaucoma is treated early and successfully. In contrast, once optic atrophy is noted the changes are irreversible and the vision is damaged permanently. Glaucoma presenting in older children often does so without the classic signs and symptoms noted above. Decreased vision, increasing myopia (especially asymmetric) and associated ocular disease (especially trauma) assume importance in suspecting the diagnosis.

Loss of vision from childhood glaucoma generally results from pathologic changes in the cornea and optic nerve and also from the development of unilateral and bilateral refractive errors resulting in amblyopia. This amblyopia can often be successfully treated if diagnosed early in the course of the disease.

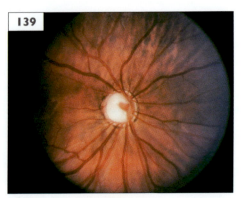

139 Disc cupping in glaucoma.

Ocular examination

The eye examination of the infant or child in the pediatric office can be challenging, but it can also be a brief and directed affair for the primary care provider. Historical details, such as aversion to lights (even indoors) and tearing are commonly noted (**140, 141**). The presence of a family history of related eye problems is important to record. Trauma history (including forceps-related birth trauma, **142, 143**), medications, systemic abnormalities, and ocular abnormalities are also important to review in some detail (see *Table 12*). If vision can be obtained, is it normal and equal in both eyes? Has there been a rapid and/or asymmetric myopic shift? Observation of the child is important: does he/she fixate and follow appropriately, is he/she uncomfortable with lights on in the exam room, or does he/she only open their eyes when the room lights are turned off? Utilizing the direct ophthalmoscope, is the cornea clear and the red reflex sharp? Are iris details easily seen and is the lens clear? These can all be assessed in seconds by the astute examiner.

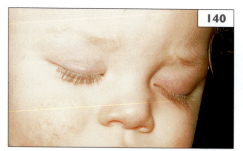

140 Corneal clouding and photophobia in congenital glaucoma. Patient presented at 10 months of age unable to open his eyes when outside or with the room lights turned on. The mother was concerned because 'he always looks down'.

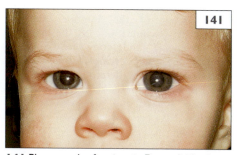

141 Photograph of patient in Figure **140** taken in total darkness demonstrating bilateral corneal enlargement and corneal opacification. IOP was in the mid-30s (infant IOP normal range 10–12 mmHg) during examination under anesthesia.

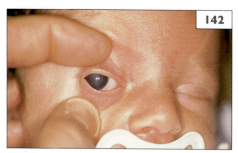

142 Perinatal forceps injury with vertical corneal opacity in right eye. IOP was normal but corneal scarring persisted with astigmatism resulting in poor vision despite patching and spectacles. Left eye was normal.

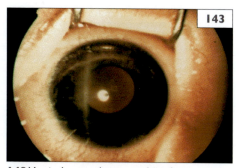

143 Vertical corneal scar resulting from perinatal forceps injury. In this case astigmatism was mild and vision recovered to the 20/30 level with spectacles and patching.

The Tonopen (**144**) has recently become available for use in a wide variety of primary care settings. It is easy to use, reasonably accurate, and can be a very useful screening device in children and even infants. Any degree of forced eyelid closure renders the results invalid, but asymmetric values in particular can be very helpful in planning subsequent referrals and diagnostic interventions. The Tonopen can be utilized in children as young as 4 years of age during office examinations, and in infants who are sleeping (**145**) or actively bottle-feeding. Lastly, the direct ophthalmoscope can be used to assess the degree of optic nerve cupping and reproduced for the chart. Once referral has been made to the ophthalmic specialist, a much more detailed examination can be undertaken, usually under general anesthesia, including IOP determination, corneal diameter measurement, biomicroscopy of the anterior segment, gonioscopy (examination of the anterior chamber angle), funduscopy (including disc examination), and cycloplegic refraction. Ultrasonic biometric determination of axial length is obtained for the serial determination of ocular growth and glaucoma pressure control.

Differential diagnosis of pediatric glaucoma

The signs of glaucoma in children are shared by a multitude of other eye diseases, most of which occur much more commonly. *Table 12* includes some of the ocular and systemic conditions involved with, and complicated by, pediatric glaucoma. Tearing is most commonly associated with nasolacrimal duct obstruction in children. Corneal enlargement can occur in the absence of glaucoma, but is uncommon and should warrant early referral to a specialist. Corneal opacification (**146**, **147**) can occur in several ocular and systemic conditions. Storage diseases, corneal dystrophies, and anterior segment inflammation all warrant careful investigation and may require prolonged ocular and/or systemic treatment, even in the absence of glaucoma. Nevertheless, it is always important to exclude glaucoma in the presence of these signs or symptoms even when a nonglaucomatous cause is initially suspected.

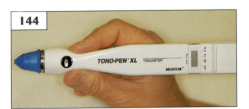

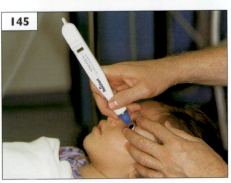

144, **145** Tonopen and its use in a sleeping child.

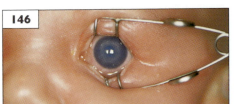

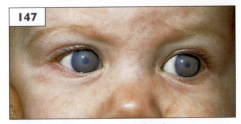

146, **147** Bilateral corneal clouding in congenital hereditary endothelial dystrophy (CHED). IOP was normal. Patient's older sister had similar corneal appearance with moderate visual compromise. Corneal transplantation was not required.

Primary infantile glaucoma

ETIOLOGY

Primary infantile glaucoma is the most common pediatric glaucoma, occurring in approximately 1 in 10,000 live births. Most cases (65–80%) are bilateral, but unilateral cases occur. Gender predilection has not been consistently described. About one-fourth of cases are diagnosed at birth, but more than 80% have onset of disease within the first year of life. Most cases of primary infantile glaucoma are sporadic without known family history, but about 10% of cases are familial, usually inherited as an AR trait. The primary defect consists of an isolated maldevelopment of the anterior chamber. The insertion of the iris can be observed to be higher than in unaffected children. The trabecular meshwork is less permeable to the passage of aqueous humor (**148**).

DIAGNOSIS

Disease severity can be variable, making early detection difficult in mild cases. Progressive corneal enlargement can occur with corneal edema caused by breaks in Descemet's membrane (**149**) during the first year of life. Corneal enlargement over 13 mm in the first year of life is unusual and should arouse suspicion for the presence of increased intraocular pressure. Asymmetric corneal enlargement occurs in unilateral glaucoma and is surprisingly obvious even when as little as 1 mm of difference in horizontal diameter is noted (**150**).

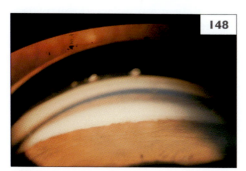

148 Gonioscopic appearance of the angle deformity present in primary infantile glaucoma. Goniotomy was required for IOP control.

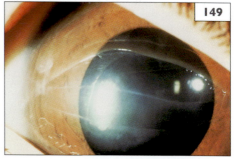

149 Haab's striae. Horizontal rupture of Descemet's membrane generally persists following normalization of IOP and is a major cause of astigmatism and amblyopia in children with congenital glaucoma.

150 Asymmetric corneal enlargement in congenital glaucoma. Patient was referred by a family physician because of apparent drooping of the right upper eyelid. She responded well to goniotomy in the left eye and now has 20/30 vision with correction 12 years later. Right eye has remained normal without IOP elevation. Current refraction is OD plano, OS + 2.00 + 2.25 × 160.

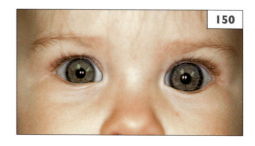

MANAGEMENT/TREATMENT

Surgical intervention is the definitive treatment for primary infantile glaucoma. Angle surgery (goniotomy or trabeculotomy) is successful in lowering pressure in the majority of cases, but is less effective in cases presenting at birth or if diagnosis (and treatment) are delayed until after 2 years of age. Topical medication is generally less effective and can be difficult to administer chronically. Other surgical modalities including filtration, cycloablation, and glaucoma Seton implantation are used in cases refractory to angle surgery with variable success in lowering pressure.

PROGNOSIS

The ultimate visual outcome in children with primary infantile glaucoma depends upon the amount of damage to the optic nerve and the cornea as well the presence of any associated amblyopia. Structural changes in the cornea (scarring or astigmatism) or the development of significant levels of myopia lead to the development of amblyopia in many children with glaucoma. It is important to remember that the most common cause of poor vision in these children is secondary to amblyopia rather than optic nerve damage due to uncontrolled IOP.

Juvenile open-angle glaucoma

ETIOLOGY AND DIAGNOSIS

Juvenile open-angle glaucoma is a rare, bilateral and acquired form of pediatric glaucoma characterized by marked IOP elevation typically beginning late in the first decade of life. The etiology of juvenile glaucoma is similar to that of primary infantile glaucoma. The anterior chamber shows a similar high insertion of the iris.

Loss of central vision and/or visual field loss often brings the patient in for initial examination. The typical signs and symptoms of primary infantile glaucoma are not present in most cases.

MANAGEMENT/TREATMENT AND PROGNOSIS

Treatment is difficult. Many cases do not respond to medical management and will require surgery. Unlike primary infantile glaucoma, angle surgery tends not to be effective. Alternative pathways for the outflow of aqueous fluid are often needed.

Because of the lack of signs and symptoms early in the disease, most children present late when significant optic nerve damage has already occurred. Therefore, the prognosis tends to be poorer in these patients.

Primary pediatric glaucoma associated with systemic disease

Lowe's syndrome

ETIOLOGY AND DIAGNOSIS

Lowe's syndrome, or oculocerebrorenal syndrome, is a rare form of congenital glaucoma which affects males with a female carrier state (X-linked recessive trait). Affected males may develop cataracts, glaucoma, aminoaciduria, and mental retardation. The syndrome can present with acidosis in infancy. The female carrier state is characterized by fine punctate lens opacities. In affected males, cataract is nearly always present, but the presence of glaucoma is more variable. Diagnosis can be made by clinical ocular findings in association with aminoaciduria. Affected patients show similar angle deformities as are seen in other forms of pediatric glaucoma.

MANAGEMENT/TREATMENT AND PROGNOSIS

Most children with Lowe's syndrome will require surgery to control the intraocular pressure. The combination of glaucoma and cataract makes this an especially difficult glaucoma to treat. Many patients experience poor outcomes due to the coexistence of glaucoma and cataracts.

Sturge–Weber syndrome

ETIOLOGY AND DIAGNOSIS

Sturge–Weber syndrome consists of facial nevus flammeus of the upper eyelid and abnormalities in the vascularity of the leptomeninges. The glaucoma is usually unilateral on the side of the nevus flammeus, but bilateral involvement has been reported (**151**). Neurologic manifestations include seizures, paralysis, and visual field defects from intracranial involvement. A choroidal hemangioma may be present and is visible on funduscopic examination.

The cause of glaucoma in Sturge–Weber syndrome is debatable. Theories include an elevation of episcleral venous pressure or angle maldevelopment. It is likely that both play some role.

MANAGEMENT/TREATMENT AND PROGNOSIS

Medical and surgical treatment may be needed in many patients. With early diagnosis and treatment, IOP can often be controlled. Because the disease is often unilateral, amblyopia occurs in many cases. Rapid choroidal expansion and hemorrhage may complicate intraocular surgical intervention and can be sight threatening.

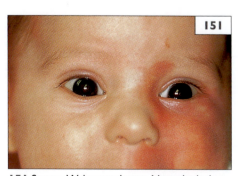

151 Sturge–Weber syndrome. Note the lack of right upper eyelid involvement. Fundus examination and IOP have remained normal.

Neurofibromatosis

ETIOLOGY AND DIAGNOSIS

Neurofibromatosis type 1 is an AD disease with variable expressivity. The cause of glaucoma in neurofibromatosis is not known. Theories include angle infiltration and angle maldevelopment similar to other forms of glaucoma that occur in children.

Café-au-lait spots are commonly noted on the trunk early in life, often within the first year (**152**). Lisch nodules of the iris are also common but typically appear later, often just prior to the onset of puberty (**153**). Both findings are often seen on routine physical examination of the otherwise well child. The glaucoma associated with this syndrome is congenital, unilateral, and typically occurs in the setting of eyelid plexiform neuroma involvement.

MANAGEMENT/TREATMENT AND PROGNOSIS

Medical therapy is usually tried first and surgical intervention is necessary if medical management fails. The response to conventional angle surgery is usually poor and more aggressive surgical measures may be required.

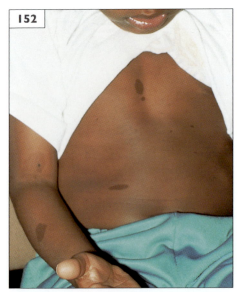

152 Café-au-lait spots in neurofibromatosis-1.

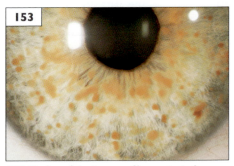

153 Lisch nodules in neurofibromatosis-1.

Pediatric glaucoma associated with ocular anomalies

As noted in *Table 12*, there are many ocular anomalies that coexist with pediatric glaucoma. Many of these anomalies occur in the setting of systemic syndromes with multisystem involvement, making early detection a priority for the primary care provider caring for these children.

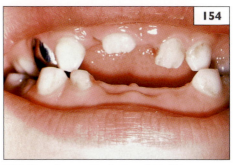

154 Dental anomalies in Axenfeld–Rieger syndrome.

Axenfeld–Rieger syndrome

ETIOLOGY AND DIAGNOSIS

Axenfeld–Rieger syndrome (A-RS) is part of the spectrum of the anterior chamber cleavage disorders (iridocorneal dysgenesis). Usage of the term A-RS implies inclusion of the systemic manifestations of this bilateral, congenital ocular developmental disorder. These include dental anomalies (**154**), skull and skeletal dysplasia, and umbilical abnormalities. Developmental abnormalities of the anterior segment lead to increased IOP. Loci on chromosomes 4q25, 6p25, and 13q14 have been linked to A-RS. Family history is common, with an AD mode of inheritance.

Bilateral ocular involvement is noted with glaucoma occurring in more than half of affected patients. Ocular defects include posterior embryotoxon (Axenfeld's anomaly), which often can be seen without magnification. Iris defects are commonly noted and include corectopia (**155**), iris stromal hypoplasia, and iridocorneal process formation (**156**). Polycoria may also be seen. Many patients appear to have previously undergone anterior segment eye surgery or to have sustained eye trauma.

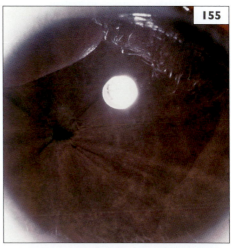

155 Corectopia in Axenfeld–Rieger's anomaly.

PROGNOSIS

Glaucoma usually occurs later in the first decade of life. With careful follow-up, it is possible to detect early rises in IOP, which allows for early treatment. Many patients will require surgery.

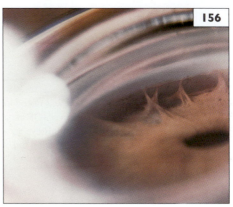

156 Iridocorneal adhesions in Axenfeld–Rieger's anomaly.

Aniridia

ETIOLOGY AND DIAGNOSIS

Aniridia is a bilateral disorder in which the iris is partially or nearly totally absent. Two forms of aniridia exist: sporadic and familial. Familial aniridia is inherited in an AD pattern with near complete penetrance. A genetic mutation in the PAX6 gene leads to the development of aniridia. The association with Wilm's tumor has been well described in sporadic aniridia and rarely reported in the familial form of the disease.

A small rudimentary stump of iris is often visible only with the microscope. The affected child appears to have extremely dilated pupils (**157**). Glaucoma occurs in at least 50% of patients with aniridia. Aniridia is a panocular disorder and not only a disorder of the iris. Multiple ocular defects also occur which include microcornea, cataracts, and macular hypoplasia with nystagmus and poor visual function.

MANAGEMENT/TREATMENT AND PROGNOSIS

Medical therapy can be tried initially, followed by surgical intervention in refractory cases. Successful control of aniridic glaucoma is often difficult to achieve. Limbal stem cell deficiency can lead to severe ocular surface abnormalities even in the absence of glaucoma (**158**). This can compromise the corneal surface in a patient with poor baseline visual function, making early diagnosis and management of dry eye and related corneal problems critical. Genetic testing should be performed on affected individuals to ascertain their risk for the development of Wilm's tumor. Patients at risk should undergo serial renal ultrasound testing.

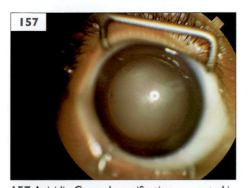

157 Aniridia. Corneal opacification was noted in the left eye with coexisting elevation of IOP at birth. Angle surgery was required in this eye at 1 week of age. Glaucoma is now controlled but vision in the left eye remains limited by corneal surface abnormalities.

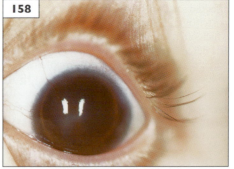

158 Ocular surface abnormalities in aniridia occur as a result of limbal stem cell deficiency and in this patient initially presented with unilateral conjunctivitis at age 8 months. Punctal occlusion and topical cyclosporine have resulted in improved patient comfort in both eyes with relative preservation of vision in the right eye (20/100). Vision is 20/400 in the left eye (shown). IOP remains normal in both eyes with topical medication.

Peters anomaly

ETIOLOGY AND DIAGNOSIS

Peters anomaly consists of central corneal opacification associated with the lack of Descemet's membrane presenting in the newborn infant (**159, 160**). Defects in the PAX6 gene lead to the development of Peters anomaly. Iris strands to the cornea are often noted and cataract commonly coexists. It may be unilateral or bilateral and generally occurs sporadically.

MANAGEMENT/TREATMENT AND PROGNOSIS

Many patients will require corneal transplantation for the corneal opacification. If glaucoma occurs, it generally requires surgical intervention. Approximately 50% of patients who undergo corneal transplantation develop glaucoma. The glaucoma in these patients is difficult to treat and often requires multiple surgeries. Glaucoma can increase the risk of corneal transplant failure. These issues have led to a debate regarding the benefit of corneal transplantation in children with unilateral disease.

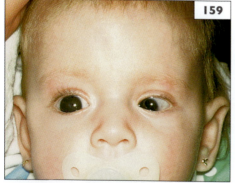

159 Peters anomaly with cataract in the right eye of a child with multiple congenital systemic anomalies. Lensectomy was required, corneal transplantation was not. The patient died of cardiac complications unrelated to eye surgery.

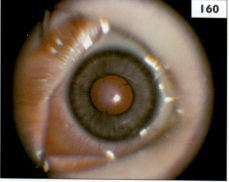

160 Mild Peters anomaly. Note corneolenticular adhesions.

Secondary childhood glaucoma

As noted in *Table 12*, pediatric glaucoma may occur as a result of a multitude of ophthalmic conditions, many of which have significant systemic implications for the primary care provider.

Trauma

ETIOLOGY AND DIAGNOSIS

The most common form of traumatic glaucoma in childhood occurs as a result of anterior chamber hemorrhage (hyphema). This typically occurs 1–3 days following a blunt, nonpenetrating injury to the globe. Rebleeding in hyphema typically occurs 3–5 days after the initial injury and can cause a significant pressure spike which can result in nausea, vomiting, and severe visual loss if not treated promptly.

The diagnosis of traumatic glaucoma is made when the IOP is found to be elevated following an injury, or suspected injury, consistent with the development of glaucoma. An assessment of IOP is important in any child who sustains a significant ocular injury.

MANAGEMENT/TREATMENT AND PROGNOSIS

Although bedrest and hospitalization are no longer considered mandatory, eye protection, cycloplegia, and avoidance of further injury are paramount. Topical therapy for elevated IOP is sometimes indicated. Anterior chamber washout is necessary in some cases of hyphema associated with glaucoma to prevent permanent blood-staining of the cornea or optic nerve damage. Children with sickle cell hemoglobinopathies are at special risk for this complication and may require earlier surgical intervention.

Most cases can be treated if identified in a timely manner. However, even in cases with spontaneous resolution of the hyphema, patients remain at long-term risk of developing glaucoma later in life secondary to damage to the anterior chamber angle structures as a result of the initial injury. All patients with hyphema should be examined not only during the acute postinjury phase but also throughout their life for signs of glaucoma.

Neoplasia

The most common cause of glaucoma secondary to ocular tumor in childhood is retinoblastoma. This may occur due to iris neovascularization (rubeosis) with consequent angle closure, infiltration of the angle with tumor cells, or secondary to a large tumor pushing the iris forward and closing off the angle. Other causes include leukemia, lymphoma, and juvenile xanthogranuloma. Treatment is usually medical along with treatment of the underlying cause as indicated. Glaucoma surgery is contraindicated in patients with retinoblastoma.

Uveitis (iritis) (161)

ETIOLOGY AND DIAGNOSIS

The most common example of uveitis causing glaucoma is seen in juvenile rheumatoid arthritis. The uveitis in the setting of HLA-B27 disease (ankylosing spondylitis) generally occurs in adolescents and young adults. Most patients with uveitis that develop glaucoma do so as a complication of chronic disease. Many of these patients are being followed by an ophthalmologist for their underlying disorder. However, some patients with uveitis initially present with coexistent glaucoma. In a smaller group of patients, the glaucoma may be responsible for symptoms leading to their presentation. Assessment of IOP is an important part of the care of the child with uveitis.

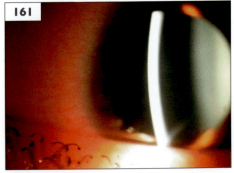

161 Ciliary flush and corneal edema in acute anterior uveitis. (Courtesy of Hasan M. Bahrani, MD.)

Chronic iritis can cause glaucoma in childhood as a result of anterior segment inflammation. This inflammation may lead to inflammation and abnormal function of the trabecular meshwork (trabeculitis), or cause scarring of the angle drainage structures (angle closure). In addition, glaucoma is a common side-effect of long-term topical corticosteroid use. For this reason, the chronic treatment of uveitis with topical corticosteroids should be avoided if possible.

MANAGEMENT/TREATMENT AND PROGNOSIS

Medical treatment is the first line of treatment in patients with glaucoma and uveitis. If possible, corticosteroids should be discontinued. Topical glaucoma medication may be helpful. Surgery is useful in those patients who fail to respond to medical management.

Early and more aggressive treatment can help to avoid the changes in the anterior segment that lead to glaucoma. Systemic therapy with corticosteroid-sparing agents will also help to decrease the incidence of glaucoma. Patients who present with glaucoma at the time of diagnosis are especially challenging.

Glaucoma following pediatric cataract surgery

ETIOLOGY AND DIAGNOSIS

Glaucoma is common following pediatric cataract surgery, developing in up to 25% or more of patients undergoing lensectomy in one study. During the immediate postoperative period, pupillary block leading to angle closure glaucoma can occur either with or without intraocular lens placement. Open-angle glaucoma is more common and may occur months to years after lensectomy. The underlying cause of this form of glaucoma is unknown.

In young infants, the signs and symptoms typical of primary infantile glaucoma may occur. Older children behave more like those with juvenile glaucoma. Because of the high risk and the fact that the signs and symptoms may be subtle, an especially high level of surveillance for the development of glaucoma must be maintained in any child undergoing cataract surgery.

MANAGEMENT/TREATMENT AND PROGNOSIS

Laser or surgical management of the iris is needed in cases that have developed pupillary block glaucoma. Medical therapy with topical agents are the preferred initial form of therapy unless rapid IOP lowering is required, in which case oral agents (i.e. acetazolamide) may be needed. Surgical intervention including Seton implantation and cycloablation (destruction of the ciliary processes which produce aqueous humor) are often required in these cases to control elevated IOP.

Glaucoma following cataract surgery in children is difficult to treat and often requires both medical and surgical treatment. Lifelong follow-up is mandatory to optimize the opportunity for early diagnosis and treatment in these patients.

Other causes of secondary glaucoma in children

There are a multitude of additional causes of secondary childhood glaucoma as noted in *Table 12*. These include lens-induced glaucoma (Marfan's and homocystinuria), secondary angle closure (retinopathy of prematurity, microphthalmos, and persistent hyperplastic primary vitreous), glaucoma associated with increased venous pressure (cavernous or dural sinus fistula), and intraocular infection (toxoplasmosis, herpetic iritis, and endogenous endophthalmitis).

Treatment of pediatric glaucoma

Traditional teaching dictated that childhood glaucoma was a surgical disease. Advances in the pharmacologic management of glaucoma have changed this dictum to some degree. However, surgery is still the primary form of treatment for many types of glaucoma that occur in children.

Angle surgery remains the first line of therapy in primary infantile glaucoma. Medical therapy is often tried first in cases of juvenile open-angle glaucoma, aphakic glaucoma, and in the treatment of secondary glaucoma. However, the implications of lifelong medical therapy (with attendant side-effects) including cost and compliance are significant and need to be considered carefully in choosing therapeutic options. Many promising drugs are now available and approved for use in children, but the long-term side-effects remain unknown. As the routine use of the miotic drugs (i.e. pilocarpine) has been largely supplanted in the treatment of glaucoma, there remain four classes of drug with which the primary care provider should be familiar in the care and treatment of pediatric patients. All four classes of these drugs are used on both a short- and long-term basis.

Drug treatment

CARBONIC ANHYDRASE INHIBITORS

The oral carbonic anhydrase inhibitor acetazolamide has been used safely and effectively for over 50 years in the treatment of pediatric glaucoma. It acts as a suppressant of aqueous humor production. The pressure-lowering achieved can be upwards of 30–40% and can in many cases clear the cornea preoperatively to allow safe angle surgery. Side-effects include decreased appetite, diarrhea, and metabolic acidosis. The latter can be problematic in infants under 12 months of age. Topical carbonic anhydrase inhibitors are now available. Brinzolamide and dorzolamide are widely used in both adult and pediatric patients. They are utilized mostly in an adjunctive role with other topical medication. All carbonic anhydrase inhibitors should be avoided in patients with sulfa allergy.

BETA BLOCKERS

The topical beta blockers have an important role in the treatment of pediatric glaucoma. The mode of action is suppression of aqueous humor production. As in adults, the side-effects include fatigue, lethargy, bradycardia, apnea, and asthma exacerbation. The initial dose may produce an adequate therapeutic effect in many cases and may obviate further topical or surgical therapy for the patient.

ADRENERGIC AGONISTS

Apraclonidine and brimonidine are both approved for the topical therapy of glaucoma in adult patients. The mechanism of action has a dual effect, producing both suppression of aqueous humor production and an increase in uveoscleral outflow. The use of apraclonidine in adults has been limited by the high incidence of topical allergy, which approached 15% in some studies. It is not used routinely to any degree in the treatment of pediatric glaucoma. Topical brimonidine has produced lethargy and somnolence in toddlers and apnea, bradycardia, and hypotension in infants. The use of brimonidine in the treatment of childhood glaucoma should therefore be restricted to older children. It should not be considered first-line therapy and the very real possibility of life-threatening side-effects should be discussed with the patient's parents prior to the initiation of treatment in all cases.

PROSTAGLANDIN ANALOGS

The prostaglandin analogs include latanaprost, bimatoprost, and travoprost. This class of drugs works by enhancing uveoscleral outflow and can produce dramatic reductions in IOP, approaching 25–30% in many cases. They are dosed once-daily, thereby improving therapeutic compliance. Systemic side-effects are minimal, but excessive eyelash growth and darkening of the iris are frequently noted. The prostaglandin drugs should be used with caution where intraocular inflammation coexists with glaucoma, due to the risk of increasing the inflammatory response.

Surgical management

Goniotomy was introduced by Barkan in the 1940s and revolutionized the therapy for primary infantile glaucoma, with cure rates today approaching 80% in experienced hands (**162–164**). A special lens is placed on the cornea which allows visualization of the angle structures. A knife is passed across the anterior chamber and an incision is made into the abnormal tissue blocking fluid passage out of the eye. A relatively clear cornea is needed to perform a goniotomy.

Trabeculotomy is an alternative form of angle surgery in which the canal of Schlemm is cannulated externally with the trabeculotome (or suture material). This is then utilized to tear

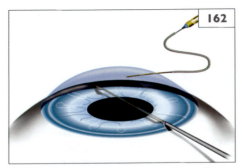

162 Goniotomy demonstrating incision of Barkan's membrane in a counter-clockwise direction. Modern technique generally includes the use of a viscoelastic agent such as Healon.

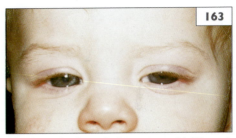

163 Severely photophobic patient with bilateral corneal opacification. IOP was 35 mmHg right eye and 37 mmHg left eye. Angle surgery was required.

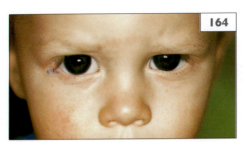

164 Patient in Figure 163 1 year following bilateral goniotomy. Corneas are clear and photophobia has resolved. After 14 years of follow-up IOP remains controlled in the right eye with topical lumigan. Vision is 20/25 with correction. Vision in the left eye is poor due to central corneal scarring from Haab's striae.

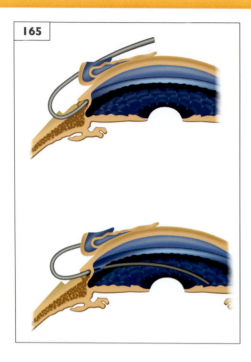

165

165 Trabeculotomy utilizing the Harm's trabeculotome.

thereby allowing an alternative outflow pathway for aqueous humor. It may be especially useful in more difficult cases. Cycloablation is used to reduce aqueous humor production. Destruction of the ciliary processes can be performed with cryotherapy or with laser. Laser can be applied externally or internally through the use of an endoscopic probe.

With these new tools now available in the armamentarium against pediatric glaucoma, progression to a blind, painful, and often unsightly eye is less likely than in preceding decades. However, in these unfortunate cases enucleation is still sometimes necessary and can be very helpful in returning the affected child to a more normal routine and appearance. Modern orbital implants can provide excellent ocular prosthesis support and very satisfactory cosmesis.

through the abnormal membrane obstructing the trabecular meshwork from the outside in, towards the anterior chamber space (**165**). Trabeculotomy can be performed when the cornea is cloudy and therefore is the preferred procedure if the cornea remains opaque, thereby making angle visualization for goniotomy impossible. Both goniotomy and trabeculotomy address the anatomic defect present in this disease, acting to clear away the abnormal tissue creating obstruction to outflow of aqueous humor through the trabecular meshwork.

Trabeculectomy (filtration surgery) is an alternative surgical approach in which a partial thickness fistula is created between the anterior chamber and the sub-Tenon's space outside the eye, thereby allowing aqueous humor outflow to bypass the abnormal trabecular meshwork. It is utilized when angle surgery fails. In children, trabeculectomy is often combined with antimetabolite medication (e.g. Mitomycin-C or 5-fluorouracil) in order to prevent the fistula from scarring closed.

Drainage implant (Seton) surgery involves the placement of a tube from an externally placed reservoir into the anterior chamber,

Summary

In summary, the pediatric patient with the signs and symptoms of glaucoma presents infrequently to the primary care provider. Most providers will see only a few of the cases described in this chapter during his/her career. Even with prompt diagnosis and referral to the appropriate ophthalmic specialist, treatment can be challenging and often less than optimal, requiring multiple surgical procedures and long-term medication administration in many cases, even in the hands of very experienced providers. The implications for lifelong visual compromise often depend upon the diagnostic acumen of the harried pediatrician or family practitioner during a busy clinic day. The importance of prompt specialty referral cannot be overemphasized.

Retinal diseases

Vicki M. Chen, MD and
Deborah K. VanderVeen, MD

- **Introduction**

- **Coats' disease**

- **Leber's congenital amaurosis**

- **X-linked congenital stationary night blindness**

- **Achromatopsia**

- **Stargardt disease**

- **Best's disease**

- **Persistent fetal vasculature**

- **X-linked juvenile retinoschisis**

- **Albinism**

- **Retinal dystrophies with systemic disorders (ciliopathies)**

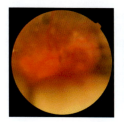
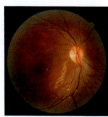
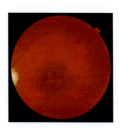
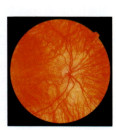

Introduction

Retinal diseases are amongst the most challenging of eye conditions for the nonophthalmologist to diagnose, due to the limited nature of the in-office, undilated eye exam. The standard hand-held direct ophthalmoscope available in most physician offices allows the examiner to see a greatly magnified view of the optic nerve and posterior retina, but offers a limited view of the remaining retina. A fully dilated examination using an indirect ophthalmoscope offers a substantially wider field of view, allowing for evaluation of other important anatomical structures within the retina (**166**).

The nonophthalmologist is often the first physician to evaluate a child and diagnose early signs of retinal disease such as poor visual attention, nystagmus, or even leukocoria. By early recognition of the possibility of these conditions and prompt referral to an ophthalmologist, the primary physician offers the patient the best opportunity for early intervention and possible treatment, when applicable.

Coats' disease

DEFINITION/OVERVIEW

Coats' disease, or retinal telangiectasia, is a relatively rare condition of congenital retinal vasculature anomalies resulting in massive external retinal and subretinal accumulation of exudate (**167**).[1-3] The classic vasculature changes are described as focal or multifocal telangiectatic vessels and microaneurysms within the arterial system of arterioles and capillaries, but these anomalies may also occur within the venular system.[2] These vascular lesions are commonly found in the peripheral retina, but may also be seen centrally. The massive exudation often found in this disease can cause retinal detachment and may lead to vision loss if detachment occurs within the macula. When extensive elevation of the retina occurs, this disease may mimic retinoblastoma or other retinal tumors, and is an important condition to differentiate when such diagnoses are being considered.

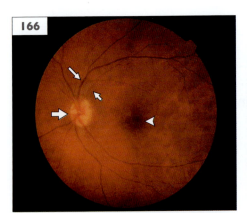

166 Normal retina, demonstrating the major anatomical structures seen with indirect ophthalmoscopy. Note that the optic nerve head (wide arrow) is pink in color, the caliber of the arterioles (small arrow) is about 2/3 that of the venules (arrow), and the retina is evenly pigmented. The fovea (arrowhead) shows a normal pigmentation pattern and reflex indicative of normal development.

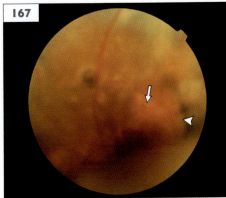

167 Coats' disease: retinal image showing characteristic telangiectatic blood vessels (arrow) and focal areas of yellow-white subretinal and intraretinal exudates (arrowhead).

ETIOLOGY

Coats' disease is a sporadic disorder, without a known inheritance pattern. Recent reports have suggested that Coats' disease may be caused by a somatic mutation in the NDP (Norrin) gene, which has been implicated in other diseases of retinal vasculogenesis. The disease is a congenital vascular disease characterized by the presence of telangiectasias of the inner retina vessels and dilated thin-walled arterioles and capillaries.

Histopathologic studies have shown that the vessel wall may consist of only endothelium, with or without a PAS-positive basement membrane. The high intravascular pressure and low vascular permeability is thought to allow for extravasation of serum, plasma, and blood cells, which accumulate within and beneath the retina. The leakage of serum is thought to allow accumulation of cholesterol and lipid in the external retina space and also stimulates retinal fibroblasts and other inflammatory cells, leading to subretinal fibrosis, further lipid deposition, and cystic changes within the retina.[2,3]

The inciting cause of this vascular thinning has been proposed to be the presence of PAS-positive mucopolysaccharides within the vascular walls or within the retina itself, but the exact etiology of this congenital vascular disease is not known.[4]

CLINICAL PRESENTATION

Children may present with strabismus, decreased vision, or leukocoria. Coats' disease is usually a unilateral disease and occurs more frequently in boys (2:1 male to female ratio). The mean age of onset is 5 years, with most cases diagnosed at ages 2–10 years. It is a sporadic disorder, with rare instances of vasculogenic retinal disease in family members. Patients with Coats' disease have no known systemic disease such as hypertension or hypercholesterolemia that might predispose them to having retinal fluid extravasation.

For the ophthalmologist, indirect ophthalmoscopy shows areas of retinal elevation with yellow-white exudate both beneath and within the retina (**168**).[3] Hemorrhages may also be seen. If fluorescein angiography is performed, telangiectatic vessels and microaneuryms are classically identified in the inner retinal layers. The disease may show

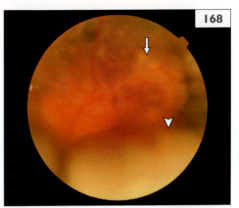

168 Coats' disease: retinal image showing confluent areas of exudates (arrow) and adjacent area of retinal detachment (arrowhead).

focal areas of exudate, or massive accumulations of confluent lipid and cholesterol deposition. Advanced cases may present with retinal detachment and leukocoria, and areas of retinal dysplasia may simulate retinal tumor.

DIFFERENTIAL DIAGNOSIS

The most important differential diagnosis to exclude in a patient with Coats' disease is retinoblastoma. The age of onset overlaps with that of retinoblastoma, and clinically differentiating between these two diseases can be challenging. Indeed, there have been multiple case reports of patients having undergone enucleation for presumed retinoblastoma who were found to have Coats' disease on histopathologic examination. Other important diseases to consider are retinal exudation due to other vascular diseases such as angiomas and macroaneurysms, toxocariasis, toxoplasmosis, and rarely retinal tumors of other types (lymphoma).

DIAGNOSIS

The diagnosis of Coats' disease is made by direct visualization of the retina using indirect ophthalmoscopy. Fluorescein angiography can be very helpful in visualizing the abnormal vasculature and identifying the classic telangiectasias and microaneurysms (and excluding other retinal anomalies). B-scan ultrasonography may also be helpful in assessing the content of the lesion (exudate has a low internal reflectivity), and the size and shape of the involved area. Computed tomography (CT) is useful to distinguish Coats' from retinoblastoma, which usually demonstrates areas of calcification within the tumor.

The exclusion of other causes of retinal exudate and elevation including tumors, infections, inflammation, retinal holes, and traction is necessary prior to making the diagnosis of Coats' disease.

MANAGEMENT/TREATMENT AND PROGNOSIS

Management of Coats' disease in the early stages is aimed at closure of telangiectatic vessels and microaneurysms by photocoagulation laser therapy. Treatment may halt the progression of the exudation, but the lipid accumulation does not usually resolve with treatment. In some cases closure of anomalous vessels may increase the intravascular pressure within collateral vessels and thereby worsen other areas by increasing the rate of vascular leakage. Once there is retinal detachment, cryotherapy may be useful, or surgery such as vitrectomy may help reattach the retina. For cases of advanced Coats' disease, damage to the retina is severe and there is little hope of restoring useful vision. Glaucoma may develop, and the eye may become painful. Conservative treatments may be employed, but many eyes diagnosed at a late stage are eventually removed.

Many cases of Coats' disease end up with a poor outcome and reduced vision. Many children present late in the course of the disease when significant retinal damage has already occurred. Prognosis is better when the disease is detected before permanent changes in the retina take place.

Leber's congenital amaurosis

DEFINITION/OVERVIEW

Leber's congenital amaurosis (LCA) is a group of recessively inherited congenital retinal dystrophies that result in severe visual impairment. Of patients with congenital blindness, the prevalence of LCA is thought to be 10–18%, making it one of the more common diagnoses of blindness in children. The incidence of this condition is 2–3 in 100,000. LCA is characterized by moderate to severe visual impairment identified at or within a few months of birth, infantile nystagmus, sluggish pupillary responses, and absent or poorly recordable electroretinographic (ERG) responses early in life.[5]

ETIOLOGY

LCA is an inherited, autosomal recessive (AR) disease, and the prevalence of LCA dramatically increases with consanguinity. LCA has been linked to numerous genes including GUCY2D (encoding RetGC-1) at 17p13.1, RPE65 at 1q31, CRX at 19q13.3, AIPLI at 17p13.1, TULP1 at 6p21.3, CRB1 at 1q31-3, and RPGRIP at 14q11.[5,6] These mutations together account for about half of LCA patients.

The exact pathophysiologic pathways that lead to absent photoreceptor function have not been elucidated. The genes identified with LCA are expressed preferentially in the retina or the retinal pigment epithelium, and their functions are quite diverse and include retinal embryonic development (CRX), photoreceptor cell structure (CRB1), phototransduction (GUCY2D), protein trafficking (AIPL1, RPGRIP1), and vitamin A metabolism (RPE65).

CLINICAL PRESENTATION

Infants with LCA present with poor visual responses and often a large amplitude, roving nystagmus. Although not always seen, the oculodigital reflex (rubbing or poking at the eyes) is an ominous sign of poor vision in an infant, and is postulated to be an attempt to stimulate the retina by manual compression of the globe.

Visual acuity in early childhood ranges from 20/120–20/200, but progressively worsens to hand-motion or light perception by adolescence or early adulthood. Other important clinical findings include minimally reactive pupils, high refractive error, and later, cataract, keratoconus, keratoglobus, and enopthalmos. By definition, LCA patients have no structural anomalies on ophthalmologic exam and have no known neurologic diseases. As the child matures, retinal changes often develop, most commonly chorioretinal pigmentation in the peripheral fundus of both eyes.

Systemic findings have been seen with higher frequency in LCA patients, including mental retardation (3–50%), medullary cystic kidney disease, cardiomyopathy, cerebellar vermis hypoplasia (10%), and neurosensory hearing loss (5–10%).[5]

DIFFERENTIAL DIAGNOSIS
The diagnosis of LCA cannot be differentiated from retinitis pigmentosa (RP), congenital stationary night blindness (CSNB) or achromatopsia on initial clinical examination. ERG is needed to determine the extent and relative decreased function of rods relative to cones; RP does not initially affect rods as severely as LCA, and both CSNB and achromatopsia affect cones more than rods.

DIAGNOSIS
LCA is diagnosed by first excluding all ocular and cerebral causes of poor vision. If the ocular exam is normal, then poor vision caused by damage to intracerebral visual pathways, including the optic tracts, optic radiations, and occipital lobe, should be evaluated by neurologic examination and magnetic resonance imaging (MRI). When ophthalmologic, neurologic, and radiographic examinations are negative ERG is indicated to determine functionality of the photoreceptors and the bipolar retinal cells. ERG typically shows nonrecordable function or severely attenuated responses of both rods and cones. Visual evoked potential (VEP) testing may reveal some response in patients with no demonstrable ERG recordings.

Some patients with LCA will have subtle abnormalities in pigmentation of the central and peripheral fundus (10%) and/or macular dysplasia (10%) in infancy. As the child matures, the chorioretinal pigmentation often progresses, and optic nerve pallor and retinal arteriolar attenuation are commonly seen (**169, 170**).

MANAGEMENT/TREATMENT AND PROGNOSIS
There are no known treatments that halt the progression or improve the vision in patients with LCA. Due to the possibility of known systemic disorders occurring in conjunction with LCA, a full pediatric physical exam should be performed. Ancillary testing such as cardiac and renal ultrasonography may also be considered. An important intervention that can be very helpful for patients with LCA and their families is referral to early vision services in infancy, with continued low-vision therapy and services for school age children. Gene therapy is currently being studied in animal models. Because of genetic heterogeneity such treatments need to be tailored to the genetically defined subgroups.[6]

The appearance of the retina may undergo marked changes with age, but vision usually remains fairly stable through young adult life.

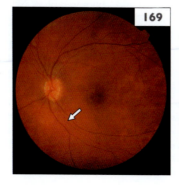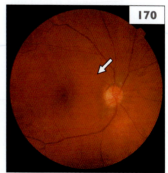

169, 170 Leber's congenital amaurosis: retinal photographs of the right (**169**) and left eyes (**170**) showing a mild dysplasia of the macula and arteriolar narrowing (arrows).

X-linked congenital stationary night blindness

DEFINITION/OVERVIEW

X-linked congenital stationary night blindness (CSNB) is a nonprogressive congenital dysfunction of rod photoreceptors leading to poor vision in dimly lit environments and varying degrees of visual impairment. It can be thought of as a problem with night vision. Three types of CSNB have been described and categorized according to the extent and type of rod photoreceptor dysfunction: complete and incomplete, and enhanced S-cone syndrome.

ETIOLOGY

As its name implies, this condition is most commonly inherited as an X-linked disorder, specifically linked to Xp11. Both AR and autosomal dominant (AD) variants have been reported; patients with AD-inherited CSNB are not visually impaired. The complete type of CSNB has been linked to the NYX (nyctalopin) gene, and the incomplete type of CSNB has been linked to CACNA1F, both found on chromosome X. Enhanced S-cone syndrome has been linked to the gene NR2E3 at 15q23.[6]

Histopathologic studies have not revealed specific anatomic or functional abnormalities in patients with CSNB. ERG studies have suggested that the problem lies in communication synapses between outer retinal cells (attenuated 'b' wave). NYX, which encodes a glycosylphosphatidyl (GPI)-anchored protein called nyctalopin, is a unique member of the small leucine-rich proteoglycan (SLRP) family. The role of other SLRP proteins suggests that mutant nyctalopin disrupts developing retinal interconnections involving the optic nerve bipolar cells, leading to the visual losses seen in patients with complete CSNB.

CLINICAL PRESENTATION

Children with poor central vision may present with a sensory, roving nystagmus and poor visual attention and tracking. Visual acuity ranges from 20/20–20/200. The oculodigital reflex is an ominous sign of poor vision. Other important clinical findings include observation of a paradoxical pupillary response (direct, bright light stimulus causes dilation as opposed to the expected constriction of the pupil), which is characteristic of CSNB and achromatopsia. Myopic refractive errors are common, and hyperopia may occasionally be observed.

By definition, patients with CSNB have no structural anomalies on ophthalmologic exam and have no known neurologic diseases. The definitive diagnosis is by ERG, which shows an absent or varying degrees of low rod-mediated 'b' wave response compared with age-matched normal patients. The cone-mediated responses on ERG are normal. In contrast to LCA, no systemic disorders have been associated with X-linked or AR CSNB.[7]

DIFFERENTIAL DIAGNOSIS

The diagnosis of CSNB cannot be differentiated from Leber's or achromatopsia on initial clinical examination of an infant. An ERG is needed to determine if the rods are affected relatively more than the cones (CSNB affects rods > cones, achromatopsia affects cones > rods), or if both types of photoreceptor are affected (LCA severely affects both rods and cones).

DIAGNOSIS

CSNB is diagnosed by first excluding all ocular causes of poor vision. Also, poor vision caused by damage to intracerebral visual pathways, including the optic tracts, optic radiations, and occipital lobe, should be evaluated by neurologic examination and MRI. When ophthalmologic (**171, 172**), neurologic, and radiographic examinations are negative, an ERG is indicated to determine relative functionality of the photoreceptors and the bipolar retinal cells. ERG typically shows nonrecordable function or severely attenuated responses of cone photoreceptors. No retinal pigmentary changes are seen in patients with CSNB.

MANAGEMENT/TREATMENT AND PROGNOSIS

There are no known treatments that improve the vision in patients with CSNB. An important intervention that can be very helpful for patients with CSNB and their families is low-vision therapy and social service referrals for infants and children with limited vision. Progression of vision loss is rarely seen in CSNB.

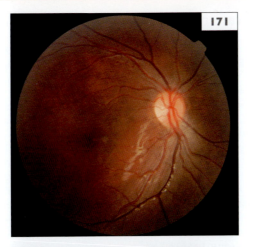

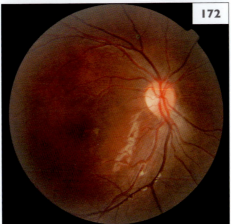

171, 172 Congenital stationary night blindness (CSNB): retinal photographs showing normal retinal vasculature, normal optic nerves, and normal maculae in both eyes of a patient with X-linked CSNB.

Achromatopsia

DEFINITION/OVERVIEW

Achromatopsia, also known as rod monochromatism, is a nonprogressive congenital dysfunction of cone photoreceptors leading to decreased central vision. It is a relatively rare condition, with an incidence of 1 in 30,000. There are three main types of achromatopsia categorized by the extent of cone photoreceptor dysfunction: complete, incomplete, and blue-cone monochromatism. Due to their relative or complete absence of cone (color) receptors, patients tend to function better under dimly lit conditions (scotopic) rather than brightly lit conditions (photopic). Because the fovea has a relatively high density of cone photoreceptors, central visual acuity is affected in this condition. The degree of visual impairment varies from mild to severe in accordance with percentage of affected cones and type of achromatopsia.

ETIOLOGY

Both complete and incomplete types of achromatopsia are AR-inherited, although incomplete achromatopsia may also be inherited in an X-linked manner. Several genes, including CNGA3 (Chr 14), CNGB3 (Chr 14), and GNAT2 (Chr 1p13), have been linked to 60% of the cases of achromatopsia.[8] Blue-cone monochromatism is also inherited via the long arm of the X chromosome, specifically on Xq28.

Histologic studies have shown that patients with achromatopsia have substantially fewer cones in both the extrafoveal and foveal areas. This reduction may be on the order of 95–100% in patients with complete achromatopsia. The morphology of the remaining cones has also been shown to be abnormal, with increased number of ectopic nuclei.[5] Blue-cone monochromatism affects only blue cones; red-green cones continue to function normally.

CLINICAL PRESENTATION

Children with poor central vision may present with a sensory, roving nystagmus and poor visual attention and tracking. Visual acuity in infancy and childhood ranges from 20/120–20/200. The oculodigital reflex is an ominous sign of poor vision. Progression of vision loss is rarely seen. Other important clinical findings include observation of a paradoxical pupillary response (direct, bright light stimulus causes dilation as opposed to the expected constriction of the pupil), which is characteristic of achromatopsia and CSNB. Refractive errors including moderate (greater than 3 diopters) hyperopia and astigmatism may also be observed.

By definition, patients with achromatopsia have no structural anomalies on ophthalmologic exam and have no known neurologic diseases (**173, 174**). The definitive diagnosis is by ERG, which shows an absent or varying degree of low cone-mediated response compared with age-matched normal patients. The rod-mediated responses on ERG are normal. In contrast to LCA, no systemic disorders have been associated with achromatopsia.

DIFFERENTIAL DIAGNOSIS

The diagnosis of achromatopsia cannot be differentiated from LCA or CSNB on initial clinical examination of an infant. An ERG is needed to determine if the cones are affected relatively more than the rods (achromatopsia affects cones > rods, CSNB affects rods > cones), or if both types of photoreceptors are affected (LCA severely affects both rods and cones).

DIAGNOSIS

Achromatopsia is diagnosed by first excluding all ocular causes of poor vision. Poor vision caused by damage to intracerebral visual pathways including the optic tracts, optic radiations, and occipital lobe, should be evaluated by neurologic examination and MRI. When ophthalmologic, neurologic and radiographic examinations are negative, an ERG is indicated to determine relative functionality of the photoreceptors and the bipolar retinal cells. ERG typically shows nonrecordable function or severely attenuated responses of cone photoreceptors.[8]

No retinal pigmentary changes are seen in patients with achromatopsia.

MANAGEMENT/TREATMENT AND PROGNOSIS

There are no known treatments that improve the vision in patients with achromatopsia. An important intervention that can be very helpful for patients with achromatopsia and their families is low-vision therapy and social service referrals for infants and children with limited vision.

Achromotopsia is a stable condition. Continued loss of vision is uncommon.

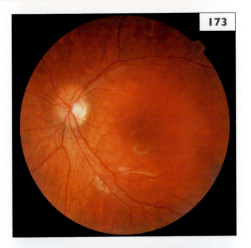

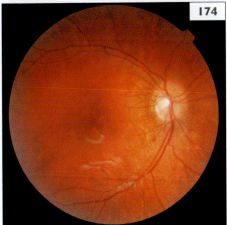

173, 174 Achromatopsia: retinal photographs of a patient with achromatopsia showing normal pigmentation, normal foveal reflexes, and normal optic nerves in both eyes.

Stargardt disease

DEFINITION/OVERVIEW

Stargardt disease, also known as Stargardt dystrophy or fundus flavimaculatus, is the most common type of juvenile-onset macular dystrophy. However, it is still a relatively rare condition, with an incidence of 1 in 30,000–50,0000 (7% of all retinal dystrophies). As the name implies, patients with Stargardt macular dystrophy demonstrate a degenerative change within the macula which ultimately affects central visual acuity. Symptoms of decreased vision do not generally occur until the second decade of life, but findings of retinal changes may be seen within the first decade of life. This type of macular dystrophy occurs significantly earlier than the adult-onset type known as age-related macular dystrophy, which generally becomes symptomatic in the 6–7th decades of life.

ETIOLOGY

This condition is inherited in an AR manner, due to a dysfunctional protein encoded by the gene ABCA4.[9,10] Stargardt disease classically demonstrates an accumulation of a retinal waste product known as lipofuscin within the subretinal space. This occurs as a result of a dysfunctional energy transport protein coded by the gene ABCA4. Lipofuscin is thought to be the waste product or perhaps an accumulation of degenerating photoreceptors, that accumulates because energy transport into the retina is not occurring normally. The deposits block the normal choroidal flush which is usually seen in the early phases of a fluorescein angiogram.

Recent genetic studies have shown that a mutation in the same gene (ABCA4) results in a varied phenotype, ranging from findings historically described as Stargardt disease to findings which had been traditionally called fundus flavimaculatus. It is now believed that these diseases are different phenotypic expressions of the same genotype. Not all of the mutation sites and alleles for the ABCA gene have been identified, and some studies have suggested that current testing for alleles may fail to diagnose or predict which patients will develop Stargardt disease.[11]

CLINICAL PRESENTATION

Children may fail a vision screening test, but the diagnosis is often not made until after vision has declined enough to affect daily visual function. The visual acuity of patients with Stargardt disease varies with the degree of involvement and the age of diagnosis. Acuities may be normal in early stages, and range from 20/100–20/400 by the 4th decade of life. A characteristic early symptom of visual dysfunction is a complaint of requiring more time to adjust to darkly lit environments after exposure to bright lights (prolonged dark adaptation).

On ophthalmoscopy, a 'beaten-bronze' appearance of the retina is classically described and seen in about 85% of cases (**175, 176**). Fluorescein angiography shows a 'silent choroid', as lipofuscin accumulation beneath the level of the retina blocks fluorescence from the choroidal circulation. Some patients show a decreased photoreceptor responses of both rods and cones on ERG testing, but this test is not always abnormal in Stargardt disease.

DIFFERENTIAL DIAGNOSIS

The diagnosis of Stargardt disease or fundus flavimaculatus is differentiated from other macular dystrophies by its classic appearance on direct retinal examination and fluorescein angiogram.

DIAGNOSIS

The diagnosis of Stargardt disease is made by clinical examination, by evaluation of visual acuity, indirect ophthalmoscopy, and fluorescein angiography. ERG, dark adaptation testing, and genetic evaluation are not necessary for the definitive diagnosis, but may be helpful in certain clinical situations.

MANAGEMENT/TREATMENT AND PROGNOSIS

There are no known treatments that improve the vision in patients with Stargardt disease. An important intervention that can be very helpful for patients with Stargardt disease and their families is low-vision therapy and social services referrals for the blind if vision falls below 20/200.

The progression of vision loss is variable and can start with a visual acuity of 20/40 and decrease rapidly (especially in children) to 20/200. By age 50, approximately half of affected people have vision of 20/200–20/400.

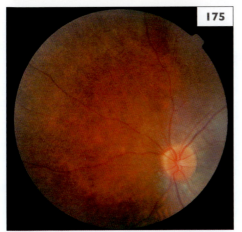

175 Stargardt disease: retinal photograph showing the characteristic 'beaten-bronze' appearance of the central retina (macula) in the right eye of a patient with Stargardt disease.

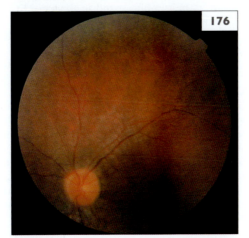

176 Stargardt disease: retinal photograph showing the irregular retinal pigmentation. Note the irregular sheen of the retinal light reflexes, which suggests an irregularity of the retinal surface due to accumulation of lipofuscin beneath the retina.

Best's disease

DEFINITION/OVERVIEW

Best's disease, also known as vitelliform macular dystrophy type 2 (VMD2), is a degenerative disorder of the central macula named for its 'egg-yolk'-like (vitelliform) appearance seen in the early stages. It is most commonly a bilateral disorder. In later stages, this condition causes retinal degeneration and atrophy leading to bilateral loss of central vision (**177**).[12,13]

ETIOLOGY

Best's disease is an AD-inherited macular dystrophy that begins with an 'egg-yolk'-like accumulation of material underneath the central macula, which later leads to degeneration and atrophy in this area and subsequent central vision loss. The gene responsible for this condition is found on Chr 11q13 and was only recently discovered (1998).[14] The gene, known as bestrophin, codes for a calcium-sensitive chloride channel protein within the retinal pigment epithelium (the cell layer underneath the retina that aids in metabolism and removal of waste products).

CLINICAL PRESENTATION

Patients with Best's disease frequently first present with mildly decreased vision or are sometimes diagnosed incidentally on a routine ophthalmologic examination. The initial presentation of this condition can be quite variable. In the early stages, a dilated fundus examination reveals a yolk-like (vitelliform) elevated, subretinal accumulation of yellowish material (lipofuscin) within the central macula of both eyes (**178**).

DIFFERENTIAL DIAGNOSIS

The diagnosis of Best's disease should be differentiated from other macular dystrophies including Stargardt disease, Sorsby's macular dystrophy, Doyne's honeycomb dystrophy, and butterfly macular dystrophy. Other non-degenerative macular diseases such as subretinal fluid (central serous chorioretinopathy) and infections (toxoplasmosis) should also be included in the differential; however, these conditions rarely present with bilateral involvement.

DIAGNOSIS

The diagnosis of Best's disease is simpler when the characteristic vitelliform lesion is seen in the early stages. In the later stages when macular atrophy is seen, the diagnosis is more difficult due to an appearance similar to other macular degenerations. ERG generally shows a normal full field retinal response, because this is a localized disease of the central macula (ERG results are a summation of the entire retinal response). The ERG readings are usually abnormal in other retinal degenerative disorders such as Stargardt disease.

The definitive test for Best's disease is an electro-oculogram (EOG). This test examines the change in voltage across the retina as the eye moves horizontally from one extreme of gaze to the other. In most degenerative retinal diseases, when the EOG results are abnormal, the ERG results are also abnormal. Best's disease is the only known retinal condition that demonstrates a normal ERG and an abnormal EOG.

MANAGEMENT/TREATMENT AND PROGNOSIS

There are no known treatments that improve the vision in patients with Best's disease. An important intervention that can be very helpful for patients with Best's disease and their families is low-vision therapy and social services referrals for the blind if vision falls below 20/200.

The vitelliform lesion may remain stable for years without causing significant vision loss. Over time, the material within the lesion may settle inferiorly, resulting in a fluid level superiorly. In the later stages of Best's disease, the lipofuscin is gradually absorbed, resulting in an appearance described as 'scrambled eggs'. These changes lead to thinning and dysfunction of the overlying retina, and ultimately atrophy of the central macula. In these later stages, central vision is slowly but progressively lost. The vision ranges depending on the stage of involvement, but final visual acuity is often in the range of 20/100–20/200.

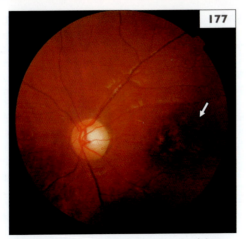

177 Best's disease: retinal photograph of the right eye showing atrophy of the central macula (arrow).

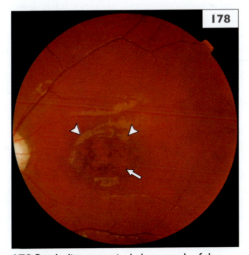

178 Best's disease: retinal photograph of the right eye showing the 'scrambled egg' appearance of the lesion in the central macula (arrow). Note the light reflexes surrounding the lesion, which suggest an elevation of the retina adjacent to the lesion (arrowheads).

Persistent fetal vasculature

DEFINITION/OVERVIEW

Persistent fetal vasculature (PFV), previously known as persistent hyperplastic primary vitreous (PHPV), is congenital persistence of normal ocular vasculature that would normally be reabsorbed prior to full-term birth.

ETIOLOGY

The etiology of this disorder is not known. As its former name implies, the primary vitreous forms the initial fetal vasculature of the eye during the 3rd–6th weeks of embryological development. The term PFV was coined in 1997 by Dr. Morton Folk Goldberg, who proposed that the term was more descriptive of the anatomic and developmental changes seen in the condition.[15] The primary vitreous is composed of mesenchymal vasoproliferative cells and ectoderm that fill the cavity between the fetal lens and retina. During this time, the hyaloid artery extends from the dorsal ophthalmic artery through the fetal fissure anteriorly to reach the lens. This artery, aided by mesenchymal elements from the primary vitreous, then forms a network of vessels, known as the tunica vasculosa lentis, that surround and nourish the developing lens.

The secondary adult vitreous begins to form during the 9th week, and is composed of sodium hyaluronic acid, hyalocytes, and collagen fibrils. The development of secondary vitreous causes regression and displacement of the primary vitreous. At full term, the vasculature that once enveloped the lens and extended from the optic nerve anteriorly, has regressed, leaving only avascular adult vitreous.

Failure of this fetal vasculature to regress is seen in only 3% of full-term infants, but is commonly seen (95%) in varying degrees of severity in patients born prior to 36 weeks gestational age. PFV is a spontaneous disorder, but several cases of genetic linkage have been reported in some families.

CLINICAL PRESENTATION

Patients with PFV are frequently diagnosed soon after birth when the pediatrician, using a direct ophthalmoscope in the nursery or office, discovers a dim red reflex or frank leukocoria. The majority of patients with PFV have unilateral disease (>90%);[16] however, careful examination of the contralateral eye may reveal clinically insignificant evidence of persistent vasculature (Mittendorf's dot or pupillary strands). The findings of PFV may be categorized according to their location of involvement: 25% of cases involve only the anterior segment, 12% of cases involve only the posterior segment, and the remaining 63% involve both anterior and posterior segments. However, significant abnormalities of the posterior segment are only present in about 10%.

The anterior form of PFV commonly shows a plaque of white, opaque fibrovascular tissue posterior to the lens (retrolental tissue) (**179, 180**). Occasionally only a small lens opacity is present, but this often progresses over time. Amblyopia is common in the setting of unilateral cataracts, warranting careful observation and treatment. Untreated PFV can lead to shallowing of the anterior chamber and angle-closure glaucoma.

The posterior form of PFV (**181**) does not involve anterior segment structures, but the posterior fibrovascular tissue commonly leads to folds or detachments of the retina (70%). Other abnormalities include poor macular development and optic nerve hypoplasia. Other ocular abnormalities seen in PFV patients include microphthalmia and strabismus.

DIFFERENTIAL DIAGNOSIS

The most important diagnoses to distinguish from PFV include retinoblastoma, retinopathy of prematurity, uveitis, and ocular toxocariasis, because these diagnoses require different and urgent treatments. Other conditions that may be confused with PFV include Norrie's disease, incontentia pigmenti, familial exudative vitreoretinopathy, and simple unilateral congenital cataract.[17]

DIAGNOSIS

Any infant with an abnormal red reflex should be referred for a complete ophthalmologic exam. PFV is diagnosed by careful direct visualization by indirect ophthalmoscopy and slit-lamp examination, as well as b-scan ultrasonography if the fundus is difficult to view. An examination under anesthesia may be required in order to establish the diagnosis and perform the appropriate treatment.

MANAGEMENT/TREATMENT

The management of PFV is surgical, specifically lens removal (lensectomy), membrane removal (membranectomy), and vitreous removal (vitrectomy). The goal of treatment in anterior PFV is to remove the cataractous lens and fibrovascular tissue that obstruct the visual axis, and to relieve any contractures that may be shallowing the anterior chamber. Management should be instituted soon after diagnosis.

PROGNOSIS

Patients who undergo early surgery for unilateral cataracts associated with PFV have a guarded visual prognosis. In the study by Anteby *et al.*, approximately 12% of patients ultimately showed visual acuity of 20/70–20/200, 47% showed visual acuity of 20/350 light perception, and 30% showed no light perception.[18] However, cases that are left untreated do not develop useful vision, and other complications such as severe glaucoma may develop as soon as 3 months after birth, and eventually, phthisis bulbi.

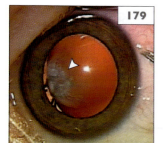
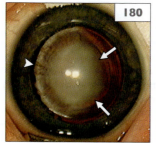
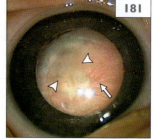

179–181 Persistent fetal vasculature (PFV). **179:** External photograph of an eye with a mild anterior PFV causing a small peripheral cataract (cloudy lens, arrowhead) that partially obscures the visual axis; **180:** external photograph of an eye with typical moderate anterior PFV causing a diffuse cataract (cloudy lens) involving 80% of the visual axis (arrows) extending to the periphery (arrowhead); **181:** external photograph of an eye with posterior PFV with a very dense plaque (arrowheads) and a thick hyaloid stalk (arrow) extending from the optic nerve (not seen) into the vitreous cavity.

Introduction

Uvea is the collective term traditionally used to describe the central vascular layer of the eye. The uvea is divided anatomically into three parts: anterior iris, intermediate ciliary body, and the posterior choroid (**188**). The ciliary body is further delineated by an anterior portion, the pars plicata, and a posterior portion, the pars plana. The functions of the uvea include thermoregulation, production of the aqueous fluid, and nutritional support for the structures of the eye. Over 95% of the blood flow to the eye is distributed throughout the uvea with a majority transported through the choroid.

Uveitis is a collective term, used to describe intraocular inflammatory diseases that affect the uveal tract. Many of these diseases also affect other ocular tissues, and many are ocular manifestations of systemic diseases. Uveitis is an uncommon disease with a prevalence of 0.5% in the general population, of which 5–10% is classified as pediatric uveitis. It is important for the pediatrician to recognize a potential case of uveitis because it is an often treatable, vision-threatening disease that has the best prognosis when discovered early in its course.

Common clinical features

The most common clinical symptoms of uveitis include blurred vision, photophobia, pain, and conjunctival/scleral redness. Some patients or parents may only notice epiphora (increased tearing). Patients with posterior or intermediate disease may complain of floaters or decreased vision from swelling of their macula (**189**). Many of these symptoms may not be present in the pediatric patient and often an asymptomatic pediatric uveitis is discovered by routine ophthalmologic screening. In some pediatric patients, the presenting complaint is decreased vision that is secondary to longstanding uveitis with cataract formation.

Early uveitis in a child may not be apparent on routine examination by a pediatrician. By the time clinical signs of uveitis become visible without a slit-lamp, significant damage may have already occurred.

External examination of a child with uveitis may show redness around the limbus, called ciliary flush (**190**), or may be normal. Ciliary flush is more commonly seen in cases of adult uveitis and frequently the external examination in pediatric uveitis is normal.

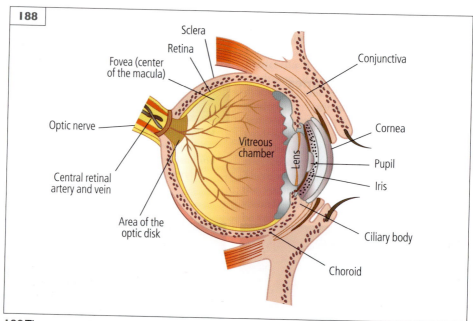

188

Sclera
Retina
Fovea (center of the macula)
Conjunctiva
Optic nerve
Vitreous chamber
Cornea
Lens
Pupil
Central retinal artery and vein
Iris
Area of the optic disk
Ciliary body
Choroid

188 The uvea.

Corneal signs common to uveitis include keratic precipitates (**191**), which are collections of white blood cells on the posterior corneal surface, and corneal edema (**192**) may be present if there is an elevation in the intraocular pressure (IOP). Keratic precipitates can often be seen in the red reflex of a direct ophthalmoscope (**193**).

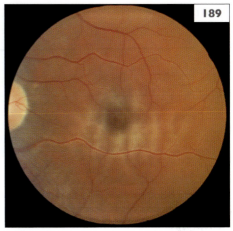

189 Uveitic swelling of the macula. (Courtesy of Peter Buch, CRA.)

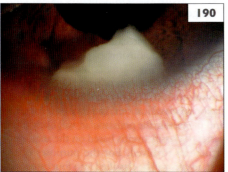

190 Ciliary flush and uveitis with retained lens fragment in the anterior chamber after cataract extraction. (Courtesy of Peter Buch, CRA.)

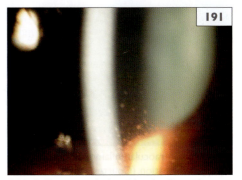

191 Collections of white blood cells on the posterior cornea (keratic precipitates). (Courtesy of Hasan M. Bahrani, MD.)

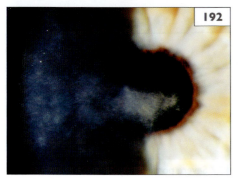

192 Corneal edema in a patient with chronic uveitis. (Courtesy of Peter Buch, CRA.)

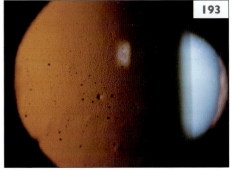

193 Retroillumination of keratic precipitates. (Courtesy of Peter Buch, CRA.)

Intermediate uveitis

Intermediate uveitis is a term created by the International Committee on Uveitis to encompass three separate entities: pars planitis, peripheral uveitis, and chronic cyclitis (inflammation of both the pars plana and pars plicata).[6] While subtle differences exist between these three entities, for the purpose of this chapter they will be considered together.

CLINICAL PRESENTATION/DIAGNOSIS

Intermediate uveitis is generally an asymptomatic disease in children, but symptoms can include mild blurring of vision and pain in more advanced cases. Occasionally children will complain of floaters or distortion of their vision. This disease is bilateral in 80% of cases but is often asymmetric. Early in the course of the disease accumulations of white blood cells are seen in the anterior vitreous and are often termed 'snowballs'.

Diagnosis is made clinically by an ophthalmologist by visualizing 'snowballs' or 'snow banks' (characteristic exudates over the pars plana). Many times diagnosis is made on routine screening of an asymptomatic child. Laboratory investigations are typically normal in these patients and often no causative agent is discovered. Testing is often directed towards Lyme disease, sarcoidosis, and tuberculosis, as each of these entities can present first with an intermediate uveitis and can be treated medically. Also, rare cases of toxocariasis have presented similarly and often an enzyme-linked immunosorbent assay (ELISA) test for *Toxocara* is performed.

MANAGEMENT/TREATMENT AND PROGNOSIS

As this is generally a benign, self-limited disease, treatment is only indicated when there is decreased vision (<20/40), or significant discomfort. Topical steroids are of little benefit, and periocular steroid injections are often used in cases of significant vision loss. In some cases, systemic immunomodulating therapy is needed. Mydriatic agents can be added to prevent scarring.

When early therapy is initiated for vision loss, most patients regain normal or near normal vision. Exceptions include cases where inflammation causes a posterior cataract to form on the lens, or cases of membrane formation on the retina secondary to chronic inflammation.[7]

Posterior uveitis

Toxoplasmosis

CLINICAL PRESENTATION/DIAGNOSIS

Toxoplasmosis is the most common form of posterior uveitis seen in children, accounting for at least 50% of cases. The infective agent is the intracellular protozoan *Toxoplasma gondii*. Cats are the definitive host, with human infection a result of ingestion of the encysted organism in undercooked meats. A large percentage of ocular toxoplasmosis infection occurs in the womb, when a previously uninfected woman is infected during pregnancy. Acquired forms occur, but ingestion of encysted protozoans in immunocompetent individuals usually does not lead to clinical disease. Active ocular toxoplasmosis appears as focal areas of inflammation over the retina and choroid (**202**). There is significant inflammation in the vitreous and this presentation is often called 'headlight in the fog'. Central lesions in the retina can cause significant traction and scarring with resulting loss of vision.[8]

Diagnosis is generally made clinically; however, a laboratory diagnosis can be made with ELISA on undiluted serum. A positive IgM suggests recent infection but a positive IgG does not confirm the diagnosis. Many normal individuals have positive IgG titers without evidence of ocular toxoplasmosis.

MANAGEMENT/TREATMENT AND PROGNOSIS

Triple therapy (pyrimethamine, a sulfonamide, and clindamycin) is initiated depending on the severity of the disease. Folinic acid is given to help prevent the myelosuppression associated with pyrimethamine. If there is severe inflammation systemic steroids can be given after 24 hours of antibiotic therapy. In immunocompetent individuals ocular toxoplasmosis is a self-limited disease and usually resolves in 1–2 months, so in many cases treatment of peripheral, nonvision-threatening lesions is unnecessary.

Prognosis depends on the location of the lesion. Peripheral lesions have an excellent prognosis and old toxoplasmosis scars are a common incidental finding on routine ophthalmic exam. Macular lesions usually result in scarring with a scotoma (lack of vision) in the

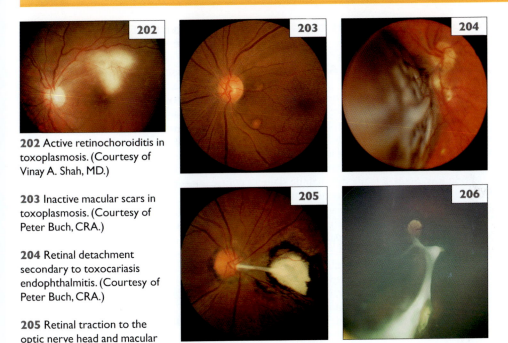

202 Active retinochoroiditis in toxoplasmosis. (Courtesy of Vinay A. Shah, MD.)

203 Inactive macular scars in toxoplasmosis. (Courtesy of Peter Buch, CRA.)

204 Retinal detachment secondary to toxocariasis endophthalmitis. (Courtesy of Peter Buch, CRA.)

205 Retinal traction to the optic nerve head and macular scarring in toxocariasis. (Courtesy of Peter Buch, CRA.)

206 Anterior traction on the optic nerve head from toxocariasis. (Courtesy of Donald Sauberan, MD.)

area of the scar (**203**). Central lesions or lesions near the optic nerve often result in legal blindness. Recurrences are fairly common and usually occur at the edge of a previous scar. No treatment has been shown to prevent recurrence.

Toxocariasis

CLINICAL PRESENTATION/DIAGNOSIS

Ocular toxocariasis is caused by the canine roundworm *Toxocara canis*. Infection commonly occurs after ingestion of soil contaminated by the roundworm eggs. Ocular toxocariasis is more common in boys and usually there is a history of geophagia. Ocular involvement is usually unilateral and presents either as endophthalmitis or as a granuloma (peripheral or central). The endophthalmitis is often quite severe and can present with leukocoria (white pupil) and hypopyon.

Accurate diagnosis is important as toxocariasis is one of the most common conditions incorrectly diagnosed as retinoblastoma (with resulting removal of the eye). The most reliable test for *Toxocara* antibodies is the ELISA test. Antibody testing of the aqueous or vitreous is more sensitive than serum testing.[9] Ultrasound can also be useful in differentiating *Toxocara* granulomas from retinoblastoma.

MANAGEMENT/TREATMENT AND PROGNOSIS

Peripheral lesions with minimal inflammation are not generally treated. Steroids have been shown to decrease the sequelae of the acute inflammation associated with posterior pole lesions and endophthalmitis. Antihelminthic agents and laser treatments generally increase the level of inflammation with the death of the worm and are not indicated.

Prognosis is poor in cases of endophthalmitis or macular involvement. Endophthalmitis often results in cataract, synechiae formation, and can result in retinal detachment (**204**).

Macular granulomas commonly cause traction on the retina and significantly decreased vision (**205**, **206**). Peripheral lesions generally do not cause significant visual loss after the inflammation has subsided.

Vogt–Koyanagi–Harada syndrome

CLINICAL PRESENTATION AND DIAGNOSIS

Vogt–Koyanagi–Harada syndrome (VKH) is a multisystem disease, seen more frequently in darker pigmented individuals, that generally presents in three stages. The first stage is commonly mistaken for a viral infection, with flu-like symptoms, headache, and tinnitus or hearing loss. Stage 2 is the ophthalmic stage where patients develop bilateral panuveitis (whole uveal tract), hyperemia of the optic disc, and serous retinal detachments (**207**). This stage is often when the patient presents with pain, photophobia, and decreased vision. During stage 3, the convalescent stage, dermatologic manifestations appear. These include poliosis (whitening/graying of a patch of hair), vitiligo (**208**), and alopecia (loss of hair). Stage 3 ophthalmic disease is characterized by retinal depigmentation, proliferation of retinal pigment epithelium, which can cause a puckering of the macula (**209**), and development of peripheral yellow/white deposits under the retina (Dalen–Fuchs nodules).

Diagnosis is made based on clinical findings since the exact cause of VKH is unknown. Systemic autoimmune response to retinal, uveal, and cutaneous melanocytes has been proposed as a mechanism of the disease, although this is currently unproven. Laboratory studies are usually not helpful in making the diagnosis, but a lumbar puncture with pleocytosis is supportive. Ophthalmic ultrasound during active inflammation shows findings consistent with panuveitis (inflammation throughout the uvea).

MANAGEMENT/TREATMENT AND PROGNOSIS

The mainstay of treatment during the active ophthalmologic stage is systemic corticosteroids. Most cases respond quite well to steroids, with rapid resolution of ocular inflammation and subretinal fluid. Cases that are only partially responsive to corticosteroids are often treated with concomitant cyclosporine.

Prognosis is guarded in these patients. Sometimes the inflammation follows a benign course and resolves entirely after steroid treatment. In others there are frequent recurrences, and the complication rates are high. Complications of chronic uveitis in VKH patients include cataracts, glaucoma, and retinal neovascularization.

Sympathetic ophthalmia

CLINICAL PRESENTATION AND DIAGNOSIS

Sympathetic ophthalmia is an uncommon bilateral panuveitis seen after penetrating ocular trauma or surgery. It presents in both eyes, with the injured eye (exciting eye) often developing inflammation first, and the uninjured eye (sympathizing eye) following weeks to months later. Sympathetic ophthalmia most frequently develops within 3 months (70%) of the original injury; however, it may develop in as short as 5 days and as long as 42 years. More than 90% of cases manifest within the first year. Patients generally present with pain, decreased vision, and photophobia in both eyes.[10]

The mechanism of disease is unknown, but the consensus is that the immune system is somehow sensitized to uveal antigens during the trauma or surgery and the immune system develops a systemic response to the entire uvea. Laboratory investigations are generally not useful. Fluorescein angiography can be performed (showing multiple foci of retinal leakage and late pooling of dye). However, the diagnosis is most often made clinically.

MANAGEMENT/TREATMENT AND PROGNOSIS

Treatment of sympathetic ophthalmia is controversial. Sympathetic ophthalmia can be prevented with early removal of the injured eye if there is no visual potential. Because of the rarity of sympathetic ophthalmia, if there is any potential vision, removal is not always recommended. High-dose systemic steroids, along with topical and periocular injections, are recommended. Cyclosporine can help in unremitting cases. Once inflammation has commenced, some studies recommend removal of the inciting eye. This is controversial, however, and other studies have shown no benefit of removal.

Visual prognosis is good with up to 75% of patients retaining good vision (>20/50). Many of those patients require long-term steroids to retain that vision, since recurrences are common. Complications of chronic inflammation in sympathetic ophthalmia include cataract, glaucoma, retinal detachment, and retinal scarring.

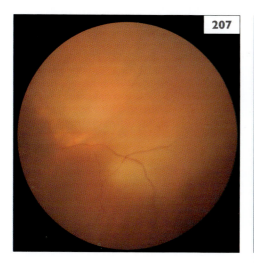

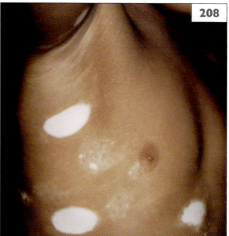

207 Panuveitis with serous retinal detachments in VKH. (Courtesy of Peter Buch, CRA.)

208 Vitiligo as a manifestation of VKH. (Courtesy of James Sanfilippo, MD.)

209 VKH-associated macular pucker from an epiretinal membrane in an otherwise quiet eye. (Courtesy of Peter Buch, CRA.)

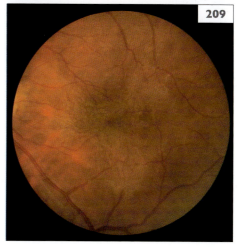

Masquerade syndromes

Retinoblastoma

CLINICAL PRESENTATION AND DIAGNOSIS

Retinoblastoma is the most common pediatric malignant ocular tumor. Retinoblastoma presents most commonly as either leukocoria (white pupil), strabismus, or with signs of ocular inflammation. The inflammation from retinoblastoma often causes a red, painful eye that is photophobic. A hypopyon may be present as well as a 'pseudohypopyon', which actually represents a layering of the tumor cells in the anterior chamber.

Diagnosis is usually suspected with direct visualization of the tumor. Ocular ultrasound and/or computed tomography (CT) may be performed to demonstrate intraocular calcification.

MANAGEMENT/TREATMENT AND PROGNOSIS

Treatment for large tumors is most often enucleation. Multiple 'eye-sparing' techniques have recently gained favor. These include scleral plaque radiotherapy, phototherapy, cryotherapy, chemotherapy, and external beam radiation.[11]

Without treatment, most children die within 2 years. However, with modern therapies, prognosis is very good, with a cure rate of greater than 95%. Early diagnosis and treatment have the best outcomes. Children with retinoblastoma that has invaded into the optic nerve, choroid, sclera, orbit, or anterior chamber often require chemotherapy, and have a poorer prognosis.

Leukemia

CLINICAL PRESENTATION AND DIAGNOSIS

The most common ocular presentation of systemic leukemia is retinal hemorrhages on fundus examination. Leukemic infiltrates within the uvea may lead to pseudoanterior iritis, which can layer out in the anterior chamber forming a hypopyon (**210**). Choroidal involvement generally presents as serous retinal detachments and optic nerve involvement presents as papilledema.[12]

Definitive diagnosis is made with bone marrow biopsy and smear. Aqueous tap may also be performed for cytology.

MANAGEMENT/TREATMENT AND PROGNOSIS

Treatment of systemic leukemia is managed by a hematologist/oncologist and is outside the scope of this book. Optic nerve infiltration is an ophthalmic emergency and requires radiation therapy to prevent permanent vision loss. With early radiation therapy, vision can often be saved in optic nerve-related disease.

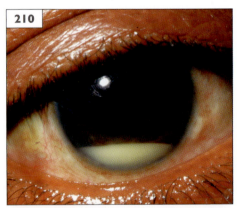

210 Leukemic pseudohypopyon. (Courtesy of Peter Buch, CRA.)

Diseases of the optic nerve

Paul H. Phillips, MD

- **Introduction**
- **Optic nerve hypoplasia**
- **Morning glory disc anomaly**
- **Optic disc coloboma**
- **Peripapillary staphyloma**
- **Congenital tilted disc**
- **Optic pit**
- **Myelinated retinal nerve fibers**
- **Papilledema**
- **Pseudopapilledema**
- **Optic disc drusen**

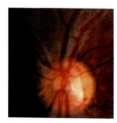
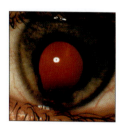
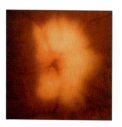
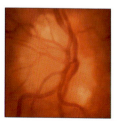

Introduction

Ophthalmologists frequently evaluate infants and children with visual loss from diseases of the optic nerve. It is essential to diagnose the cause of the optic neuropathy accurately, not only for treatment and prognosis regarding vision, but also to detect associated neurologic and systemic disorders.[1]

Several clinical principles apply to children with optic nerve dysfunction. Children with bilateral optic neuropathy acquired prior to 2 years of age often present with nystagmus. Children with unilateral optic neuropathy often present with strabismus due to loss of vision (sensory strabismus). Color vision is typically normal in children with visual loss from a congenitally anomalous optic nerve. This is in contrast to the dyschromatopsia that occurs in children with acquired optic neuropathies.[1]

It should be remembered that a structural ocular abnormality in infants and children may lead to superimposed amblyopia.[2] Therefore, a trial of occlusion therapy is often warranted in children with unilateral optic neuropathies and decreased vision. Vision may improve with occlusion therapy even among children who have a relative afferent pupillary defect.[1]

Optic nerve hypoplasia

DEFINITION/OVERVIEW

Optic nerve hypoplasia is a developmental anomaly in which there is a subnormal number of axons within the affected nerve, although the mesodermal elements and glial supporting tissue of the nerve are normal.

ETIOLOGY

Certain prenatal pharmacological insults may be associated with the development of optic nerve hypoplasia. Drug associations include exposure to phenytoin, quinine, lyseric acid diethylamide, meperidine, diuretics, and corticosteroids. The presence of maternal diabetes mellitus has also been implicated in some cases.

CLINICAL PRESENTATION

Children present with unilateral or bilateral reduction in vision. Children with a significant impairment of vision in both eyes will present early with nystagmus. Patients with unilateral optic nerve hypoplasia often present after failing a vision screening test or with strabismus.

The hypoplastic optic disc appears abnormally small and is often gray or pale in color (**211, 212**). The disc may be surrounded by a yellowish peripapillary halo bordered by a dark pigment ring (double ring sign) (**213**).[3] Associated retinal vascular tortuosity may occur. Histologically, optic nerve hypoplasia is characterized by a subnormal number of optic nerve axons with normal mesodermal elements and glial supporting tissue.[3] Magnetic resonance imaging (MRI) will often show a small optic nerve and chiasm in children with optic nerve hypoplasia.[4]

Visual acuity may range from 20/20 to no light perception and does not necessarily correlate with the overall size of the optic disc. Visual fields often have localized defects as well as general constriction.[5]

Optic nerve hypoplasia is associated with multiple central nervous system (CNS) malformations. Septo-optic dysplasia (de Morsier's syndrome) refers to the combination of small anterior visual pathways, absence of the septum pellucidum, and agenesis or thinning of the corpus callosum.[6] Cerebral hemispheric migration anomalies (schizencephaly, cortical heterotopias) or intrauterine or perinatal

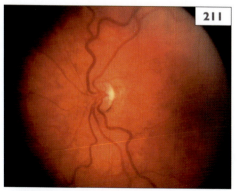

211 Optic nerve hypoplasia, left eye. Note associated retinal vessel tortuosity.

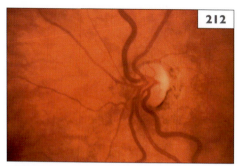

212 Close-up view of left optic nerve hypoplasia.

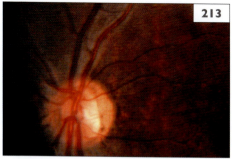

213 Optic nerve hypoplasia, left eye. Note double ring sign.

hemispheric injury (periventricular leuko-malacia, encephalomalacia) occur in 45% of patients with optic nerve hypoplasia. These abnormalities are highly predictive of neuro-developmental deficits.[7]

DIAGNOSIS

MRI demonstrates neurohypophyseal abnormalities in approximately 15% of children with optic nerve hypoplasia.[1,7] In normal children, MRI delineates the pituitary infundibulum, anterior pituitary gland, and the posterior pituitary gland, which appears as a 'bright spot' located in the sella (**214**). In children with optic nerve hypoplasia, absence of the infundibulum, or posterior pituitary ectopia may occur (**215**). Posterior pituitary ectopia denotes the abnormal location of the posterior pituitary in the hypothalamus. These pituitary abnormalities are associated with endo-crinologic dysfunction.[7–9] Some children have an absent pituitary infundibulum and no 'bright spot' (**216**). These children are at high risk for anterior and posterior pituitary dysfunction with diabetes insipidus.[9]

MANAGEMENT/TREATMENT

There is no treatment available to improve the vision that is decreased due to the hypoplastic optic nerve(s). If there is a possibility of superimposed amblyopia, treatment should be initiated. Low-vision services are warranted for those patients with significantly reduced vision.

The detection of endocrinologic dysfunction is an essential component of the evaluation of children with optic nerve hypoplasia. Growth hormone insufficiency is the most common endocrinologic abnormality associated with optic nerve hypoplasia.[10,11] However, hypothyroidism, hypocortisolism, panhypopituitarism, diabetes insipidus, and hyperprolactinemia may also occur.[3,12–14] Children with undiagnosed endo-crinologic deficiency are at risk for impaired growth, hypoglycemia, seizures, and death.[15] Early pituitary hormone replacement may prevent or ameliorate these complications. Therefore, parents should be questioned regarding the presence of protracted neonatal jaundice (associated with hypothyroidism) and previous episodes of neonatal hypoglycemia (associated with hypocortisolism). As noted above, MRI is helpful for the detection of endocrinologic dysfunction in children with optic

nerve hypoplasia.[8] Children with either a history suggestive of pituitary dysfunction or neurohypophyseal abnormalities on cranial MRI (such as absence of the infundibulum or posterior pituitary ectopia), should undergo diagnostic endocrinologic evaluation.

SPECIAL FORMS OF OPTIC NERVE HYPOPLASIA

Children with periventricular leukomalacia often have a special form of optic nerve hypoplasia characterized by a large cup and a thin, narrow retinal rim within a normal sized optic disc.[16,17] This appearance has been attributed to bilateral injury to the optic radiations with retrograde trans-synaptic degeneration of retinogeniculate axons after the scleral canals have developed to a normal diameter.

Superior segmental optic nerve hypoplasia with an inferior visual field defect occurs in some children of insulin-dependent diabetic mothers (**217**).[18,19]

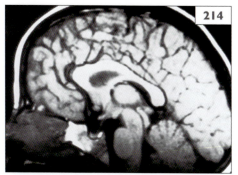

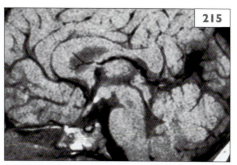

214 Cranial magnetic resonance imaging: T1 weighted, sagittal view of a patient with optic nerve hypoplasia and normal endocrinologic function. Note presence of the infundibulum and the bright spot denoting the posterior pituitary located in the sella. (From Phillips PH, Spear C, Brodsky MC (2001). Magnetic resonance diagnosis of congenital hypopituitarism in children with optic nerve hypoplasia. *J AAPOS* **5**(5):275–280, with permission.)

215 Cranial magnetic resonance imaging: T1 weighted, sagittal view of a patient with optic nerve hypoplasia and anterior pituitary dysfunction. There is absence of the infundibulum and posterior pituitary ectopia. (From Phillips PH, Spear C, Brodsky MC (2001). Magnetic resonance diagnosis of congenital hypopituitarism in children with optic nerve hypoplasia. *J AAPOS* **5**(5):275–280, with permission.)

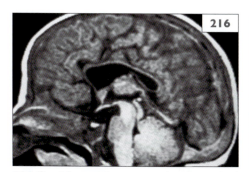

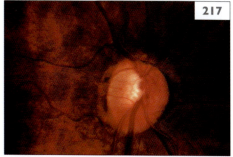

216 Cranial magnetic resonance imaging: sagittal view of a patient with optic nerve hypoplasia and panhypopituitarism. The patient has diabetes insipidus. There is absence of the infundibulum and no detectable posterior pituitary gland (absence of the posterior pituitary bright spot). (From Phillips PH, Spear C, Brodsky MC (2001). Magnetic resonance diagnosis of congenital hypopituitarism in children with optic nerve hypoplasia. *J AAPOS* **5**(5):275–280, with permission.)

217 Fundus photograph, right eye, of a 14-year-old girl who presented with a right inferior visual field deficit. Her mother was a Type I diabetic. This figure denotes superior segmental optic nerve hypoplasia.

Morning glory disc anomaly

DEFINITION/OVERVIEW AND ETIOLOGY

The morning glory disc anomaly is a congenital, funnel-shaped excavation of the posterior fundus that incorporates the optic disc.[20]

The etiology is uncertain, but it possibly arises from a failure of posterior scleral development during gestation.

CLINICAL PRESENTATION

The disc is enlarged, orange or pink in color, and situated within a funnel-shaped excavation (218). A white tuft of glial tissue often overlies the central portion of the disc. The blood vessels appear increased in number and arise from the periphery of the disc. The retinal vessels are abnormally straight and tend to branch at acute angles. Arterioles may be indistinguishable from venules. The fundus excavation is often surrounded by an elevated annular zone of retinal epithelial pigmentation. The macula may be incorporated into the excavation. The morning glory disc anomaly was named by Kindler (Kindler 1970) because of its resemblance to a morning glory flower.[21]

Visual acuity is generally less than 20/200, although it may range from 20/20 to no light perception. Most cases are unilateral although bilateral cases have been reported.[22] Morning glory discs occur more frequently in females and in Caucasians.[23] Serous retinal detachments occur in 26–38% of eyes with morning glory discs and often involve the peripapillary retina.[20] The source of the subretinal fluid is unknown. Contractile movements of the optic disc have been documented. These may occur from fluctuations in subretinal fluid volume and the degree of retinal separation within the excavation.[20]

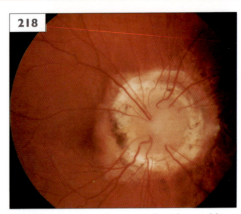

218 Morning glory disc anomaly, right eye. Note central glial tuft, peripapillary retinal pigment epithelial changes, and peripheral origin of disc vessels.

DIAGNOSIS

Neuroimaging may show a funnel-shaped enlargement of the distal optic nerve at its junction with the globe.[22,24] In addition, morning glory optic discs are associated with basal encephaloceles in patients with midfacial anomalies (hypertelorism, cleft palate, cleft lip, depressed nasal bridge, midline upper lid notch).[22] Therefore, children with morning glory discs and midfacial anomalies should be evaluated by MRI in order to detect associated basal encephaloceles.

MANAGEMENT/TREATMENT

With unilateral cases in young children, amblyopia therapy may be indicated to ameliorate nonorganic visual loss.

Optic disc coloboma

DEFINITION/OVERVIEW AND ETIOLOGY

The term 'coloboma' is used to describe any congenital notch, gap, or fissure of the ocular structures. Optic disc colobomas occur bilaterally in approximately 50% of patients. All ocular colobomas may occur sporadically or with autosomal dominant (AD) inheritance.[25] Colobomas occur from incomplete coaptation of the embryonic fissure.

CLINICAL PRESENTATION

An optic disc coloboma appears as a white, bowl-shaped excavation that occurs in an enlarged optic disc. The excavation is decentered inferiorly such that the superior neuroretinal rim is relatively spared. In cases of complete excavation of the entire disc, the excavation is deeper inferiorly. The defect may extend inferiorly to involve the adjacent choroid and retina (**219**). Chorioretinal colobomas are associated with microphthalmia.[26] Iris and ciliary body colobomas often coexist (**220**).

Visual acuity impairment may be mild or severe and is difficult to predict from the optic disc appearance. Visual acuity has been associated with the appearance of the fovea.[27] Optic disc colobomas are associated with serous macular detachments. In addition, rhegmatogenous retinal detachments may occur with retinochoroidal colobomas.[28] Retinal detachments may require surgical treatment.

DIAGNOSIS

Ocular colobomas may be accompanied by multiple systemic abnormalities and conditions such as the CHARGE association, Walker–Warburg syndrome, Goldenhar sequence, and linear sebaceous nevus syndrome.[29] Therefore, children with ocular colobomas should be evaluated for associated genetic syndromes. Family members should have an ophthalmologic evaluation to identify subclinical ocular colobomas and establish AD inheritance.

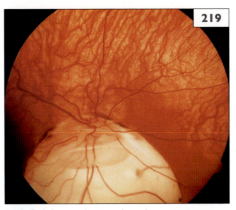

219 Coloboma that involves the optic nerve, choroid and retina.

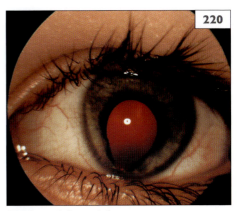

220 Iris coloboma, left eye.

Peripapillary staphyloma

DEFINITION/OVERVIEW AND ETIOLOGY

Peripapillary staphyloma is a generally sporadic, rare, usually unilateral optic disc anomaly in which a deep fundus excavation surrounds the optic disc. A peripapillary staphyloma is usually an isolated finding. There are typically no associated ocular or systemic abnormalities.

CLINICAL PRESENTATION

The disc, which is generally normal appearing, is at the bottom of the excavated defect (**221**). The walls and margin of the excavated defect may show atrophic pigmentary changes in the retinal pigment epithelium and choroid. In contrast to the morning glory disc, there is no central glial tuft overlying the disc and the retinal vascular pattern is normal.

Visual acuity may be mildly or severely decreased. Affected eyes usually have mild myopia, although high myopia has been reported.[30] Peripapillary staphylomas are associated with basal encephalocele in patients with midfacial anomalies.[31] Therefore, MRI is indicated for children with peripapillary staphylomas and midfacial anomalies.

Congenital tilted disc

DEFINITION/OVERVIEW AND ETIOLOGY

Congenital tilted disc is known as the nasal fundus ectasia or a Fuch's coloboma, occurring in 1–2% of the population. The congenitally tilted optic disc is a generally sporadic anomaly. It most likely arises from partial nonclosure of the embryonic fissure and is a variant of a colobomatous defect.

CLINICAL PRESENTATION

The superotemporal optic disc is elevated and the inferonasal disc is posteriorly displaced. The optic disc appears oval with the long axis obliquely oriented (**222, 223**). The tilted optic disc is accompanied by situs inversus of the retinal vessels and thinning of the inferonasal retinal pigment epithelium (RPE) and choroid. The optic disc appearance occurs from posterior ectasia of the inferonasal fundus and optic disc. The fundus ectasia results in myopic astigmatism in affected patients.

DIAGNOSIS AND MANAGEMENT/TREATMENT

Patients with tilted optic discs may have an artifactual bitemporal hemianopia that does not reflect chiasmal dysfunction.[32] The bitemporal hemianopia is typically incomplete and involves the superior quadrants. This visual field defect occurs partially from a refractive scotoma, secondary to regional myopia in the inferonasal retina. Therefore, placement of a –3.00 lens over the patient's glasses will often eliminate the visual field abnormality, confirming the refractive nature of the deficit. In some cases, retinal sensitivity may be decreased in the area of ectasia, so that the defect persists despite appropriate refractive correction.[33] Unlike the visual field loss accompanying chiasmal lesions, the visual field defects associated with tilted disc do not respect the vertical meridian and mostly affect the medium-sized isopters, owing to the marked ectasia of the midperipheral fundus.

Children with tilted optic discs and visual field deficits that do not respect the vertical meridian do not require neuroimaging. However, tilted discs have been reported in patients with suprasellar tumors.[34–36] Therefore, intracranial MRI is indicated in a child with tilted disc syndrome and a bitemporal hemianopia that respects the vertical meridian. Tilted discs have also been associated with X-linked congenital stationary night blindness in patients with nystagmus.[37] Therefore, children with tilted discs and nystagmus should be evaluated with an electroretinogram.

In unilateral cases, amblyopia therapy may improve nonorganic visual loss.

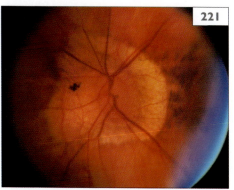

221 Peripapillary staphyloma, left eye. Optic nerve is contained within a posteriorly excavated fundus.

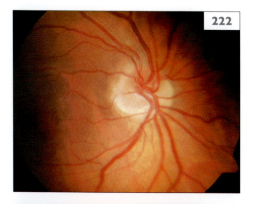

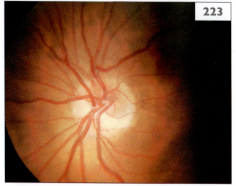

222, 223 Bilateral tilted optic nerves. **222:** Right eye; **223:** left eye. There is inferonasal fundus ectasia accounting for the superior temporal visual field deficit that did not respect the vertical meridian.

Optic pit

DEFINITION/OVERVIEW AND ETIOLOGY

An optic pit is a round oval depression in the optic disc (**224**). Optic pits are generally sporadic, although familial cases of AD inheritance have been reported.[38] They are most likely due to a defect in development of the primitive epithelial papillae.

CLINICAL PRESENTATION

The pit may appear gray, white, or yellow. Optic pits may be located in any sector of the optic disc, although the temporal disc is commonly involved.[30] Optic pits located temporally are often accompanied by adjacent peripapillary pigment epithelial changes. Cilioretinal arteries are common in eyes with optic pits. Although optic pits are typically unilateral, bilateral pits occur in 15% of cases.[30] In unilateral cases, the involved disc is slightly larger than a normal disc. Histologically, the lamina cribrosa is defective in the area of the pit and some optic pits extend into the subarachnoid space.

DIAGNOSIS AND MANAGEMENT/TREATMENT

Visual acuity is typically normal unless there is subretinal fluid. Approximately 45% of eyes with congenital optic pits develop serous macular elevations.[1] These elevations represent both retinoschisis and retinal detachment.[39] Optic pit-associated macular retinoschisis/detachments often occur in the third and fourth decades of life. The risk of an eye developing retinoschises or detachment is greater with large pits and with temporally-located pits.[40] These retinal elevations have been treated with laser photocoagulation, internal gas tamponade, and vitrectomy with variable success.[41,42]

Myelinated retinal nerve fibers

DEFINITION/OVERVIEW AND ETIOLOGY

During development, myelination starts at the lateral geniculate nucleus and stops at the lamina cribrosa. In some patients, retinal nerve fibers acquire a myelin sheath, and may arise from abnormal nests of oligodendrocytes within the retina and the optic nerve.

CLINICAL PRESENTATION AND MANAGEMENT/TREATMENT

Myelinated retinal nerve fibers (MRNFs) appear as a white area in the nerve fiber layer with frayed, feathered edges that follow the same orientation as a normal retinal nerve fiber layer (**225**). The myelinated nerve fibers may occur as an isolated patch or in several noncontiguous spots. MRNF are most commonly located along the optic disc margin (**226**). Retinal vessels are often obscured. Visual acuity ranges from normal to severe visual impairment. Some patients have associated unilateral high myopia as well as a hypoplastic macula.

If unilateral high myopia and amblyopia are present, appropriate optical correction and amblyopia therapy should be instituted.

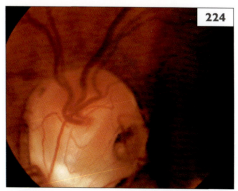

224 Optic nerve coloboma that contains a temporal optic nerve pit, left eye. Note the cilioretinal vessel emanating from the optic nerve pit.

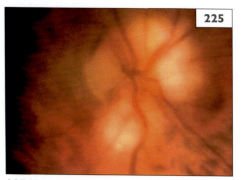

225 Myelinated nerve fibers, right optic nerve. Myelinated nerve fibers obscure the disc and the disc margin, as well as some of the disc vessels. The feathery edges are illustrated.

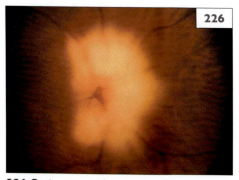

226 Optic nerve with severe myelinated nerve fibers that obscure the disc and the disc vessels, right eye.

Papilledema

DEFINITION/OVERVIEW AND ETIOLOGY

Papilledema is a sign of increased intracranial pressure (ICP). Because it is a sign and not a diagnosis in itself, the discovery of papilledema should lead to neuroimaging. The term papilledema should be reserved for disc edema that occurs from ICP. The ICP is transmitted to the optic nerve head through the subarachnoid space resulting in the disc appearance described below.

CLINICAL PRESENTATION

Disc edema occurs from an insult at the optic nerve head that causes impaired intra-axonal transport. This causes swelling of the optic nerve axons at the disc. The disc appears elevated with obscuration of the retinal vessels at the disc margins and peripapillary retinal wrinkling (Paton's lines) (**227**). The swollen disc may increase central retinal venous pressure, resulting in retinal venous dilation and tortuosity, disc hyperemia, intraretinal hemorrhages, and cotton-wool spots. Fluorescein angiography shows extracellular dye leakage at the disc.

DIAGNOSIS

Clinical characteristics that suggest (but do not prove) papilledema include spared visual acuity, and intact color vision, as well as bilateral involvement. Papilledema initially impairs the peripheral visual field causing constriction, arcuate defects, and nasal steps. Peripheral visual field loss may eventually involve fixation resulting in loss of visual acuity. Some patients have loss of visual acuity from retinal edema or hemorrhage. Patients may have 'a graying out' or loss of vision that lasts several seconds, so-called transient visual obscurations.

MANAGEMENT/TREATMENT

Papilledema is a medical emergency. The differential diagnosis of papilledema includes an intracranial mass, meningitis, venous sinus thrombosis, and hydrocephalus. ICP may shift the brain stem resulting in a cranial nerve VI palsy and consequent diplopia. Associated systemic signs of elevated ICP include headache, nausea, and vomiting. Cranial MRI is indicated to detect any intracranial abnormality. If neuroimaging does not reveal an intracranial mass or hydrocephalus, a lumbar puncture is indicated to measure the ICP as well as to examine the cerebrospinal fluid content.

Pseudotumor cerebri is a syndrome defined by the presence of elevated ICP, normal cranial MRI and normal cerebrospinal fluid content. In contrast to adults, pseudotumor cerebri in children is not associated with obesity and occurs with equal frequency in males and females.[43] Pseudotumor cerebri in children has been associated with drug use (tetracycline, doxycycline, and vitamin A), viral infections, growth hormone use, and thyroid medications. Treatment options, including acetazolamide, topiramate, optic nerve sheath fenestration, and shunting procedures are similar to those of adults.

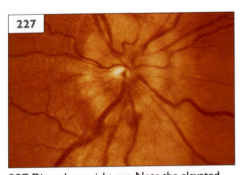

227 Disc edema, right eye. Note the elevated disc, obscuration of disc vessels, Paton's lines, venous dilation and tortuosity, and nerve fiber layer retinal hemorrhage.

Pseudopapilledema

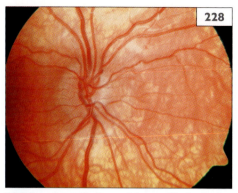

228 Pseudopapilledema, right eye. Optic disc is elevated, however, there are no vessel obscuration, disc hyperemia, retinal hemorrhages, or cotton-wool spots. There is abnormal branching of the large retinal vessels.

DEFINITION/OVERVIEW AND ETIOLOGY

Pseudopapilledema is an elevated disc anomaly that may be confused with papilledema (**228**). Pseudopapilledema is often bilateral and familial. Etiologies include buried optic disc drusen and prominent glial tissue.

CLINICAL PRESENTATION AND DIAGNOSIS

Pseudopapilledema can be differentiated from papilledema by the absence of disc hyperemia, vessel obscurations, nerve fiber layer hemorrhages, and cotton-wool spots (**229**). There is often abnormal branching of the large fundus vessels.

Ultrasonography or CT may show buried disc drusen. Fluorescein angiography does not show the disc leakage that occurs with true papilledema.

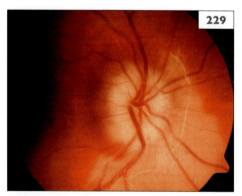

229 Pseudopapilledema, right eye. The optic nerve is elevated. There are no disc hyperemia, obscuration of disc vessels, retinal hemorrhages, or cotton-wool spots. The large retinal vessels have an anomalous branching pattern. The nerve fiber layer has a shiny light reflex with no opacification.

Optic disc drusen

DEFINITION/OVERVIEW AND ETIOLOGY

The majority of cases of anomalous elevations of the optic disc (pseudopapilledema) are associated with hyaline bodies of the optic nerve called drusen. Drusen are frequently bilateral and are inherited in an AD pattern.

CLINICAL PRESENTATION

Drusen may initially occur beneath the optic disc surface, so-called buried drusen. Subsequently, the drusen may enlarge and the disc axons may degenerate, resulting in visible drusen at the optic disc surface. The drusen appear as shiny refractile bodies with a gray-yellow translucent appearance. They may cause an irregular optic disc border. They do not obscure the retinal vessels overlying the disc (**230**).

Central visual acuity is generally normal. However, asymptomatic peripheral visual field defects such as constriction, arcuate defects, and nasal steps, commonly occur.

DIAGNOSIS

Optic disc drusen must be differentiated from papilledema. In contrast to papilledema, disc drusen occur without disc hyperemia, vessel obscuration, nerve fiber layer hemorrhages, or exudates. Optic disc drusen may be associated with subretinal hemorrhages as well as peripapillary subretinal avascular membranes.

Fluorescein angiography shows autofluorescence of the drusen without disc leakage. B-scan ultrasonography and CT may demonstrate drusen as noted above. These modalities are helpful for the detection of buried disc drusen that are not clearly visible on clinical examination.

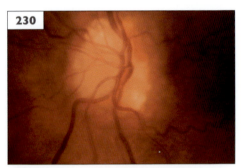

230 Optic nerve with visible drusen, left eye. The drusen are particularly visible at the 5 o'clock and 11 o'clock positions.

Disorders of the lacrimal system

Donald P. Sauberan, MD

- **Introduction**
- **Dacryocele**
- **Nasolacrimal duct obstruction**
- **Lacrimal sac fistula**
- **Decreased tear production**
- **Dacryoadenitis**

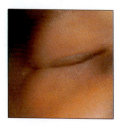
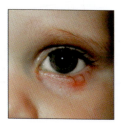
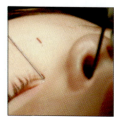

Introduction

Disorders of the nasolacrimal system are among the most common ocular disorders that a pediatrician will encounter. Knowledge of the natural history of various abnormal conditions of the nasolacrimal system and their associated treatment options will allow for assured discussion with parents to alleviate fears and increase awareness of the child's condition. It can also act as a guide to ascertain when more serious conditions may be present, and when further ophthalmologic evaluation may be necessary.

The nasolacrimal system consists of both a secretory portion (lacrimal and accessory lacrimal glands) and a drainage portion (the puncta, canaliculi, lacrimal sac, and nasolacrimal duct). Abnormalities at any point along the system can manifest clinically. The lacrimal gland is the main producer of reflex tear secretion, and is generally functional between birth and 2 months of age. The accessory lacrimal glands are responsible for basal tear secretion, and are functional at birth. The puncta are openings at the medial eyelid margin which the tears enter. They are usually situated on a mildly elevated area of eyelid called the ampulla. Absence of both punctum and ampulla suggests complete agenesis as opposed to simply an imperforate punctum. The eyelid puncta begin to open at approximately 6 months gestation.[1] The canalicular system takes the tears from the punctal opening into the nasolacrimal sac. The upper and lower canaliculi usually (~90%) connect into a common canaliculus just prior to entering the nasolacrimal sac. The nasolacrimal duct exits the nasolacrimal sac and traverses through bony canal into the inferior meatus beneath the inferior turbinate. The nasolacrimal duct begins as a cord of surface ectoderm. It cannulates from the proximal end to the distal end. It is most common for the distal end to open at about term, though about 6% of neonates will have an imperforate nasolacrimal duct.[2]

Dacryocele

ETIOLOGY

A dacryocele is formed when the nasolacrimal duct is obstructed at both the proximal and terminal ends, both at the valve of Rosenmuller (at the level of the common canaliculus entering into the nasolacrimal sac) and the valve of Hasner (at the level of the nasolacrimal duct entering the inferior meatus in the nose). Blockage of both the inlet and the outlet of the duct leads to sequestration of mucus which can become secondarily infected.

CLINICAL PRESENTATION

The presentation of a dacryocele (sometimes called amniotocele, lacrimal sac mucocele, dacryocystocele) is usually at birth. A bluish mass is noted inferior to the medial canthal angle (**231**). In the case of infection, the skin overlying the lacrimal sac can be erythematous. Schnall and Christian (1996) found that 4/21 (19.0%) dacryoceles had evidence of infection, with three occurring at the time of presentation.[3] Becker (2006) found a much higher percentage of secondary infection, with 21/29 (72.4%) developing dacryocystitis and/or cellulitis.[4] A dacryocele may also exhibit intranasal extension, causing respiratory distress in the newborn. Paysse *et al.* (2000) found a concurrent intranasal mucocele in 23/30 (~77%) dacryoceles, with respiratory distress present in seven patients.[5]

DIAGNOSIS

The diagnosis of a dacryocele is usually clinical. As noted above, it is usually a bluish elevation occurring below the medial canthal tendon. The differential diagnosis for such a lesion includes meningoencephalocele (which are normally located superior to the medial canthal tendon), dermoid cyst, or hemangioma. Imaging is not normally necessary. MRI can be performed to assess the area should an atypical lesion be present.[6] Suggestions of an atypical presentation include an elevation occurring above the medial canthal tendon, hypertelorism, pulsation, and known CNS abnormality.[6] Prenatal diagnosis of dacryocele has also occurred using ultrasound.[7] Nasal examination using a nasal speculum or endoscope can be performed to evaluate for the presence of an intranasal mucocele.

MANAGEMENT/TREATMENT

There are differing opinions regarding the treatment of dacryoceles. Current conservative measures include digital massage of the lacrimal sac in an attempt to hydrostatically decompress the lacrimal sac. Infrequently, the dacryocele can decompress through the canalicular system, but the nasolacrimal duct can remain blocked distally at the valve of Hasner.[4] Schnall and Christian (1996), in a prospective study, found that 16/21 (76%) resolved with conservative treatment consisting of antibiotics (topical and/or systemic based on presence of infection), digital massage, and warm compresses.[3] In addition, 4/4 dacryoceles that were infected at presentation or became infected after presentation resolved with conservative therapy. All dacryoceles resolved within 1 week, thus a recommendation was made that 1 week of conservative therapy is indicated in these patients prior to nasolacrimal duct probing. Becker (2006), however, found that 7/7 (100%) of patients without infection who had a nasolacrimal duct probing had resolution, whereas only 10/19 (~53%) who had infection had resolution following a nasolacrimal duct probing.[4] He advocated early probing in an attempt to open the system prior to the development of thickened cyst wall and turbid purulent fluid, which can lead to early closure. The failure rate of initial probing was highest in those patients who had an infection. Should initial probing fail, repeat probing with or without silicone tube intubation, balloon dacryoplasty, or marsupialization of the intranasal cyst can be undertaken.[4]

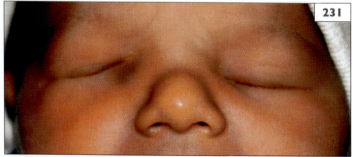

231 Dacryocele of the right eye. (Courtesy of Bruce Schnall, MD.)

Nasolacrimal duct obstruction

ETIOLOGY

Approximately 6% of all neonates have nasolacrimal duct obstruction.[2] The number is as high as 75% when fetal autopsies are performed. The most common etiology is failure of the valve of Hasner to open. The valve of Hasner is located at the distal end of the nasolacrimal duct where it enters the inferior meatus lateral to the inferior turbinate. The nasolacrimal duct normally canalizes from proximal to distal, so the distal end is often last to open. Thus, premature infants probably have much higher rates of nasolacrimal duct obstruction. However, because tear production does not occur until near term, these infants often do not exhibit the symptoms of epiphora.

CLINICAL PRESENTATION AND DIAGNOSIS

Most infants present with tearing and/or mattering of the involved eye. Depending on the level of obstruction, the symptoms may be more tearing than mattering or *vice versa* (**232**). Mucopurulent discharge can sometimes be expressed from the lacrimal sac through the punctum with digital massage. Symptoms are often worse in the cold or wind, or when the child has an upper respiratory infection. The presentation may be unilateral or bilateral. There is usually not concurrent conjunctival injection, which differentiates it from more typical conjunctivitis.

The diagnosis of nasolacrimal duct obstruction is a clinical one. One must be diligent in looking for other, less common causes of tearing. The most important diagnosis on the differential is infantile glaucoma. Increased intraocular pressure (IOP) can lead to corneal epithelial edema and breakdown, resulting in tearing. Other signs and symptoms consistent with infantile glaucoma include increased corneal diameter, optic nerve cupping, photophobia, and increased axial length resulting in myopia. The combination of epiphora with any of these other signs or symptoms should lead one to consider the diagnosis of infantile glaucoma. Other causes of infantile epiphora include keratitis, foreign body, or agenesis of the lacrimal puncta. The dye disappearance test can be used to assess the presence of nasolacrimal duct obstruction. One drop of fluorescein is placed into each conjunctival sac. After 5 minutes, the conjunctival tear lake is assessed using cobalt blue light. The normal infant will not have fluorescein remaining in the conjunctival sac, whereas the infant with nasolacrimal duct obstruction will show a varying amount of fluorescein depending on the degree of stenosis.[1]

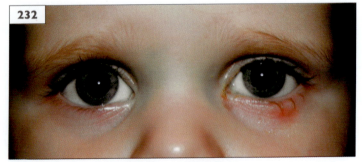

232 Nasolacrimal duct obstruction of the left eye.

MANAGEMENT/TREATMENT

The treatment of nasolacrimal duct obstruction is, at first, conservative. Peterson and Robb (1978) evaluated the natural history of nasolacrimal duct obstruction, and found that 44/50 (88%) resolved spontaneously using conservative treatment.[8] Conservative treatment usually consists of some mixture of nasolacrimal massage, warm compresses, and antibiotics if needed for secondary infection. Crigler in 1922 described massage of the lacrimal sac in an attempt to open the distal nasolacrimal duct by creating an increase in hydrostatic pressure within the sac to break open the distal membrane. This is still the method of choice for nasolacrimal massage.

Surgical intervention consists of the introduction of a flexible metallic probe into the nasolacrimal duct to open it. While classically the obstruction is located at the valve of Hasner, the location of obstruction may be anywhere along the route. A probe is placed into the nasolacrimal duct and passed into the nose (**233**). The nasolacrimal system can also be irrigated to assess patency following probing. This can be done by using fluorescein-stained balanced salt solution to irrigate with nasal suction to collect the fluid. One must remember, however, that this test does not mimic physiologic tear drainage, and that an open system to irrigation may not stay patent. Various opinions remain as to the most beneficial timing to pursue surgical intervention. Some argue that early intervention will have a higher success rate and allow for probing in the office, eliminating the need for general anesthesia. Others state that the procedure should be delayed as long as possible to allow for maximum spontaneous resolution. Classically, it is thought that the older a patient is at the time of probing, the less successful the probing will be. Katowitz and Welsh (1997) found a decreasing level of success after the first year of life.[9] This led to the use of 1 year of age as an ideal time to perform the initial surgical procedure. Various studies show a success rate of 90–95% after initial probing.

Should the initial probe fail, one must decide whether to perform a secondary probing or an ancillary procedure. The two main secondary procedures are balloon dacryoplasty and silicone tube intubation. Balloon dacryoplasty involves the insertion of a balloon catheter on a flexible

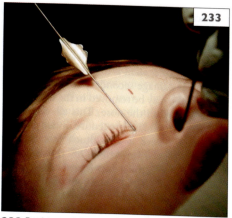

233 Probing of the nasolacrimal duct. A second metal probe is placed into the nose to confirm passage through the nasolacrimal system.

guidewire into the nasolacrimal duct, and inflation of the catheter to a predetermined pressure for a predetermined time. Success rates for balloon dacryoplasty as a primary procedure have been quoted to be as high as 94%;[10] however, the extra cost associated with its usage may preclude its use for common nasolacrimal duct obstructions. It may be useful in recalcitrant cases where other modalities have failed.

Silicone intubation of the nasolacrimal duct can be used as a secondary or primary procedure. Silicone tubes can be bicanalicular or monocanalicular. Bicanalicular silicone tubes consist of the silicone tube with a flexible metal probe on each end. Each separate end is introduced into the upper or lower punctum and then retrieved from the nose. The tube endings are tied in knots to prevent premature removal, and are often secured into the nasal vestibule via a suture. The tubes are kept in for a varying amount of time (surgeon preference), and then removed under general anesthesia. The disadvantages to this system include the possibility of punctate/canalicular tearing secondary to a tight tube and injury to the nasal mucosa while removing the tube from the inferior meatus. The other type of tube is the

Introduction

The eyelids are important accessory structures to the eye and can directly impact on vision. They are derived from surface ectoderm and fused together until the sixth month of gestation. With the exception of certain rare conditions such as ankyloblepharon, separation usually occurs before birth. Eyelid movement, or blinking, plays a key role in supporting the anterior ocular surface, and subsequent development of useful vision. In children, even benign appearing eyelid maldevelopment or pathology can lead to loss of vision by causing amblyopia.

Two different cranial nerves are responsible for eyelid opening and closing. The levator palpebrae superioris is responsible for eyelid opening and is innervated by the superior division of the third cranial nerve. The orbicularis oculi is served by the temporal branch of the facial nerve and closes the eyelid. Muller's muscle, located posterior to the levator muscle, is sympathetically innervated and can affect eyelid position in cases of Horner's syndrome or thyroid eye disease. The tarsal plates, made of firm connective tissue, provide structure to the eyelid margins and contain glands that contribute to the tear film. The upper eyelid tarsus is approximately 10 mm in height, while the lower eyelid tarsus is 5 mm in vertical height.

The eyelids are served by a delicate anastomotic arterial network from both the internal and external carotid circulations. Two clinically important arcades are the marginal and peripheral arcades of the upper eyelid. The marginal arcade is a superficial, horizontal arterial supply that lies just 2 mm above the eyelid margin. The peripheral arcade, while also horizontal, lies deeper, and just superior to the tarsal plate. It serves as a surgical landmark between the levator and Muller's muscles. The eyelid crease is created by the attachment of strands of the underlying orbicularis oculi muscle to the skin and can show varying positions in cases of ptosis.[1]

Anophthalmia/ microphthalmia

Just as eyelid structure is important to ocular development, normal eye development is similarly critical to eyelid development. Anophthalmos is a rare condition where the optical vesicle fails to form and there is no globe in the orbit (**234**). More common is microphthalmos, which is the development of a small but disorganized globe. In both cases, eye socket growth is impaired and the eyelids may show shortened horizontal palpebral fissures. In many cases proper growth can be stimulated by the placement of expanding conformers. Surgical correction may involve expanding the orbital volume with dermis fat grafts or synthetic material.

Cryptophthalmos and ankyloblepharon

Cryptophthalmos is a rare condition where there is complete failure of the development of eyelid folds. This is nearly always accompanied by abnormal development of the anterior segment of the eye. Ankyloblepharon is failure of the eyelids to separate. Ankyloblepharon fili forme adnatum occurs when fine bands of tissue connect the upper and lower eyelids. The treatment involves surgical division and possible lid margin repair.

Coloboma of the eyelid

This cleftlike deformity may vary from a small indentation or notch of the free margin of the eyelid to a large defect involving almost the entire lid (**235**). If the gap is extensive, ulceration and corneal damage may result from exposure. Early surgical correction of the lid defect is recommended in such cases. Other deformities frequently associated with eyelid colobomas

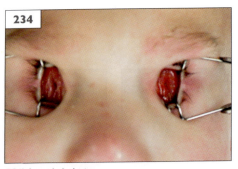

234 Anophthalmia.

include dermoid cysts or dermolipomas on the globe; they often occur in a position corresponding to the site of the lid defect. Eyelid colobomas may also be associated with extensive facial malformation, as in mandibulofacial dysostosis (Franceschetti or Treacher–Collins syndrome). Upper eyelid colobomas are characteristically seen in cases of Goldenhar syndrome.

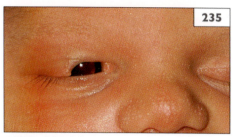

235 Eyelid coloboma.

Blepharoptosis

DEFINITION/OVERVIEW AND ETIOLOGY

In blepharoptosis, the upper eyelid droops below its normal level. Congenital ptosis is usually a result of a localized dystrophy of the levator muscle in which the striated muscle fibers are replaced with fibrous tissue. The condition may be unilateral or bilateral and can be familial, transmitted as an autosomal dominant (AD) trait.

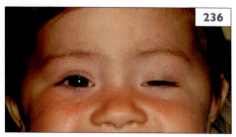

236 Blepharoptosis with absent lid crease.

CLINICAL PRESENTATION AND DIAGNOSIS

Parents often comment that the eye looks smaller because of the drooping eyelid. The lid crease is decreased or absent where the levator muscle would normally insert below the skin surface (**236**). Because the levator is replaced by fibrous tissue, the lid does not move downward fully in downgaze (lid lag). If the ptosis is severe, affected children often attempt to raise the lid by lifting their brow or adapting a chin-up head posture to maintain binocular vision. Marcus–Gunn jaw-winking ptosis accounts for 5% of ptosis in children. In this syndrome, an abnormal synkinesis exists between the 5th and 3rd cranial nerves; this causes the eyelid to elevate with movement of the jaw. The wink is produced by chewing or sucking and may be more noticeable than the ptosis itself.

Although ptosis in children is often an isolated finding, it may occur in association with other ocular or systemic disorders. Systemic disorders include myasthenia gravis, muscular dystrophy, and botulism. Ocular disorders include mechanical ptosis secondary to lid tumors, blepharophimosis syndrome, congenital fibrosis syndrome, combined levator/superior rectus maldevelopment, and congenital or acquired third nerve palsy. A small degree of ptosis is seen in Horner's syndrome. A complete ophthalmic and systemic examination is therefore important in the evaluation of a child with ptosis.

Amblyopia may occur in children with ptosis. The amblyopia may be secondary to the lid's covering the visual axis (deprivation) or induced astigmatism (anisometropia). When amblyopia occurs, it should generally be treated before correcting the ptosis.

MANAGEMENT/TREATMENT

Treatment of ptosis in a child is indicated for elimination of an abnormal head posture, improvement in the visual field, prevention of amblyopia, and restoration of a normal eyelid appearance. The timing of surgery depends on the degree of ptosis, its cosmetic and functional severity, the presence or absence of compensatory posturing, the wishes of the parents, and the discretion of the surgeon. Surgical treatment is determined by the amount of levator function that is present. In cases of congenital ptosis, levator function is often decreased, and requires that a suspension material (usually silicone or fascia lata) be placed between the frontalis muscle and the tarsus of the eyelid. This then allows the patient to use their brow and frontalis muscle more effectively to raise the eyelid. Amblyopia remains a concern even after surgical correction and should be monitored closely. This frontalis sling approach to congenital ptosis is reliant on visual stimulation, and therefore is not as effective in cases where patients have no visual potential.

Epicanthal folds and euryblepharon

These vertical or oblique folds of skin extend on either side of the bridge of the nose from the brow or lid area, covering the medial canthal region. They are present to some degree in most young children and become less apparent with age. The folds may make the eyes appear crossed (pseudoesotropia) (**237**). Epicanthal folds are a common feature of many syndromes, including chromosomal aberrations (trisomies) and disorders of single genes. Epicanthal folds may be further described as epicanthal tarsalis, epicanthus inversus, epicanthus palpebralis, and epicanthus supraciliaris depending on where the skin fold begins.

Euryblepharon occurs when there is increased vertical separation of the temporal eyelid opening such that the inner surface of the lower eyelid is not in apposition with the eye. The lateral canthus may be inferiorly displaced and there is increased risk of exposure keratopathy. The treatment involves surgical lid tightening.

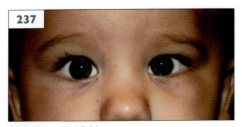

237 Epicanthal folds.

Lagophthalmos

This is a condition in which complete closure of the lids over the globe is difficult or impossible. It may be paralytic, because of a facial palsy involving the orbicularis muscle, or spastic, as in thyrotoxicosis. It may be structural when retraction or shortening of the lids results from scarring or atrophy consequent to injury (burns) or disease. Infants with collodion membrane may have temporary lagophthalmos caused by the restrictive effect of the membrane on the lids. Lagophthalmos may accompany proptosis or buphthalmos when the lids, although normal, cannot effectively cover the enlarged or protuberant eye. A degree of physiologic lagophthalmos may occur normally during sleep, but functional lagophthalmos in an unconscious or debilitated patient can be a problem.

In patients with lagophthalmos exposure of the eye may lead to drying, infection, corneal ulceration, or perforation of the cornea; the result may be loss of vision, even loss of the eye. In lagophthalmos protection of the eye by artificial tear preparations, ophthalmic ointment, or moisture chambers is essential. Gauze pads are to be avoided, because the gauze may abrade the cornea. In some cases, surgical closure of the lids (tarsorrhaphy) may be necessary for long-term protection of the eye.

Lid retraction

Pathologic retraction of the lid may be myogenic or neurogenic. Myogenic retraction of the upper lid occurs in thyrotoxicosis, in which it is associated with three classic signs: a staring appearance (Dalrymple sign), infrequent blinking (Stellwag sign), and lag of the upper lid on downward gaze (von Graefe sign).

Neurogenic retraction of the lids may occur in conditions affecting the anterior mesencephalon. Lid retraction is a feature of the syndrome of the sylvian aqueduct. In children, it is commonly a sign of hydrocephalus. It may occur with meningitis. Paradoxical retraction of the lid is seen in the Marcus–Gunn jaw-winking syndrome. It may also be seen with attempted eye movement after recovery from a third nerve palsy, if aberrant regeneration of the oculomotor nerve fibers has occurred.

Simple staring and the physiologic or reflexive lid retraction ('eye popping'), in contrast to pathologic lid retractions, occur in infants in response to a sudden reduction in illumination or as a startle reaction.

Ectropion, entropion, and epiblepharon

Ectropion is eversion of the lid margin; it may lead to overflow of tears (epiphora) and subsequent maceration of the skin of the lid, to inflammation of exposed conjunctiva, or to superficial exposure keratopathy. Common causes are scarring consequent to inflammation, burns, or trauma, or weakness of the orbicularis muscle as a result of facial palsy; these forms may be corrected surgically. Protection of the cornea is essential. Ectropion is also seen in certain children who have faulty development of the lateral canthal ligament; this may occur in Down syndrome. Congenital ectropion may be seen in association with congenital ichthyosis,[2] Treacher–Collins syndrome, or blepharophimosis syndrome. The blepharophimosis syndrome, or Kohn–Ramono syndrome, is an AD condition which also includes blepharoptosis, epicanthus inversus (epicanthal folds that extend from the lower eyelid), and telecanthus (a wide intercanthal distance).[3]

Entropion is inversion of the lid margin, which may cause discomfort and corneal damage because of the inward turning of the lashes (trichiasis). A principal cause is scarring secondary to inflammation such as occurs in trachoma or as a sequela of Stevens–Johnson syndrome. There is also a rare congenital form. Surgical correction is effective in many cases.

Epiblepharon is commonly seen in childhood, more often in Asian children, and may be confused with entropion (**238**). In epiblepharon, a roll of skin beneath the lower eyelid lashes causes the lashes to be directed vertically and to touch the cornea. Unlike entropion, the eyelid margin itself is not rotated toward the cornea. Epiblepharon usually resolves spontaneously. If corneal scarring begins to occur, surgical correction may be necessary.

Blepharospasm

This spastic or repetitive closure of the lids may be caused by irritative disease of the cornea, conjunctiva, or facial nerve; fatigue or uncorrected refractive error; or common tic. Thorough ophthalmic examination for pathologic causes, such as trichiasis, keratitis, conjunctivitis, or foreign body, is indicated. Local injection of botulinum toxin may give relief but frequently must be repeated.

Blepharitis

This inflammation of the lid margins is characterized by erythema and crusting or scaling; the usual symptoms are irritation, burning, and itching. The condition is commonly bilateral and chronic or recurrent. The two main types are staphylococcal and seborrheic. In staphylococcal blepharitis, ulceration of the lid margin is common, the lashes tend to fall out, and conjunctivitis and superficial keratitis are often associated. In seborrheic blepharitis, the scales tend to be greasy, the lid margins are less red, and ulceration usually does not occur. The blepharitis is often of mixed type.

Thorough daily cleansing of the lid margins with a cloth or moistened cotton applicator to remove scales and crusts is important in the treatment of both forms. Staphylococcal blepharitis is treated with an antistaphylococcal antibiotic applied directly to the lid margins. When a child also has seborrhea, concurrent treatment of the scalp is important.

Pediculosis of the eyelashes may produce a clinical picture of blepharitis. The lice can be

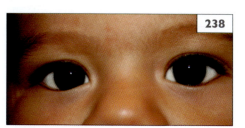

238 Epiblepharon.

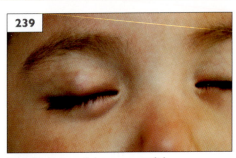

239 Chalazion of the upper eyelid.

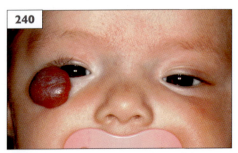

240 Capillary hemangioma of the eyelid in an infant twin #1, managed with observation as it did not obstruct visual acuity.

smothered with ophthalmic-grade petrolatum ointment applied to the lid margin and lashes. Nits should be mechanically removed from the lashes. It should be remembered that pediculosis represents a sexually transmitted disease.

Hordeolum

Infection of the glands of the lid may be acute or subacute; tender focal swelling and redness are noted. The usual agent is *Staphylococcus aureus*. When the meibomian glands are involved, the lesion is referred to as an internal hordeolum; the abscess tends to be large and may point through either the skin or the conjunctival surface. When the infection involves the glands of Zeis or Moll, the abscess tends to be smaller and more superficial and points at the lid margin; it is then referred to as an external hordeolum or stye.

Treatment is frequent warm compresses and, if necessary, surgical incision and drainage. In addition, topical antibiotic preparations are

often used. Untreated, the infection may progress to cellulitis of the lid or orbit, requiring the use of systemic antibiotics.

Chalazion

A chalazion is a granulomatous inflammation of a meibomian gland characterized by a firm, nontender nodule in the upper or lower lid (**239**). The meibomian glands are located in the tarsal plates and are normally responsible for producing a component of the tear film. This lesion tends to be chronic and differs from internal hordeolum in the absence of acute inflammatory signs. Although many chalazia subside spontaneously, excision may be necessary if they become large enough to distort vision (by inducing astigmatism by exerting pressure on the globe) or to be a cosmetic blemish. Patients who experience frequent chalazia formation, or those who have significant corneal changes secondary to the underlying blepharitis, may benefit from systemic erythromycin treatment.

Tumors of the eyelid

A number of eyelid tumors arise from surface structures (the epithelium and sebaceous glands). Nevi may appear in early childhood; most are junctional. Compound nevi tend to develop in the prepubertal years and dermal nevi at puberty. Malignant epithelial tumors (basal cell carcinoma, squamous cell carcinoma) are rare in children, but the basal cell nevus syndrome and the malignant lesions of xeroderma pigmentosum and of Rothmund–Thomson syndrome may develop in childhood.

Capillary hemangiomas (**240**) are the most common eyelid and orbital tumors in the infant. Many tend to regress spontaneously, although they may show alarmingly rapid growth in infancy. In many cases, the best management of such hemangiomas is patient observation, allowing spontaneous regression to occur. Examination by a pediatric ophthalmologist will help rule out any astigmatic effects that may not be as obvious as direct obstruction of the visual axis. In the case of a rapidly expanding lesion, or one potentially causing amblyopia, corticosteroid, propranolol, or surgical treatment should be considered. These treatment options, whether oral or percutaneous, are not benign and include systemic risks as well as eyelid necrosis, subcutaneous fat atrophy, or very rarely embolic occlusion.[4]

Nevus flammeus (port-wine stain), a non-involuting hemangioma, occurs as an isolated lesion or in association with other signs of Sturge–Weber syndrome. Affected patients should be monitored for the development of glaucoma (see Chapter 9, Glaucoma). Lymph-angiomas of the lid appear as firm masses at or soon after birth and tend to enlarge slowly during the growing years or following an upper respiratory infection. Associated conjunctival involvement, appearing as a clear, cystic, sinuous conjunctival mass, may provide a clue to the diagnosis. In some cases there is also orbital involvement. The treatment for these lesions is usually observation, with the rare need for surgical excision. Plexiform neuromas of the lids (**241**) occur in children with neurofibromatosis, often with ptosis as the first sign. The lid may take on an S-shaped configuration and has a characteristic 'bag of worms' consistency. The eyelids may also be involved by other tumors, such as retinoblastoma, neuroblastoma, and rhabdomyosarcoma of the orbit.

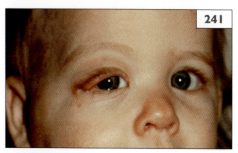

241 Plexiform neuroma.

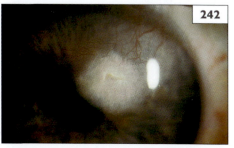

242 Chronic herpes simplex keratitis with corneal scarring and deep and superficial vascularization. (From Vernon S, *Differential Diagnosis in Ophthalmology*, Manson Publishing.)

Preseptal and orbital cellulitis

Both preseptal and orbital cellulitis may cause eyelid edema, even to the point that ocular examination is difficult. Examination of the eye in these situations is still vital to the diagnosis and can be vision or life saving. Visual acuity assessment, ocular motility, pupillary evaluation, fever, and leukocytosis are key clinical findings that help distinguish these two entities. In children with orbital cellulitis, a single organism is usually the cause, with *Staphylococcus* and *Streptococcus* species being the most common. Hospital admission with intravenous coverage for methicillin-resistant *S. aureus* (MRSA) is warranted in cases of orbital cellulitis.[5] Younger patients with even mild infections may also require admission for intravenous antibiotics and monitoring. Infections that do not resolve with intravenous antibiotics should raise suspicion of a subperiosteal abscess, and may need surgical drainage. Otolaryngology or oculoplastic consultation early in these cases facilitates the surgical decision-making process.

Herpes simplex, molluscum contagiosum, and verruca vulgaris

Herpes simplex is a deoxyribonucleic acid (DNA) virus that can present with vesicles along the eyelid. The virus can spread to the cornea, at which time significant visual compromise can occur (**242**). Beyond careful ophthalmic evaluation for the presence of dendrites, the treatment is oral or topical antiviral therapy. A topical antibiotic to prevent secondary bacterial infection may also be warranted. Most cases of herpes simplex are self-limited although corneal scarring can lead to loss of vision through the scar itself or by producing amblyopia.

Molluscum contagiosum is a common skin disease in children, caused by a DNA pox virus, and shows multiple raised lesions with central umbilication in the periocular area. These central areas contain intracytoplasmic 'molluscum bodies', which may enter the tear film. As such, the presenting symptom is often a follicular conjunctivitis. Symptomatic patients or those at risk for corneal injury benefit from surgical excision.

Verruca vulgaris, or a wart, is caused by the human papillomavirus and can be seen on the eyelid. Similar to molluscum, lesions near the lid margin may cause a secondary conjunctivitis. Most cases are also self-limiting, but those that persist can be surgically removed with or without cryotherapy.

Allergic conjunctivitis

The most common cause of chronic conjunctivitis is allergy. The eyelid may show secondary lichenification or scaling dermatitis in such cases. Allergic conjunctivitis in children may be due to vernal or perennial causes.

Trauma

Eyelid trauma can result in consequences that last a lifetime. Lid margin involvement that is not appropriately approximated can result in notching with secondary compromise of the ocular surface. Ophthalmology consultation is recommended for repair of these lacerations. Injury to the medial canthus must be examined carefully for involvement of the lacrimal system. Tactile crepitus of the eyelid in cases of orbital fracture is sometimes noted due to communication with the aerated sinuses. In cases of acute blunt trauma, the superior rectus and levator complex may be 'stunned', resulting in inability to elevate the eyelid or look up and therefore giving the appearance of muscle entrapment. Forced duction testing, in which manual movement of the globe with forceps is attempted, in these cases would rule out any entrapment. Penetrating trauma to the eyelid with exposed orbital fat is a sign that the septum has been violated, and increases the risk of damage to the levator muscle, requiring surgical exploration. True dehiscence of the medial canthus from its attachments requires complex repair by an experienced orbital surgeon. Finally, several studies have shown that any eyelid or surrounding bone trauma

mandates a careful ophthalmologic examination and may reveal underlying pathology not seen at the skin surface.

Summary

Pathology of the human eyelid can affect the development of vision in several ways. Various congenital syndromes include eyelid malformations as part of the constellation of findings. Tumors involving the eyelid or orbit can potentially be fatal. Trauma to the eyelid may indirectly result in subsequent injury to the eye, surrounding structures, or lacrimal system. Infectious etiologies require prompt recognition and follow-up before central dissemination occurs. As such, careful evaluation of the eyelids and ocular adnexa is a key component in ophthalmic evaluation of a child and may demonstrate the sentinel signs of visual compromise or systemic disease.

CHAPTER 15

Ocular manifestations of systemic disorders

Merrill Stass-Isern, MD and Laurie D. Smith, MD, PhD, FAAP Diplomate, ABMG

- **Introduction**

- **Cystinosis**

- **Marfan's syndrome**

- **Homocystinuria**

- **Wilson's disease**

- **Fabry disease**

- **Osteogenesis imperfecta**

- **The mucopolysaccharidoses**

- **Sickle cell disease**

- **Albinism**

- **Congenital rubella**

Introduction

Ocular abnormalities may primarily involve the eye or represent findings secondary to systemic disease. In either case, ocular disease can negatively impact on vision and the quality of life. Because the internal anatomy of the eye may be easily and rapidly evaluated, an ocular examination should always be included in the assessment of the pediatric patient. A delay in diagnosis of the ocular component of systemic diseases may be significant, resulting in permanent vision loss and also compromising the early academic years. At times, even a prompt diagnosis will not ensure a good outcome, as there may be few therapeutic options available to improve vision. In severe cases, we may be limited to prescribing proper visual aids, guiding parents to select the scholastic path that will best meet their child's needs, and also helping them to manage the implications of their child's visual disability. It is therefore imperative to maintain good communication between the pediatrician and ophthalmologist in order to optimize the proper medical care of these children.

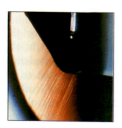
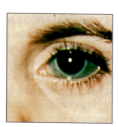
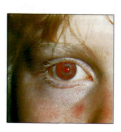
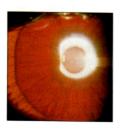

Marfan's syndrome

DEFINITION/OVERVIEW AND ETIOLOGY

This disorder was first described in France by A.B. Marfan in 1896.[16] He described a family with four affected individuals with dolichostenomelia (very long extremities and bones). It was recognized as a connective tissue disorder in 1979,[17] and the diagnostic criteria were published in 1996.[18] Although it is now known to result from a mutation in the fibrillin (FBN1) gene,[19] diagnosis remains clinical as this gene is large and most mutations are private. Fibrillin is a glycoprotein and is a major constituent of microfibrils and elastic fibers in the extracellular matrix.

The clinical diagnosis of Marfan's syndrome requires criteria in at least two major systems (skeletal, ocular, cardiovascular, dura, or family history) and also the involvement of a third system (which can be major or minor and can also include pulmonary and skin findings). Affected individuals tend to have tall stature with long, thin extremities with scoliosis being a common complication (**244**). Major skeletal findings may include pectus carinatum, pectus excavatum requiring surgery, reduced upper segment to lower segment ratio or arm span to height ratio of >1.05, wrist and thumb signs, scoliosis >20° degrees or spondylolistesis, elbow extension of <170°, pes planus, or protrusio acetabulae. Minor skeletal findings may include moderate pectus excavatum, joint hypermobility, a high arched palate with crowded teeth, and a characteristic facial appearance (dolichocephaly, malar hypoplasia, downslanting palpebral fissures, and enophthalmos). Ocular findings are discussed below. Cardiovascular findings may include a dilated ascending aorta, dissection of the ascending aorta, mitral valve prolapse, dilatation of the main pulmonary artery or descending aorta (which is unrelated to age), or calcification of the mitral annulus (which is also unrelated to age). Pulmonary findings that can be used to support the diagnosis include spontaneous pneumonthorax and/or apical blebs. Minor skin findings include striae atrophicae or recurrent and incisional hernias. Lumbosacral dural ectasia is considered a major criterion and a first-degree relative of the diagnosis.

The major cause of death is related to vascular complications and can occur at any age. The rate of cardiac complications has been reduced with the introduction of treatment with beta blockers. Health supervision guidelines have been established by the American Academy of Pediatrics.[19]

Marfan's syndrome is inherited in an autosomal dominant (AD) manner. The fibrillin gene is located on chromosome 15. Again, although the gene has been identified, diagnosis is usually based on specific diagnostic criteria.[18]

CLINICAL PRESENTATION

The most characteristic ocular feature of Marfan's syndrome is ectopia lentis (lens subluxation), which occurs in 60% of patients.[20] The FBN1 fibrillin gene on chromosome 15 is defective. Fibrillin is a major component in multiple parts of the eye, including the lens zonules and lens capsule. These structures give support to the lens and also maintain its position behind the pupil and in front of the vitreous. Fibrillin fibers in the zonules and lens capsule are abnormal, allowing for movement and subluxation of the lens.[21–23] The defective fibrillin is more prone to degradation by matrix metalloproteinases (MMPs) or proteolytic enzymes, which are present in the aqueous humor of the eye.[24] Subluxation of the lens most commonly occurs superiorly and posteriorly (**245**). As subluxation increases, the lens can position itself such that the bottom edge straddles the visual axis. This location is most disturbing to the patient because looking through the superior aspect of the pupil through the subluxed lens usually requires a high myopic astigmatic correction, whereas the inferior (or reading) part of the pupil with the missing lens requires a high hyperopic correction. This biphasic correction is impractical to achieve in glasses or contact lenses. Even at the early stages of lens subluxation, high degrees of myopia and astigmatism are produced.

Subluxation into the vitreous, the pupil or the anterior chamber is less likely to occur in children. If the lens subluxates into the pupil, pupillary block glaucoma can occur which constitutes an ocular emergency. As the lens subluxates, the iris starts to tremble (also known as iridodenesis). This is best observed at the slit-lamp. Atrophy of the dilator muscle of the iris can also occur, resulting in poor dilation.

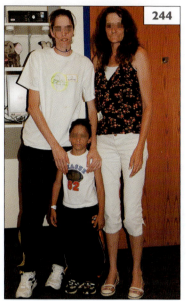

244 Family with Marfan's syndrome.

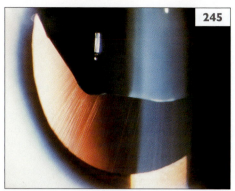

245 Ectopia lentis in Marfan's syndrome.

Microspherophakia, which is a lens that is shaped more spherically rather than the usual disc shape, occurs in 15% of patients. This condition results in high myopia. The cornea can be flat, larger than normal (megalocornea), or of normal diameter. Retinal detachment occurs more frequently and is thought to be secondary to an increased axial length; it can also occur following lens extraction.

MANAGEMENT/TREATMENT

Once a child has been identified as having Marfan's syndrome, it is essential that they have regular eye exams to detect any myopia or astigmatism. Without prompt and adequate correction of these refractive errors, amblyopia may develop. If vision is good with optical correction, then there is no need to rush surgery. Once the lens starts to subluxate into the visual axis, and proper optical correction is impossible, surgery should be considered.

Surgery is also necessary for anterior or posterior subluxation that is causing corneal damage, pupillary block glaucoma, or uveitis.

Recent advances in surgical techniques have decreased the complication rate and have achieved better surgical results. Kim *et al.* (2008) recently reported a series of 78 eyes using a microincision and an ocutome vitrectomy probe in order to remove a subluxed lens within the capsular bag.[25] Hydrodelineation was used to lessen surgical trauma to the zonules. This technique resulted in a very low rate of retinal detachment. Glasses and contact lenses were then used for visual rehabilitation. Several small studies have used intraocular lens implantation for visual rehabilitation in children.[26,27] Satisfactory results were obtained; however, the number of patients and the length of follow-up are too short to advocate this as the gold standard of care.

Homocystinuria

DEFINITION/OVERVIEW AND ETIOLOGY

Classic homocystinuria due to a deficiency of cystathionine beta synthase (CBS) was first described in 1962 by Carson and Neill.[28] Soon after the clinical entity was described, the biochemical defect was identified and the natural history of the disease was described.[29,30] The most easily recognized symptom, and often the only manifestation, is the ocular finding of ectopia lentis. Other clinical symptoms include lighter pigmentation than found with the rest of the family (i.e. hair, skin, irides) and a malar flush. Vascular instability is also a finding. Skeletal abnormalities including genu valgum, ankle vagus and pes planus, along with a tall, thin, 'marfanoid' habitus are also described. Arachnodactyly is rare. Platyspondyly, kyphoscoliosis, and compression fractures of the spine are also features of the disorder. Mental retardation is variable, depending on thromboses and vascular disease. Seizures may also be present and are probably also related to vascular accidents, as are psychiatric symptoms. Pyridoxine-responsive individuals have been identified and often have a somewhat milder clinical course.[31]

Homocystinuria is identified on expanded newborn screen as an elevated methionine level. Biochemical features include increased plasma homocysteine, homocystine, and methionine, increased urinary homocystine, and reduced CBS activity. CBS activity is tested in fibroblasts. Molecular genetic testing is available to identify mutations in the CBS gene. The disorder is inherited in an AR fashion. Management includes pyridoxine (vitamin B6) supplementation, a low protein/methionine diet, betaine treatment, and folate and B12 supplementation. The therapeutic goal is to keep plasma homocystine levels less than 11 µmol/L and to decrease plasma homocysteine levels. Aspirin therapy can also be used as an adjunct to prevent strokes.

Several other inborn errors of metabolism can present with homocystinuria. Methylene tetrahydrofolate reductase (MTHFR) deficiency and disorders of intracellular cobalamin metabolism have also been described. MTHFR deficiency was first described in 1972 and results from the inability to interconvert methylene tetrahydrofolate to methyl tetrahydrofolate.[32] Methyl tetrahydrofolate is necessary as a methyl donor for the conversion of homocysteine to methionine. Thus, plasma homocysteine is elevated while plasma methionine is decreased.

There is variability in symptoms and age of onset. The most common presentation in the pediatric population is developmental delay. Microcephaly is often noted. Neurologic involvement includes gait disturbances, seizures, and mental retardation. Ocular findings have not been described, and although subacute degeneration of the spinal cord has been described, it is not associated with megaloblastic anemia. Genetic testing is currently not available for MTHFR deficiency. It is inherited in an AR fashion.

Disorders of intracellular cobalamin metabolism have recently been described.[33,34] Several complementation groups have been identified. The most common of the disorders is cobalamin C deficiency; however, there are at least nine identified complementation groups which can be differentiated by biochemical phenotype. Complementation groups cblA, B, and D (variant 2) have the findings of methylmalonic acidemia/aciduria. cblC, D, and F have, in addition to methylmalonic acidemia/aciduria, hyperhomocysteinemia and homocystinuria. Complementation groups cblD (variant 1), E, and G have hyperhomocysteinemia and homocystinuria. All of these have low methionine, which differentiates them from CBS deficiency. Clinically, megaloblastic anemia is a defining feature. Other clinical findings include failure to thrive, mental retardation, seizures, behavioral problems, and psychiatric disturbances. Ophthalmic findings are seen in cblC, cblE, and cblG.

After the disorder is suspected, diagnostic testing includes urine organic acid analysis, plasma amino acid analysis, total homocysteine levels, urine homocystine levels, and plasma vitamin B12 levels. Genetic testing is available for CBS deficiency, cblC (MMACHC-methylmalonic aciduria and homocystinuria type C protein), cblE (MTRR-methionine synthase reductase) and cblG (MTR-methionine synthase). All are inherited in an AR fashion.

Treatment includes hydroxycobalamin injections, betaine, pyridoxine, folate or folinic acid, and methionine supplementation. Carnitine supplementation is used if methylmalonic acidemia is present. Dietary protein restriction is implemented, particularly for those with methylmalonic aciduria. Even with treatment, prognosis is poor, with most patients dying young or being severely handicapped.[33]

CLINICAL PRESENTATION

The hallmark ophthalmic feature of homocystinuria is lens dislocation or ectopia lentis. It is present in 90% of patients and has been detected as early as 3 years of age.[35] The zonules in patients with homocystinuria undergo degeneration.[36] Normal zonular structure maintains the suspended lens behind the iris and in front of the vitreous body. Abnormal zonules interrupt this suspension and predispose a lens to dislocation. Typically, it is bilateral and inferior. Dislocation anteriorly has been documented with rates of 18–50%.[37] Dislocation into the anterior chamber can traumatize the cornea and cause opacification and a bullous keratopathy. The most significant complication of anterior dislocation is pupillary block glaucoma, which is a true ophthalmic emergency. Pupillary block causes a sharp rise in the intraocular pressure (IOP), along with corneal edema and pain. If left untreated, the high pressure will cause central retinal artery occlusion, and eventual optic atrophy with visual acuity and field loss.

Iris atrophy has been reported and is likely secondary to iris ischemia from recurrent episodes of pupillary block glaucoma. Nonvisually significant cystoid retinal degeneration has been found, which worsened with age.[38] Anterior staphyloma, an extreme thinning of the cornea, is unusual, but has been reported both pre- and postoperatively.[39] Myopia is common.

The important ophthalmic feature associated with cblC, cblE and cblG is a pigmentary degenerative retinopathy that primarily affects the macula (central vision), resulting in poor vision and nystagmus. Systemic treatment appears to have little effect on the retinal disease.

MANAGEMENT/TREATMENT

Treatment falls into two main categories: preventative treatment and the treatment of ocular complications.

Preventative

The ophthalmic benefit of treatment with pyridoxine and/or a diet low in methionine and supplementation with cystine remains unclear. A clear-cut benefit without development of ectopia lentis was demonstrated in 14 patients treated over a mean follow-up of 8.2 years.[38] Other studies suggest that therapy may benefit pyridoxine responders, but showed no statistical benefit with pryridoxine unresponsive patients.

Cyloplegic refraction to detect and treat myopia is imperative. Early conservative prophylactic treatment methods (surgical or laser iridectomy) have failed to prevent lens dislocation into the anterior chamber.[37]

Ocular complications

Once dislocation of the lens into the anterior chamber has occurred, surgical treatment is necessary. Nonsurgical lens manipulation with pupillary dilatation, manual lens repositioning, and pupillary constriction fails in the long term. With newer microinstrumentation, lensectomies are safer with lower complication rates. The risk of postoperative retinal detachment has declined with newer microsurgical techniques. Prophylaxis for thromboembolic events should always be considered with general anesthesia. Most patients are visually rehabilitated with spectacle correction. If the child's mental capacity and dexterity are good, contact lenses can be considered.

Wilson's disease

DEFINITION/OVERVIEW AND ETIOLOGY

Although Kayser and Fleischer first described the corneal ring associated with Wilson's disease in 1902 and 1903,[40,41] Wilson published what is considered to be the landmark clinical description of the disease in 1912.[42] Wilson's disease is now known to be a disorder of copper transport caused by mutations in the P-type ATPase transporter that is specific to the liver.[43] This copper transporter functions in the liver and regulates copper excretion into the bile. If its function is impaired, copper cannot be incorporated into ceruloplasmin and thus accumulates in the liver, cornea, and brain.

Clinically, affected individuals have a highly variable presentation[44] with an asymptomatic period. During this time, hepatic copper deposition is occurring. Children can present with hepatic disease, even though presentation can be either hepatic or neurologic. Although it can also present as an acute hemolytic crisis in infants and young children, it more typically presents between the ages of 8 and 16 years with hepatic dysfunction. Neurologic presentation can be dystonia with rigidity, tremors, and contractures, pseudosclerotic with tremors, or psychiatric with intellectual deterioration and behavioral changes.[45]

Diagnosis relies on demonstration of copper levels in liver biopsy samples, elevated serum nonceruloplasmin-bound copper levels, and decreased serum ceruloplasmin levels. Measurement of 24-hour urinary copper can also be helpful.[46] Wilson's disease is inherited in an AR fashion and results from a defect in biliary copper excretion related to mutations in the ATP7B gene. Molecular genetic testing is available. Treatment revolves around removing excess copper from the system,[46] using penicillamine, trientine and zinc. Fulminant liver failure is treated by transplantation; however, chelation therapy must be continued afterwards in order to avoid liver failure of the transplanted liver. Because prognosis is good if treatment is initiated early, there is a current push for the inclusion of this disorder on all expanded newborn screening panels.

CLINICAL PRESENTATION

The Kayser–Fleischer ring, found in 95% of patients, is the most important ophthalmic feature of Wilson's disease (**246**). It is a deposition of copper and sulfur-rich granules in the Descemet's membrane of the peripheral cornea that appear as gold or gray-brown opacities. It appears first in the superior peripheral cornea and spreads horizontally, eventually spreading inferiorly. The width and density increase as the disease progresses and the severity of the disease correlates with the density of the ring. There are no visual aberrations produced from its presence. It is not pathognomonic of the disease, and it can be seen with intraocular copper foreign bodies and also in liver diseases such as hepatitis and cirrhosis.

A sunflower cataract can develop. This cataract develops in the anterior capsule of the lens and is likened to a sunflower with a spherical center and satellite extensions. Oculomotor problems with saccadic pursuit movements and losses of accommodation and near responses have been described.[22]

MANAGEMENT/TREATMENT

No treatment is needed for the corneal deposits; however, these tend to fade with chelation therapy. Successful liver transplantation has also resulted in the fading and disappearance of the Kayser–Fleischer ring. Cataract surgery is rarely needed for the sunflower cataract.

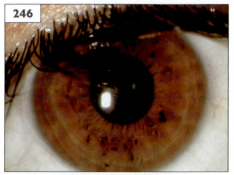

246 Wilson's disease. Kayser-Fleischer ring in a child. (From Strobel S et al. Paediatrics and Child Health – The Great Ormond Street Colour Handbook, Manson Publishing.)

Fabry disease

DEFINITION/OVERVIEW AND ETIOLOGY

Fabry disease is an inborn error of metabolism that results from a deficiency of ceramide trihexosidase (α-galactosidase A) and leads to an accumulation of glycosphingolipids. The disease was first described independently by two dermatologists: Anderson in England and Fabry in Germany.[47,48] Nonocular cardinal features of this disorder are episodic pain (particularly of the extremities), angiokeratomas of the skin, hypohydrosis, postprandial pain, and diarrhea. Due to the enzymatic defect, renal disease, along with coronary and cerebral vascular disease, typically develops over time. Intermittent and burning pain, often beginning in the first decade, is the primary complaint. Pain crises tend to be self-limited, although they can last from days to weeks. Recurrent fevers may also be present. Dark red punctate skin lesions, which microscopically are found to be angiokeratomas, appear at puberty and are commonly seen in a 'swim trunk' distribution, especially on the scrotum and buttocks. The disease is inherited in an X-linked fashion, but due to random X inactivation, carrier females may also be symptomatic. In one study, up to 70% of carrier females described pain episodes.[49] Enzyme replacement therapy with α-galactosidase is available and has helped to reverse storage of glycosphingolipids in lysosomes and alleviate some of the symptoms.[50] Renal failure is a long-term consequence of the disease. Transplantation cures the kidney disease, but does not affect accumulation of glycosphingolipids in other tissues. Molecular analyses of the GLA gene are clinically available to confirm the diagnosis after deficient enzyme activity is identified. Since heterozygous females may have normal levels of enzyme activity, this is the most reliable method of determining carrier status in females.

CLINICAL PRESENTATION AND MANAGEMENT/TREATMENT

Eye findings related to Fabry disease are subtle and rarely affect the vision. The most well known are cornea verticulatta, which are bilateral whirl-like opacities that are located in the inferior cornea. Their colors range from white to golden brown and they do not affect the vision. Although these deposits have been identified at as early as 3 years of age, there is no correlation with the progression of the disease, the deterioration of renal function, or the increase in cardiac size.[51] They bear some resemblance to the lesions produced by the systemic administration of chloroquines, indomethacin, and amiodarone.[22] This ocular finding may be seen in isolation and, therefore, is a reliable marker of the disease.

Tortuosity with aneurysmal dilatations of the conjunctival vessels, as well as retinovascular tortuosity, is also seen in Fabry disease. This tortuosity does have positive predictive value for the severity of the systemic disease. It usually does not occur in isolation, and therefore by itself is not diagnostic of Fabry. Cataracts were shown to be present in 9.8% of females and 23.1% of males in the European database for Fabry disease.[51] They are typically diagnosed before 10 years of age and have two distinct forms. One has a whirl-like appearance in the subcapsular level of the lens, while the other presents as multiple minute dots along the nuclear suture lines.[22] Both forms usually do not impair vision; slit-lamp examination is needed for visualization.

Treatment is not needed for the corneal, lenticular, conjunctival or retinal disease.

Osteogenesis imperfecta

DEFINITION/OVERVIEW AND ETIOLOGY

Osteogenesis imperfecta (OI) is a disorder of collagen synthesis.[52] The descriptive term 'osteogenesis imperfecta' was introduced in 1849 by Vrolik in his *Handbook of Pathological Anatomy*.[52] Because there are no specific diagnostic criteria for OI as are available for other connective tissue disorders, such as Marfan's syndrome or Ehlers–Danlos syndrome, a classification scheme of type I–IV was introduced in 1979.[53] This scheme, along with the identification of different bony disorders with similar clinical findings, has been widely accepted and modified. The diagnosis is dependent upon clinical presentations which include: fractures with minimal or no trauma, short stature often associated with bony deformities, blue to gray tinged sclerae, progressive hearing loss (usually after puberty), ligamentous laxity, and dentinogenesis imperfecta (which can also be seen as an independent entity not associated with OI). There can be phenotypic variability within and between families.

Types I–IV are all related to mutations in either the COL1A1 or COL1A2 genes which code for type 1 collagen. The less severe forms tend to result from mutations that result in premature chain termination or decreased chain production. This causes normal, albeit fewer, collagen fibers to be formed. The moderate and severe types are more likely to be caused by structural defects in the type I collagen, resulting in abnormal collagen molecules. The genes involved in types V and VI have not yet been identified. Type VII is caused by a mutation in the cartilage-associated protein gene, the function of which is required for prolyl 3-hydroxylation of collagens I and II. Type VIII is caused by a mutation in the leprecan protein, which is another collagen prolyl hydroxylase that is required for proper collagen biosynthesis folding and assembly.

After the diagnosis is suspected, confirmation can be done by either molecular analysis or collagen studies in fibroblasts. Mutation analysis can be quite sensitive if the diagnosis is highly suspected. Collagen studies in fibroblasts remain the gold standard of diagnosis. If no biosynthesis abnormalities or mutations are identified, then urinary collagen N-telopeptide excretion can be helpful, especially in the diagnosis of OI V.

Treatment of OI tends to be supportive. The ultimate goal is to minimize fractures and maximize function using a combination of physical therapy and orthopedic interventions. Dental surveillance is also important. Conductive hearing loss is usually related to fracture of the bones in the middle ear. With age, sensorineural hearing loss becomes apparent and is not amenable to surgery. Cochlear implantation has been performed in a limited number of patients.[54] The introduction of bisphosphonates has been heralded as a promising therapy. Some symptomatic improvements have been reported with the use of IV pamidronate, although there is a paucity of randomized, placebo-controlled clinical trials. More recently, oral alendronate has shown promising results and is quickly becoming the gold standard of care.[55] Growth hormone has been used to improve linear growth and bone formation.

CLINICAL PRESENTATION

Blue sclera is a well known clinical finding of OI (**247**). Chan *et al*. (1982) found the thickness of collagen fibers to be reduced by 25% in the cornea and 50% in the sclera.[56] They also demonstrated a lack of the typical cross striations found in these fibers. These abnormalities make the sclera near translucent and allow the underlying uveal pigment to become more clinically visible, resulting in a blue/gray appearance of the sclera. The region of sclera adjacent to the cornea often maintains a whiter appearance and is commonly referred to as a 'Saturn's ring'. Individuals affected with OI type I maintain this blue intensity throughout life, but those with types III and IV show a marked fading, typically resulting in a normal appearing sclera by adolescence and adult life.[57] This scleral abnormality does not impact on the vision; however, it does lower ocular rigidity and therefore renders the eye more susceptible to minor trauma.

Corneal thickness is reduced, which also increases the risk of injury with minor trauma. The thickness of the cornea negatively correlates with the blueness of the sclera.[58] This corneal thickness can artificially lower the IOP. Retinal hemorrhages and subdural hematomas secondary to minor trauma were found during routine work-ups for shaken baby syndrome.[59] Additional ocular findings include myopia, glaucoma, and kerataconus.

MANAGEMENT/TREATMENT

The most important role of the ophthalmologist in caring for children with OI is that of prevention. The decreased ocular rigidity and decreased corneal thickness make these children more susceptible to major eye injuries from minor trauma. Protective eyewear should be prescribed for all children that are not bed-bound. Once an injury has occurred, the ophthalmologist must be aware that repair by conventional means is not always possible; corneal grafting and scleral patching may be necessary. Pirouzian *et al.* (2007) reported a case of scleral perforation secondary to chronic rubbing that required a scleral patch.[60]

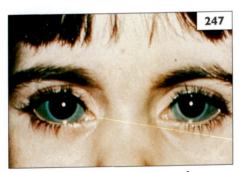

247 Blue sclera in osteogenesis imperfecta.

The mucopoly-saccharidoses

DEFINITION/OVERVIEW AND ETIOLOGY

The mucopolysaccharidoses (MPSs) are a diverse group of disorders which, due to different enzymatic defects, result in the inability to break down glycosaminoglycans (GAGs).[61,62] For the most part, affected individuals will appear normal at birth with progressive physical changes slowly becoming apparent. To date, six different MPSs have been identified including MPS I (Hurler syndrome) (**248**), MPS II (Hunter syndrome), MPS III (Sanfilippo A syndrome), MPS IV (Morquio syndrome), MPS VI (Maroteaux–Lamy syndrome), and MPS VII (Sly syndrome) (*Table 15, see page 206*).

The clinical presentation of MPS I ranges from a severe form (with the onset of clinical findings in the first year of life) to an adult variant (formerly called Scheie's disease). Most have recurrent otitis media, sinusitis, and pharyngitis starting in the first year of life. Developmental delays are common. Over time, coarse facial features, along with thickening of the skin, macrocephaly, corneal clouding, and bony abnormalities (especially gibbus deformity, kyphosis, or scoliosis) also become more apparent. Hepatosplenomegaly is a common finding. Dysostosis multiplex becomes apparent on radiologic examination (large skull, deep elongated sella, hook-shaped lower thoracic and lumbar vertebrae, pelvic dysplasia, and shortened tubular bones). Cardiac valve involvement is common. Although all of the MPSs involve some coarsening of facial features, it is important to remember that there are some distinctions. For example, patients with milder forms of MPS I, MPS II, MPS IV, and MPS VI can have normal or near normal intelligence. In fact, both MPS IV (Morquio) and MPS VI (Maroteaux–Lamy) may have very little CNS involvement. MPS III (Sanfilippo A), on the other hand, can have severe behavioral issues and hearing loss as its major presenting features.

Biochemically, all forms have excessive urinary excretion of quantitative mucopolysaccharides. The pattern of mucopolysaccharide excretion depends on the disorder and the affected enzyme. Molecular analyses are not necessary to make the diagnosis; however, they can be helpful in confirming the diagnosis and useful for prenatal diagnosis, if desired. All of the mucopolysaccharidoses, with the exception of MPS II (Hunter), are inherited in an AR fashion; MPS II is an X-linked trait.

In the past, the only treatment for the MPSs was supportive. With the identification of the enzymatic defect and the subsequent technology to produce the enzyme that can be targeted to the appropriate intracellular compartment (the lysosome), enzyme replacement therapy has now become available for several of these disorders.[63] MPS I (Hurler) is initially treated with enzyme replacement therapy (Aldurazyme) followed by bone marrow transplantation. There is evidence that bone marrow transplantation helps to slow the course of the disease[64] and may even have a positive CNS effect;[65] however, bone marrow transplantation has not been shown to be effective for any of the other MPSs. Enzyme replacement therapy is now available for MPS II (Elaprase) and MPS VI (Naglazyme). Both have been shown to improve quality of life by decreasing liver and spleen size and increasing exercise tolerance. Enzyme replacement therapy is still in the experimental stages for MPS III (Sanfilippo A).

CLINICAL PRESENTATION

This heterogeneous group is characterized by a spectrum of ophthalmic findings, including corneal clouding, pigmentary retinopathy, glaucoma, chronic papilledema, and optic atrophy.

Corneal clouding is the most common feature for which an ophthalmic consultation is sought. It results from an accumulation of GAGs (both intra- and extracellular) in the cornea with subsequent disruption of the optically important arrangement of collagen fibrils. These fibrils are essential for clear vision. It appears early in life and continues to progress. This finding is best documented in MPS I (Hurler).

The pigmentary retinopathy that occurs is also felt to be secondary to the accumulation of GAGs in the retinal pigment. This retinal dysfunction is progressive and can lead to an extinguished electroretinogram (ERG) and blindness as early as 5 years of age.

MPS IV (Morqui

A: N-acetyl-gala
6-sulfatase
B: β-galactosida

Keratan sulfate

A: GALNS (yes
B: GLB1 (yes)

Autosomal r

Corneal clou

Decreased
enzyme ac
Disproport
joint contr
kyphoscol

Supporti

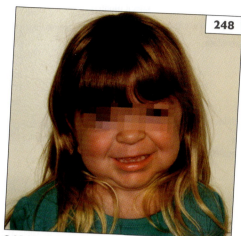

248 Hurler's syndrome.

Glaucoma and ocular hypertension can occur due to GAG accumulation within the anterior chamber structures and lead to outflow difficulties. A correlation has been shown between increased corneal thickness and IOP in patients with MPS I (Hurler) following bone marrow transplantation.[66] Increased corneal thickness can give an erroneously high intraocular reading and lead to a misdiagnosis of glaucoma. Special attention needs to be paid to all diagnostic features of glaucoma, including optic disc appearance, before starting antiglaucoma medications.

In a study of 108 patients with all types of MPS, optic nerve head swelling (chronic papilledema) was found in each type, with the exception of MPS I (Hurler).[67] This is thought to be secondary to the compression of the optic nerve by a posterior sclera thickened by the accumulation of GAGs.[22] Chronic papilledema eventually leads to optic atrophy and vision loss. Amblyopia and strabismus occur more frequently in patients with MPS than in the average population.

MANAGEMENT/TREATMENT

Enzyme replacement therapy does not appear either to significantly improve or to worsen the ocular complications of patients with MPS I (Hurler).[68] The long-term benefit of bone marrow transplantation on the evolution of ophthalmic manifestations remains controversial. If bone marrow transplantation is performed, then secondary complications such as cataracts or ocular hypertension can occur. Corneal grafting can be considered in children with MPS I (Hurler), and even though it has been associated with good outcomes, it should be approached cautiously because of the high rejection rate among children.

Table 1

Name

Enzyme

MPS

Gene
testi

Inhe

Ocu

Cl

Sickle cell disease

DEFINITION/OVERVIEW AND ETIOLOGY

Sickle cell disease was first described by James Herrick in 1910 when he found that one of his patients from the West Indies had an anemia with sickle-shaped red blood cells.[69] Sickle cell has the distinction of being the first genetic disease to be molecularly characterized, after the discovery that it was caused by a point mutation in the beta globin gene that alters the protein structure so that low oxygen concentrations lead to sickling. It is also one of the first genetic disorders to be used as an example of a heterozygote advantage, as having one copy of the hemoglobin S gene along with one copy of the normal beta hemoglobin gene (sickle cell trait) confers relative resistance to infection by malaria.[70] Sickle cell disease originally denoted homozygosity for hemoglobin S (HbSS), which accounts for the majority of sickle cell disease in the US. Subsequently, several other forms of sickle cell disease have been described, all of which involve inheritance of the Hb S gene with another abnormal copy of the beta globin gene.[71] These other forms are known as sickle-hemoglobin C disease (HbSC), HbSb+-thalassemia, HbSb°-thalassemia, HbSD-Punjab, and HbSO-Arab.

Clinically, the onset of symptoms is in childhood. Severe anemia, caused by sickling of the red blood cells with subsequent hemolysis, leads to shortness of breath, fatigue, and jaundice. Poor growth and development can also result from recurrent attacks. Pain crises result from oxygen deprivation to tissues and organs. These episodes occur when the stiff and sickled red blood cells cannot move easily through the capillaries. These episodes not only cause pain, but can also result in organ damage. The lungs, spleen, kidneys, and brain are particularly susceptible to damage. Pulmonary hypertension as a result of oxygen deprivation has been determined to be a cause of heart failure in about one-third of affected adults.[72] This diagnosis is often suspected after the presentation of dactylitis. Pallor, jaundice, pneumococcal sepsis and/or meningitis, splenomegaly with severe anemia, and acute chest syndrome are also clinical conditions that would lead toward suspecting this diagnosis.

Since the sequelae of sickle cell disease can be so dramatic and incapacitating, screening for this disease is usually performed at birth. Both newborn screening and confirmatory testing use isoelectric focusing or hemoglobin electrophoresis to demonstrate the presence of aberrant beta globin chains. This can also be done with high-performance liquid chromatography. Mutation analyses or complete gene sequencing (especially in cases with the b-thalassemia variants) can also be used to confirm the diagnosis.

Sickle cell anemia is inherited in an AR fashion. The disease can result from either homozygosity for hemoglobin S or from compound heterozygosity with the hemoglobin S gene and other abnormal beta hemoglobin genes. The most common forms are HbSS, HbSC, and sickle beta thalassemia (HbSb+-thalassemia, HbSb°-thalassemia).

Treatment for sickle cell disease is mostly supportive during acute crises and includes hydration, analgesics, oxygen, antibiotics, and transfusions.[73] Immunization with the pneumococcal vaccine is very important since splenic sequestration often leads to autosplenectomy and increased susceptibility to infection with pyogenic bacteria. Treatment with hydroxyurea can improve survival and also result in fewer symptomatic pain crises and a decreased need for transfusions. Bone marrow transplantation, although not the standard of care, has been shown to be curative.[74]

CLINICAL PRESENTATION

Patients with homozygous sickle cell anemia (SS) generally exhibit more severe systemic complications of the disease than patients with SC or S-Thal disease. The converse is true for ocular manifestations. Ocular disease results from intravascular sickling and thrombosis with the retina being primarily affected. Retinal vascular changes can be divided into nonproliferative (non-PSR) and proliferative (PSR). Major vision loss is usually the result of vitreous hemorrhage or retinal detachment, both of which are consequences of PSR. Although uncommon, PSR does occur in adolescents and it should be considered in their medical care.[75]

Changes of non-PSR include venous tortuosity and salmon patch hemorrhage, an intraretinal hematoma from sickled erythrocyte occlusion of arterioles and a subsequent blow-out of the vessel wall. It is found in the mid-periphery of the retina and undergoes a color change from bright red to orange, and then finally salmon. Black sunburst is a pigmented, chorioretinal scar in the peripheral retina; it is secondary to scarring from a previous hemorrhage. Finally, angioid streaks, pigmented striae representing breaks in Bruch's membrane of the retina, are found in non-PSR.

PSR is secondary to repeated episodes of ischemia from peripheral arterial occlusions, which then give rise to neovascularization. Neovascularization commonly occurs in the peripheral retina, but can also be seen on the optic disc. The five stages of change are:

- Stage 1: a graying appearance to the retina (retinal ischemia), which is secondary to peripheral arterial occlusion.
- Stage 2: arteriolar–venular anastomsis.
- Stage 3: neovascular fronds grow on the retinal surface. They resemble a marine invertebrate, hence their name 'sea fan neovascularization'.
- Stage 4: vitreous hemorrhage caused by neovascular traction on the retinal vessels.
- Stage 5: retinal detachment. This usually occurs as a result of traction from the neovascular tufts. Retinal ischemia can also cause retinal thinning, hole formation, and subsequent retinal detachment.

Other changes that occur are:

- Conjunctiva vessel tortuosity, which conveys a comma-shaped appearance to the capillaries.
- Iris atrophy.
- Branch and central retinal artery occlusion.
- Pseudotumor cerebri has been reported [76] and should be suspected in sickle cell patients who present with severe headaches that are unexplained by their disease.

MANAGEMENT/TREATMENT

Monitoring for changes with sickle cell disease should start by 10 years of age. A complete peripheral fundus examination is imperative. Fluorescein angiography may be necessary to delineate the early stages of the disease. Once PSR has been identified, laser photocoagulation helps stop the complications of vitreous hemorrhage and the subsequent retinal detachment. Laser photocoagulation does not, however, stop the progression of new PSR, so careful monitoring is imperative.

The presence of sickle cell hemo-globinopathies, including sickle cell trait, is a significant risk factor for complications associated with traumatic hyphema.[77] Increased IOP occurs secondary to obstruction of the aqueous outflow by the sickled erythrocytes. If uncontrolled, it can lead to central retinal artery occlusion, and optic atrophy. Re-bleeds also occur more frequently. Surgical intervention or topical antifibrinolytic therapy with aminocaproic acid may be necessary.

Albinism

DEFINITION/OVERVIEW AND ETIOLOGY

There are several genetic conditions that result in the phenotype of oculocutaneous albinism (*Table 16, see page 212*). All of these conditions affect pigmentation of the hair, skin, and eyes (**249**). Genetically, there is variability in the amount of residual pigment formed by melanocytes, which can be used to distinguish the different syndromes;[78] these result from mutations that affect the formation of the pigment. Hermansky–Pudlak syndrome[79] and Chediak–Higashi syndrome[80] result from defective intracellular organelle formation and lysosomal trafficking, respectively. These lead to abnormal pigment production. A number of different genes are involved and all conditions are inherited in an AR manner.

The management of these disorders revolves around sun avoidance, skin protection, and routine ophthalmologic care. Hermansky–Pudlak syndrome has an associated bleeding dyscrasia because of platelet dysfunction. Desmopressin has been used, as has vitamin E. Chediak–Higashi syndrome is generally fatal, and without bone marrow transplantation, death will usually occur before the age of 7 years. This is related to increased susceptibility to infection and malignant lymphoma. Although bone marrow transplantation improves survival by decreasing the frequency and severity of infection, it does not prevent progression of neurologic symptoms.[81]

CLINICAL PRESENTATION

Visual acuity and nystagmus vary according to the type of albinism. The spectrum ranges from poor vision (worse than 20/200) in the tyrosinase-negative albino to minimally impaired (20/40–20/60) in brown albinos. In the past, the degree of visual impairment was thought to correlate with the amount of pigment in the eye. However, recent studies have shown that diminished vision is more closely related to the severity of the foveal hypoplasia.[82] Nystagmus is present within the first few months of age and its severity is also dependent upon the type of albinism, ranging from severe to observable only at the slit-lamp. It usually begins with a pendular form that changes to a jerk form as fixation improves.

Both foveal hypoplasia and nystagmus contribute to these children's visual impairment.

Foveal hypoplasia is always present. Clinically, it is identified by the absence of the foveal pit, absence of the macula lutea pigment, absence of the normal hyperpigmentation of the foveal pigment epithelium, and failure of the retinal vasculature to wreath the fovea. Grading of the fovea with optical coherence tomography (OCT) has provided better predictive values for vision than iris transillumination and macular transparency.[82] Multifocal ERG has shown results suggesting a homogeneous density of cone photoreceptors across the central retina consistent with anatomic studies showing arrest of postnatal macular development.[83]

Hypopigmentation of the fundus varies with the type of albinism and the race of the child (**250**). At the extreme end, complete choroidal vasculature is visible because of the absence of retinal pigment. Less affected patients will have minimal retinal pigment dilution.

Transillumination of the iris occurs in all forms of albinism, but varies in degree (**251, 252**). In tyrosinase-negative albinos, the iris trans-illumination can be visualized by applying a light source to the lower lid, which will produce the classic 'pink eyed' appearance. With lesser degrees of iris transillumination, examination at the slit-lamp will be necessary. Iris transillumination is often the only identifiable feature that aids in the diagnosis of albinism in children with nystagmus and minimally decreased hair and skin pigment. The color of the iris varies from pale blue to brown. Photophobia is typically present and secondary to the iris hypopigmentation.

Visual pathway abnormalities are also known to occur. There is misrouting of temporal axons to the contralateral visual cortex, secondary to reduced melanin biosynthesis. The normal ratio of crossed to uncrossed fibers is 53:47.[84] Patients with albinism have fibers of 20% or more originating from the temporal retina-crossing at the chiasm that project to the contralateral hemisphere. This hemispheric asymmetry becomes evident in monocular visually evoked cortical potentials (VECPs) and, if the typical clinical features are lacking, can help in the diagnosis of albinism.

Binocular vision is reduced. Guo *et al.* (1989) proposed that the abnormal decussation of the optic nerve fibers may be the cause of this reduction.[84] Because albinos have reduced

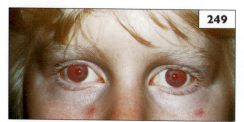

249 Albinism.

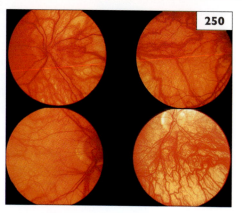

250 Hypopigmentation of the fundus in albinism.

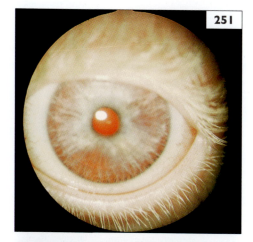

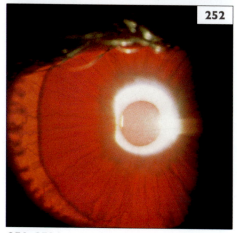

251, 252 Iris transillumination defects in albinism.

Table 16 Albinism

Name	Oculocutaneous albinism Type1A Tyrosinase-related oculocutaneous albinism [Tyrosinase-negative oculocutaneous albinism]	Oculocutaneous albinism Type 1B Tyrosinase-related oculocutaneous albinism [Oculocutaneous albinism Type 1B Yellow cutaneous albinism Temperature-sensitive OCA Minimal pigment oculocutaneous albinism]	Oculocutaneous albinism Type 2 Brown OCA May be seen with deletion forms of Prader–Willi and Angelman sydromes	Oculocutaneous albinism Type 3 [Rufous oculocutaneous albinism]
Ocular findings	Iris markedly transilluminates Retinal pigment absent Vision >20/200	Iris transillumination gradually improves Retinal pigment decreased/improves Vision = 20/30–20/400	Iris transillumination can improve Retinal pigment decreased may improve Vision = 20/30–20/400	Iris transillumination mild reduction Retinal pigment normal Vision = 20/60–20/400
Clinical findings	White hair White skin that does not tan	White or light yellow hair at birth that darkens with age White skin that develops some generalized pigment that may tan with sun exposure	Pigmented hair at birth No tanning but may develop nevi or freckling Increased risk of skin cancer	Affects those of darker skin Pigment is present but decreased
Gene	TYR (tyrosinase completely inactive)	TYR (tyrosinase partially active)	OCA2/P (P protein)	TYRP1 (tyrosinase-related protein 1)

Oculocutaneous albinism Type 4	X-linked ocular albinism	Hermansky–Pudlak syndrome	Chediak-Higashi
Iris transillumination very variable Retinal pigment variable Vision = normal to 20/400	Iris transillumination mild reduction Retinal pigmentation reduced Vision = 20/40–20/400	Iris transillumination mild Retinal pigmentation mild reduction Vision = 20/30–20/400	Iris transillumination present Retinal pigmentation reduced Vision = 20/30–20/400
At birth, hair color ranges from silvery white to light yellow More common in Japanese population Hypopigmentation of skin Increased risk of skin cancer	Absence of clinically systemic involvement No skin or hair hypopigmentation Affected males may be more lightly pigmented than unaffected siblings	Skin and hair hypopigmentation Bleeding diathesis (platelet deficiency) easy bruising, frequent epistaxis, gingival bleeding, postpartum hemorrhage, colonic bleeding, prolonged bleeding with menses or after tooth extraction, circumcision, and other surgeries Pulmonary fibrosis Granulomatous colitis Cardiomegaly Renal failure	Nonpigmented skin (patchy distribution, blonde hair, blue eyes) Abnormal gait, clumsiness, seizures, paresthesia, mental retardation, and peripheral neuropathy Recurrent skin pyodermic skin infections, enterocolitis
MATP (membrane-associated transporter protein)	GPR143 (G-protein coupled receptor 143)	8 genes HPS1 (Hermansky–Pudlak syndrome 1 protein) AP3B1 (AP-3 complex subunit beta-1) HPS3 (Hermansky–Pudlak syndrome 3 protein)	CHS1 (LYST)

Continued overleaf

Table 16 Albinism (*continued*)

Name	Oculocutaneous albinism Type1A	Oculocutaneous albinism Type 1B	Oculocutaneous albinism Type 2	Oculocutaneous albinism Type 3
Gene (*continued*)				
Inheritance	Autosomal recessive	Autosomal recessive	Autosomal recessive	Autosomal recessive
Molecular testing available?	Yes	Yes	Yes	Yes

stereopsis and binocular vision, which primarily provide a feedback signal that helps establish and maintain proper alignment, strabismus is common with an overall prevalence of 40%.

High refractive errors are common with myopia, hyperopia, and astigmatism being described.

Torticollis or anomalous head positions (AHPs) occurs. Children adopt these head positions to facilitate their null point (the position of gaze with the least nystagmus and best visual acuity). Children with albinism have relatively normal neurodevelopmental behavior and academic performance, regardless of the degree of visual impairment; however, they did have a higher prevalence of attention deficit hyperactivity disorder (ADHD) in one study.[85]

MANAGEMENT/TREATMENT

Typically, infants are directed to the ophthalmologist when nystagmus is noted and vision is not age appropriate. The diagnosis can be quite obvious if the child's skin and hair are hypopigmented, while at other times iris transillumination needs to be confirmed at the slit-lamp. Occasionally, a VECP is necessary to establish the diagnosis. Genetic referral is appropriate for the benefit of the child and the parents. Spectacle correction of high refractive errors is also appropriate and has been proven to improve visual acuity as well as binocular alignment and torticollis.[86] Separate sunglasses or photochromic lenses will help the photophobia.

Oculocutaneous albinism Type 4	X-linked ocular albinism	Hermansky–Pudlak syndrome	Chediak-Higashi
		HPS4 (Hermansky–Pudlak syndrome 4 protein) HPS5 (Hermansky–Pudlak syndrome 5 protein) HPS6 (Hermansky–Pudlak syndrome 6 protein) DTNBP1 (Dysbindin) BLOC1S3 (Biogenesis of lysosome-related organelles complex-1 subunit 3)	
Autosomal recessive	X-linked	Autosomal recessive	Autosomal recessive
Yes	Yes	Currently available for HPS1, HPS3, HPS4	No

Surgical correction of strabismus should be undertaken. Previous investigations have confirmed the efficacy of horizontal muscle recession, resections, or both (Anderson–Kestenbaum procedure), to treat the anomalous head positions produced by nystagmus.[87] Four-muscle horizontal tenotomy has also been shown to improve nystagmus waveforms and broaden the range of gaze angles, or null points.[88,89] These studies have led to more recent investigations which have shown the benefit of combining tenotomies with nystagmus or strabismus recession procedures.[90] Although these studies have focused primarily on infantile nystagmus, the benefits can be extrapolated to albinos with nystagmus.

Finally, the role of the pediatrician and ophthalmologist in directing the parents to seek help in school is very important. Albinos typically have average intelligence; however, their ability to learn may be hampered by their visual disability. An individual education plan will identify each child's needs and provide them with special services to help them succeed.

Congenital rubella

DEFINITION/OVERVIEW AND ETIOLOGY

Since the introduction of the vaccine, rubella is rare in the US. It does, however, remain a major cause of blindness in developing countries. Transplacental infection occurs during the viremic phase in the mother. The incidence of congenital infection is dependent on the month of gestation of the viremia.[91] The diagnosis is confirmed by the presence of IgM antibodies in the cord blood. *Table 17* presents the incidence and rate of infection with gestational age.

Systemic manifestations include:

- Hearing loss.
- Intrauterine growth retardation.
- Heart disease.
- Microcephaly.
- Mental retardation.
- Hepatitis/hepatomegaly.

CLINICAL PRESENTATION OF OPHTHALMOLOGIC MANIFESTATIONS

Microcornea or microphthalmia occurs in 10% of affected individuals. Bilateral cataract formation is the most visually significant complication and, if left untreated, leads to amblyopia. A 'salt and pepper' retinopathy is the classic retinal finding; its effect on vision is variable. Glaucoma is present in less than 10% of cases. The mechanism of glaucoma is multiple, including malformation of the aqueous outflow, chronic uveitis, or postcataract surgery. Keratoconus, chronic uveitis, iris coloboma, persistant pupillary membrane, and anisocoria have all been reported. Nystagmus may develop secondary to the amblyopia from the presence of a cataract. Strabismus commonly occurs after cataract surgery.

MANAGEMENT/TREATMENT

Prevention, with the use of the RA-27 vaccine, is the mainstay. If cataracts are present, early lensectomies and visual rehabilitation with aphakic spectacles or contact lenses is appropriate. With early surgery, even in the presence of nystagmus and retinopathy, visual outcome can be as good as 20/60.

Table 17 Incidence and rate of congenital rubella infection with gestational age

Gestational age at time of viremia	Risk of developing congenital infection (%)	Risk of developing a congenital defect if an infection occurs (%)
1–11 weeks	90	100
11–20 weeks	50	30
20–35 weeks	37	None
35+ weeks	100	None

Oculoneurocutaneous syndromes ('phakomatoses')

Jerry A. Shields, MD and Carol L. Shields, MD

- **Introduction**
  Genetics
  Malignant potential
  Formes frustes

- **Tuberous sclerosis complex (Bourneville's syndrome)**

- **Neurofibromatosis (von Recklinghausen's syndrome)**

- **Retinocerebellar hemangioblastomatosis (von Hippel–Lindau syndrome)**

- **Racemose hemangiomatosis (Wyburn-Mason syndrome)**

- **Encephalofacial cavernous hemangiomatosis (Sturge–Weber syndrome)**

- **Oculoneurocutaneous cavernous hemangiomatosis**

- **Organoid nevus syndrome**

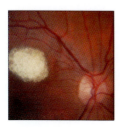
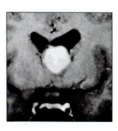

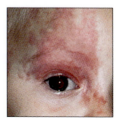

Introduction

The oculoneurocutaneous syndromes (ONCS) are a group of disorders characterized by systemic hamartomas and/or choristomas of the eye, brain, skin, and sometimes the viscera.[1–38] The term 'phakomatoses', previously used to designate these entities, is nonspecific and is used less often in the literature. As a result, we have chosen to group these entities under the rubric ONCS, which more accurately reflects their true nature. However, we realize that other terminology may be adopted in the future when the genetics of these conditions is better understood. The syndromes described include tuberous sclerosis complex (TSC), neurofibromatosis (NF), von Hippel–Lindau (VHL) syndrome, Sturge–Weber (SW) syndrome, Wyburn-Mason (WM) syndrome, oculoneurocutaneous cavernous hemangiomatosis, and organoid nevus syndrome. This chapter covers these syndromes with emphasis on their ocular manifestations. The authors also discuss and illustrate the clinical and histopathologic features of these syndromes in more detail in recent textbooks.[1–3]

Genetics

Most of the ONCS have an autosomal dominant (AD) mode of inheritance, often with incomplete penetrance. Specific chromosomal abnormalities are continually being recognized in association with these entities. Notable exceptions are SW, WM, and organoid nevus syndrome, in which heredity does not appear to play a role and genetic abnormalities are not yet clearly delineated.[3]

Malignant potential

The tumors that develop in the ONCS are generally benign.[1–3] Some of these syndromes, however, can be associated with malignant neoplasms. Examples include the increased incidence of malignant schwannomas of the peripheral nerves in patients with NF. Hypernephroma and pheochromocytoma occur with greater frequency in patients with VHL.[3]

Formes frustes

Patients with the ONCS may manifest only some of the clinical features of a particular syndrome, referred to as a forme fruste.[3] Furthermore, patients can occasionally exhibit lesions characteristic of one entity and other lesions characteristic of another, referred to as the crossover phenomenon. One example, among several, is the café au lait spots seen in patients with NF that can occasionally be seen in patients with TSC.

Tuberous sclerosis complex (Bourneville's syndrome)

DEFINITION/OVERVIEW AND ETIOLOGY

Tuberous sclerosis complex (TSC) is characterized by retinal astrocytic hamartomas, cutaneous abnormalities, central nervous system (CNS) astrocytomas, and internal tumors such as cardiac rhabdomyoma, renal angiomyolipoma, and other tumors[1–9] (*Table 18*). It is best known for producing a triad of adenoma sebaceum (cutaneous angiofibromas), seizures, and mental deficiency.

The incidence of TSC is about one in 10,000.[5] Although TSC usually is diagnosed during the first few years of life, it has occasionally been recognized in patients as young as 1 month of age or as old as 50 years. This syndrome has been identified in all races and there is no predilection for gender.

Most evidence suggests that TSC is transmitted by an AD mode with incomplete penetrance. In many cases, the family history is unremarkable and examination of family members is normal. In such patients, the disease is considered to be due to sporadic mutations. About half of the families show linkage of chromosome 9q34 and about half to chromosome 16p13.[1]

CLINICAL PRESENTATION

The retinal astrocytic hamartoma is the characteristic fundus lesion of TSC (**253, 254**).[1–3] However, an identical lesion is occasionally found in patients who have no other clinical or genetic evidence for TSC. In either case, a small noncalcified tumor can be extremely

Table 18 Clinical features of tuberous sclerosis complex

Eyelid
Angiofibroma (adenoma sebaceum), depigmented macules (ash leaf sign)

Retina
Astrocytic hamartoma, peripheral depigmented areas, atypical coloboma, optic trophy

Brain
Astrocytic hamartoma

Skin
Angiofibroma (adenoma sebaceum), ash leaf macules, shagreen patches, ungual/subungual fibromas

Other

Heart	Rhabdomyoma
Kidney	Angiomyolipoma, renal cysts
Lung	Pleural cysts
Teeth	Pitted enamel hypoplasia
Bone	Irregular cortical thickening

Liver, thyroid, pancreas, testes, and other organs can develop hamartomas

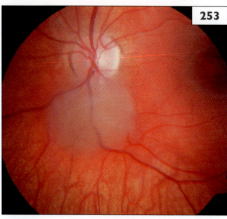

253 Tuberous sclerosis complex. Noncalcified retinal astrocytic hamartoma.

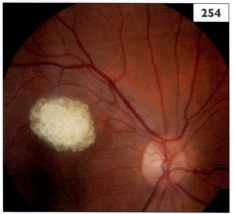

254 Tuberous sclerosis complex. Calcified retinal astrocytic hamartoma.

subtle and appear only as ill-defined translucent thickening of the retinal nerve fiber layer (**253**). A slightly larger tumor is more opaque and appears as a sessile white lesion at the level of the nerve fiber layer of the retina. The calcified variant contains characteristic dense yellow, refractile structures that resemble fish eggs or tapioca (**254**). Although it is generally stable and does not usually cause serious complications, it can occasionally produce retinal traction or vitreous hemorrhage. Retinal astrocytic hamartoma generally is a small, asymptomatic lesion that does not show enlargement. However, an aggressive variant has recently been identified in which the lesions show marked progression, which produce total exudative retinal detachment and neovascular glaucoma, sometimes necessitating enucleation of the eye.[9]

Occasionally ancillary studies, such as fluorescein angiography and ultrasonography, assist in the diagnosis of retinal astrocytic hamartoma. With fluorescein angiography, the tumor is relatively hypofluorescent in the arterial phase. A network of fine blood vessels is apparent in the venous phase. Typically, these vessels leak in the recirculation phase and stain the mass in the late angiograms. Ultrasonography is most important for the larger retinal astrocytic hamartoma. With A- and B-scan ultrasonography, the mass appears as a sessile or dome-shaped retinal mass with acoustic solidity and orbital shadowing if there is calcification in the lesion.

The uveal tract is rarely affected in TSC. A depigmented iris sector, seen in some patients with TSC, is believed to be the equivalent of the depigmented cutaneous lesions.[6] Irregular areas of atrophy of the retinal pigment epithelium (RPE) are occasionally seen with TSC.

The differential diagnosis of retinal astrocytic hamartoma includes retinoblastoma, hemangioblastoma, retinal granuloma, focal or massive gliosis of the retina, myelinated retinal nerve fibers, and optic disc drusen. Retinoblastoma is perhaps the most difficult and important tumor to differentiate from astrocytic hamartoma. The fine differentiating features of these other conditions are discussed elsewhere.[1,2]

The retinal astrocytic hamartoma has rather typical pathologic features. It is a lightly eosinophilic lesion located mainly in the nerve fiber layer of the retina and is composed of fibrillary astrocytes. The nuclei are round and mitoses are extremely rare. The more calcified tumors show fossilization, larger round cells, and basophilic laminated structures resembling psammoma bodies.[1,3,9]

OTHER FEATURES

The characteristic brain findings in patients with TSC include subependymal and paraventricular astrocytomas (**255**).[1–9] Both can demonstrate cystic and calcific changes that account for the name tuberous sclerosis (potato-like masses). These lesions may contribute to the seizures and mental deficiency, but severe mental deficiency is not necessarily a part of this syndrome. It is now recognized that many patients are of normal or near normal intelligence.

The main cutaneous manifestations of TSC include adenoma sebaceum, depigmented macules, and café au lait spots.[1–9] Adenoma sebaceum is a misnomer, since the lesions are actually angiofibromas. It is characterized clinically by multiple slightly elevated, rubbery, yellow-red papules (**256**). The lesions are often found on the face in a butterfly-shaped distribution. Similar angiofibromas can occur beneath or adjacent to the fingernails or toenails in patients with TSC. Depigmented macules resembling vitiligo are commonly present on the skin of patients with TSC (**257**). Because this characteristic lesion frequently resembles the leaf of an ash tree, it is often referred to as the 'ash leaf sign'.

MANAGEMENT/TREATMENT AND PROGNOSIS

The majority of retinal astrocytic hamartomas are asymptomatic and nonprogressive and do not require treatment. Ocular examination should be performed yearly and the patient followed for other manifestations of TSC. If there should be associated subretinal fluid that extends into the foveal area, then laser photocoagulation or photodynamic therapy can be employed in order to bring about resolution of the subretinal fluid.[1–3]

The astrocytic hamartoma of the retina has an extremely low tendency to undergo malignant change and has no recognized tendency to metastasize. The visual prognosis is also excellent, except in the rare instances in which exudation, subretinal fluid, or vitreous hemorrhage occurs. The renal lesion of TSC commonly predisposes the patient to recurrent nephritis and elevated blood urea nitrogen. Histopathologically it is a benign angiomyolipoma, with no tendency to undergo malignant transformation or to metastasize. The characteristic cardiac rhabdomyoma is composed of large spider cells with prominent vacuoles containing glycogen. Some patients with TSC develop slowly progressive subpleural cysts that result from anomalous development of pulmonary tissue.[8] These cysts can rupture, leading to spontaneous pneumothorax. Irregular cortical thickenings of bones, particularly the metatarsals and metacarpals, as well as hamartomas of the liver, thyroid, pancreas, testes, and other organs have been recognized.[8]

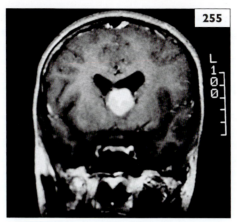

255 Tuberous sclerosis complex. MRI of
paraventricular astrocytoma.

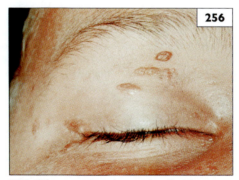

256 Tuberous sclerosis complex. Facial
angiofibromas (adenoma sebaceum) involving
the upper eyelid.

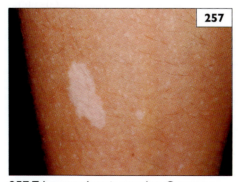

257 Tuberous sclerosis complex. Cutaneous
depigmented macule (ash leaf sign).

Neurofibromatosis (von Recklinghausen's syndrome)

DEFINITION/OVERVIEW AND ETIOLOGY

Neurofibromatosis (NF) is an ONCS characterized by multisystem involvement that can lead to a wide variety of clinical symptoms and signs.[10–17] von Recklinghausen published a classic monograph on this disease in 1882 and the condition is now known as von Recklinghausen's syndrome.[11] More recently, NF has been subcategorized into type 1 (NF-1) and type 2 (NF-2).[12] Since there is some overlap in the two types, they are discussed together in this chapter.

The frequency of a new mutation for NF is estimated to be about 1 in 2,500 to 3,000 births; there appears to be no appreciable predilection for gender.[12]

NF is transmitted by an AD mode of inheritance with about 80% penetrance. NF-1 is also known as peripheral neurofibromatosis or von Recklinghausen's syndrome. It is recognized to occur from an abnormality of chromosome 17. NF-2 is called central or bilateral acoustic neurofibromatosis. It is characterized by CNS tumors and early onset of posterior subcapsular cataract, and is recognized to be related to an abnormality in chromosome 22.[12,13]

CLINICAL PRESENTATION

NF has the most diverse systemic and ocular findings among the ONCS (*Table 19*).[1–3,12,13] Ocular changes include abnormalities in the uveal tract (80%), eyelid (25%), optic nerve (12%), retina (9%), and conjunctiva (4%).[11] The plexiform neurofibroma of the orbit and eyelid produces a typical S-shaped curve to the upper eyelid, a finding that is believed to be highly characteristic of NF-1. Plexiform or localized neurofibroma, histopathologically similar to those that appear on the skin, can also occur in the orbit in patients with NF-1. Neurilemoma (schwannoma) can also develop in the orbit of patients with NF-1 and NF-2. They arise from the Schwann cells of the ciliary nerves. Bilateral schwannoma of the auditory nerves (acoustic neuroma) is considered to be pathognomonic for NF-2.[12]

Patients with NF-2 have been recognized to have early onset of posterior subcapsular cataract.[12] Patients with NF-1 have an increased incidence of congenital glaucoma. It appears to occur more commonly in patients who have neurofibromatous involvement of the eyelids or ipsilateral facial hemihypertrophy. It can be secondary to obstruction of aqueous outflow by diffuse neurofibromatous thickening of the trabecular meshwork, angle closure from forward displacement of the iris by a ciliary body tumor, or from iris neovascularization.

Uveal tract involvement has been recognized in about 80% of patients with NF.[13] Multiple iris hamartomas, known as Lisch nodules, are the most common uveal abnormality in NF-1 (**258**).[13] They first appear in childhood around age 5 years or later as discrete, multiple, lightly pigmented elevations of the anterior border layer. Relatively flat pigmented choroidal lesions, presumably melanocytic hamartomas identical to choroidal nevi, are often seen in NF-1. Some patients with NF have a diffuse thickening of the uveal tract due to an increased number of neurofibromatous and melanocytic elements. Other choroidal tumors that rarely are associated with NF are choroidal melanoma and schwannoma. Most cases of choroidal schwannoma, however, are isolated and not associated with NF-1 or NF-2.[15] The retinal findings of NF are less common and include retinal astrocytic hamartoma, retinal vasoproliferative tumor, myelinated nerve fibers, multifocal congenital hypertrophy of the RPE ('bear tracks'), and a lesion similar to combined hamartoma of the retina and RPE. The latter typically occurs in patients with NF-2 but can be seen with NF-1. The astrocytic hamartoma is relatively rare in NF but is very common in TSC.

Table 19 Clinical features of neurofibromatosis (von Recklinghausen's syndrome)

Eye

Eyelids	Neurofibroma, neurilemoma, café au lait spots
Conjunctiva	Neurofibroma
Cornea	Possible prominent corneal nerves
Lens	Posterior subcapsular cataract
Iris	Lisch nodules
Choroid	Melanocytic hamartoma, neurilemoma (schwannoma) malignant melanoma
Retina	Astrocytic hamartoma, combined hamartoma retina/retinal pigment epithelium (RPE) myelinated nerve fibers, congenital hypertrophy RPE
Optic disc	Drusen
Optic nerve	Pilocytic hamartoma (glioma), meningioma, dysgerminoma
Orbit	Asymmetry, sphenoid bone dysphasia

Brain

Cerebrum	Glioma, meningioma, acoustic neuroma
Pituitary	Tumors
Spinal cord	Meningioma

Skin

Café au lait spots, neurofibroma, neurilemoma

Other

Breast, genitourinary, and gastrointestinal organs can develop benign and malignant tumors

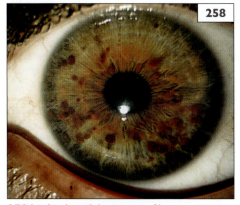

258 Iris Lisch nodules in neurofibromatosis.

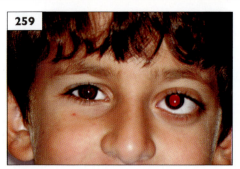

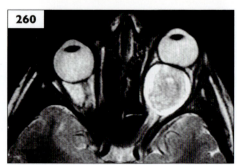

259 Neurofibromatosis. Axial proptosis of left eye due to juvenile pilocytic astrocytoma of optic nerve (optic nerve glioma).

260 Axial MRI of patient shown in **249**. T2 weighted image with gadolinium enhancement, showing optic nerve pilocytic astrocytoma.

The optic nerve can be involved with pilocytic astrocytoma (glioma) (**259, 260**) or meningioma.[2,3] In patients with pilocytic astrocytoma, the reported incidence of NF has ranged from 9% to 30%.[17] Both juvenile pilocytic astrocytoma and meningioma of the optic nerve are benign, slowly progressive lesions that often cause visual loss, proptosis, optic disc edema, retinal venous obstruction, and optic atrophy.

For differential diagnosis, the diffuse hamartomatous thickening of the uveal tract in NF should be differentiated from diffuse uveal melanoma, ocular melanocytosis, and uveal metastases. Other differentiating features are discussed elsewhere.[3]

OTHER FINDINGS

The CNS manifestations of NF vary with the size and extent of the associated tumors.[11] Acoustic neuromas, particularly if bilateral, are considered to be pathognomonic of NF-2. Other NF-2-associated tumors include gliomas in the region of the third ventricle, pituitary tumors, and spinal cord meningiomas.

The most important cutaneous manifestations of NF include subcutaneous benign nerve sheath tumors, pigmented macules (café au lait spots) and nevi.[2] Many of these skin lesions become clinically apparent at puberty, although in some instances they have been noted at birth. The benign cutaneous and subcutaneous nerve sheath tumors (neurofibromas and schwannomas) are particularly pronounced in the facial area (**260**).

The pigmented macule (café au lait spot) is characterized clinically as a patch of light brown pigmentation with fairly well-defined borders (**261**). It can occur anywhere on the skin and can assume a variety of sizes and configurations. Café au lait spots are highly characteristic of NF. Strict criteria should be met before making the diagnosis of NF-1 or NF-2 (*Table 20*).

A number of other benign and malignant systemic tumors have been associated with NF including malignant peripheral nerve sheath tumors, breast carcinoma, genitourinary tumors, gastrointestinal tumors, and cutaneous melanoma. Patients with NF are recognized to have a slightly higher incidence of pheochromocytoma.

Histopathologically, Lisch nodules are focal aggregates of melanocytes and glial cells on the anterior border layer of the iris. The choroidal hamartoma is similar to the iris lesion histopathologically. The retinal astrocytic hamartoma is apparently identical to that seen with TSC.

MANAGEMENT/TREATMENT

Management of the ocular lesions of NF varies with the location and the extent of the disease. Treatment can be very complex. In general, the fundus tumors including diffuse choroidal hamartoma, retinal astrocytic hamartoma, myelinated nerve fibers, and combined hamartoma of the retina and RPE require no treatment. Choroidal neurilemoma and malignant melanoma are managed with one of several methods, depending on many factors.[1]

261 Cutaneous café au lait macule in neurofibromatosis.

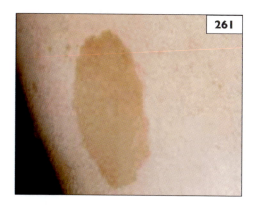

261

Table 20 Diagnostic features of neurofibromatosis (NF)

NF-1

Confirmed if three of the below criteria are found:

1. Six or more café au lait spots measuring
   >5 mm in prepubertal children
   >15 mm in adults
2. Two or more cutaneous neurofibromas or one plexiform neurofibroma
3. Lisch nodules
4. Café au lait spots (small) in axillary, inframammary, inguinal, or gluteal creases
5. Osseous lesions
6. Glioma of anterior visual pathway
7. First-degree relative (sibling, parent, offspring) with NF-1 by these same criteria

NF-2

The diagnosis of NF-2 is made by the presence of bilateral acoustic neuroma. Otherwise NF-2 is confirmed if two of the below criteria are found:

1. First-degree relative with NF-2
2. Unilateral acoustic neuroma
   or two of the following:
      neurofibroma
      meningioma
      glioma
      schwannoma
      juvenile central posterior subcapsular cataract

Retinocerebellar hemangioblastomatosis (von Hippel–Lindau syndrome)

DEFINITION/OVERVIEW AND ETIOLOGY

In 1895, von Hippel reported the clinical findings of so-called retinal angiomatosis and in 1926, Lindau made a study of cerebellar lesions and pointed out their relationship to the retinal tumors previously described by von Hippel.[18,19] Consequently, the combination of retinal and cerebellar involvement has been called the von Hippel–Lindau (VHL) syndrome. VHL syndrome has since been recognized to have several other components in addition to the eye and CNS findings, including renal cell carcinoma, pheochromocytoma, endolymphatic sac tumors, and other less common cystic lesions (*Table 21*).[20–24]

The incidence of VHL syndrome is about 1 in 40,000 live births. There is no clear-cut predilection for race or gender, although all our patients have been Caucasians.[3] The VHL syndrome is recognized to be a hereditary disorder, with an AD mode of inheritance and incomplete penetrance. Many cases seen by the ophthalmologist, however, occur as spontaneous mutations with no apparent family history of the disease. Probably about 20% of cases have a positive family history. The condition is related to a partial deletion of the short arm of chromosome 3.[3,24]

CLINICAL PRESENTATION

The ocular manifestations of VHL syndrome are not so diversified as they are in the other systemic hamartomatoses. Hemangioblastoma ('retinal capillary hemangioma') of the retina and/or optic disc are the only intraocular hamartomas that are known to occur. When associated with the VHL syndrome, the retinal and optic disc tumors are often multiple and bilateral.[1,3,24] The diagnosis of the ocular lesions is usually made in the second or third decade of life.

The ophthalmoscopic appearance of a retinal hemangioblastoma varies with the location of the lesion in the fundus. In the earliest stages, a tumor in the peripheral retina is often subtle ophthalmoscopically. A somewhat larger tumor appears as a distinct red nodule with a typical dilated tortuous afferent artery and an efferent vein that come from the optic disc to the tumor, and yellow lipoproteinaceous exudation (**262**). Retinal hemangioblastoma can eventually assume either an exudative form or a vitreoretinal form or a combination of the two.[1]

The exudative form is characterized by localized or intraretinal and subretinal yellow exudation. The exudation with larger tumors may be contiguous with the tumor or it may be remote from the tumor in the foveal area as stellate-shaped exudation. The vitreoretinal form of hemangioblastoma is characterized by fibrosis of the overlying vitreous, and traction bands elevating the retina may be visible. Flat preretinal fibrosis, especially in the macular area, are typical of this form of hemangioblastoma.[1] The tumors located on the optic disc itself do not usually develop the well-defined feeding and draining blood vessels (**263**).

Table 21 Clinical features of retinocerebellar hemangioblastomatosis (von Hippel–Lindau syndrome)

Eye	
Retina	Hemangioblastoma, twin vessels
Optic nerve	Hemangioblastoma
Brain	
Cerebellum	Hemangioblastoma
Medulla	Hemangioblastoma, syringobulbia
Spinal cord	Hemangioblastoma, syringomyelia
Skin	
No consistent findings	
Other	
Kidney	Renal cell carcinoma, hemangioblastoma, cysts
Adrenal	Pheochromocytoma, paraganglioma
Sympathetic chain	Pheochromocytoma, paraganglioma
Pancreas	Hemangioblastoma, cysts
Epididymis	Cysts

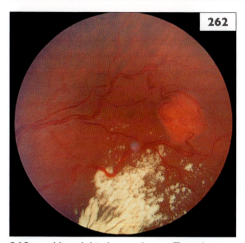

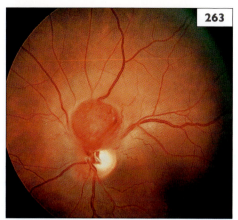

262 von Hippel–Lindau syndrome. Typical retinal hemangioblastoma, showing red tumor with dilated afferent and efferent retinal blood vessels and lipoproteinaceous exudation.

263 von Hippel–Lindau syndrome. Hemangioblastoma adjacent to optic disc, with mild surrounding exudation.

OTHER FEATURES

The cerebellar or spinal cord hemangioblastoma is the classic CNS lesion in VHL syndrome.[1,21,24] It can be small and asymptomatic but it usually enlarges slowly and can eventually produce profound cerebellar signs and symptoms. The cerebellar symptoms usually occur in the fourth decade of life, and patients with known ocular disease should have periodic neurologic evaluation and brain imaging to detect their early onset. Identical lesions can occasionally occur in the medulla oblongata and in the spinal cord. Like retinal hemangioblastoma, cerebellar hemangioblastoma characteristically has large blood vessels that supply and drain the lesion. The vascular tumor frequently occurs within a cerebellar cyst. Histopathologically, the tumor is a hemangioblastoma with features identical to the vascular tumor that occurs in the retina.[1,21]

In contrast to the other systemic hamartomatoses, VHL syndrome usually has no major cutaneous involvement.

DIAGNOSIS

Fluorescein angiography is the most helpful ancillary study in confirming the diagnosis of a hemangioblastoma.[1] In the early arterial phase, the dilated retinal feeder arteriole appears prominent. Within 2–3 seconds the retinal tumor is fluorescent as the fine capillaries that comprise the tumor fill with fluorescein. In the venous phase, the dilated draining vein fills with dye and the tumor maintains its bright fluorescence. In the late phase the tumor generally remains fluorescent and leaks dye into the vitreous. The intrinsic rapid fluorescence of the optic disc hemangioma assists in differentiating these tumors from other optic disc lesions.

Histopathologically, retinal hemangioblastoma consists of a proliferation of retinal capillaries that replace the architecture of the sensory retina.[3,25] There is a proliferation of endothelial cells, pericytes, and vacuolated interstitial cells called stromal cells. The nature of the stromal cells is still uncertain, but they may be the cell of origin of the tumor.[25]

MANAGEMENT/TREATMENT AND PROGNOSIS

The management of retinal hemangioblastoma is difficult and controversial. No active treatment may be necessary for small asymptomatic retinal tumors because some of them remain stable for many years and some even regress spontaneously. The patient should be examined periodically and treatment instituted if the tumor grows or if there is accumulation of exudation or subretinal fluid. In such instances, several methods of treatment have been advocated including argon laser, cryotherapy, photodynamic therapy, and intravitreal injection of angiostatic agents. No single treatment has emerged as the treatment of choice. If a hemangioblastoma has caused an extensive retinal detachment with subretinal exudation, a vitrectomy and/or a scleral buckling procedure may be necessary to reattach the retina. The authors have used plaque radiotherapy for selected tumors with extensive retinal detachment.

Analysis of the deoxyribonucleic acid (DNA) of the patient and all family members can be performed in an attempt to identify markers indicating VHL disease. The gene for VHL syndrome has been mapped to the short arm of chromosome 3. All patients with VHL syndrome should be followed carefully with yearly testing for systemic tumors. Furthermore, relatives of patients with VHL disease may benefit from a screening protocol depending on the results of DNA testing (*Table 22*). The retinal hemangioblastoma is often the initial sign of VHL disease and the various other systemic tumors found in this disease are best treated at an early stage. Therefore, it is important to evaluate these patients systemically.

Various systemic hamartomas can occur in patients with VHL syndrome (*Table 21*).[21] These include hypernephroma, pheochromocytoma, and cysts of the kidney, pancreas, and epididymis. A detailed medical and family history should be taken from all patients with retinal hemangioblastoma and, if indicated, appropriate studies be undertaken to detect any of the systemic components of VHL syndrome.

Table 22 Systemic evaluation for von Hippel–Lindau syndrome

Affected patient

Testing performed every year:
- Physical examination
- Eye exam (indirect ophthalmoscopy)
- Urinanalysis
- Urine 24 hour collection for vanillylmandelic acid (VMA)
- Renal ultrasound

Testing performed every 3 years:
- MRI (or CT) of brain
  (after age 50 years, brain scan is performed every 5 years)
- CT of kidneys

At-risk relative

Testing performed every year:
- Physical examination
- Eye examination (indirect ophthalmoscopy)
- Urine analysis
- Urine 24 hour collection for VMA
- Renal ultrasound

Testing performed every 3 years:
- MRI (or CT) of brain (brain scan recommended every 3 years between ages 15 and 40 years and then every 5 years until age 60 years)
- CT of kidneys
  (abdominal scan recommended every 3 years between ages 20 and 65 years)

Racemose hemangiomatosis (Wyburn-Mason syndrome)

DEFINITION/OVERVIEW AND ETIOLOGY

Racemose hemangioma of the midbrain and ipsilateral retina is called the Wyburn-Mason (WM) syndrome (*Table 23*). Wyburn-Mason described this relationship in 1943.[31] It consists of an abnormal congenital arteriovenous communication that can involve any combination of lesions in the retina, midbrain, and sometimes other areas including the orbit, mandible, maxilla, and pterygoid fossa.[1,3] This congenital condition does not appear to be familial and does not exhibit a hereditary pattern.

CLINICAL PRESENTATION

The classic ocular finding is the racemose (cirsoid) hemangioma of the retina.[31,32] It is actually a retinal arteriovenous (AV) communication, and can range from a very subtle asymptomatic lesion (**264**) to a more extensive one that consists of tumor-like vascular masses. The lesion has been divided into three groups that are detailed in the literature.[32]

OTHER FEATURES

AV communications similar to those in the retina can also occur in the midbrain. They can cause spontaneous intracranial hemorrhage that can produce stroke-like symptoms, oculomotor palsies, and seizures.[1,3] The bones of the skull, including the mandible and maxilla, can frequently be involved with the vascular malformation and abnormal bleeding can follow dental treatment.

There are no significant cutaneous changes associated with racemose hemangiomatosis, except for the rare occurrence of small facial angiomas.

DIAGNOSIS

The diagnosis of the retinal racemose hemangioma is made ophthalmoscopically, but fluorescein angiography can be of assistance. The affected artery fills rapidly with fluorescein and transit to the venous side is quick due to the lack of an intervening capillary network.

Table 23 Clinical features of racemose hemangiomatosis (Wyburn-Mason syndrome)

Eye	
Retina	Racemose hemangioma
Brain	
Midbrain	Racemose hemangioma
Skin	
No consistent findings	
Other	
Bone	Racemose hemangioma

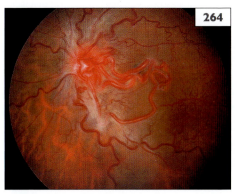

264 Retinal racemose hemangioma in Wyburn-Mason syndrome.

The retinal racemose hemangioma has not been studied extensively histopathologically. The affected vessels develop acellular fibrohyaline adventitial coverings and the retina is thin and degenerated.[1,3]

MANAGEMENT/TREATMENT AND PROGNOSIS

In general, no dermatologic or ophthalmic treatment is necessary for patients with racemose hemangiomatosis. If the retinal lesions produce persistent vitreous hemorrhage that does not resolve, then the blood can be removed by vitrectomy. WM syndrome generally exhibits no systemic manifestations other than those mentioned above.

Encephalofacial cavernous hemangiomatosis (Sturge–Weber syndrome)

DEFINITION/OVERVIEW AND ETIOLOGY

In 1879, Sturge described a syndrome composed of a facial hemangioma with ipsilateral buphthalmos and contralateral seizures.[26] Later, Weber studied the clinical manifestations in greater detail and the fully expressed entity became known as the Sturge–Weber (SW) syndrome.[27] The SW syndrome is now recognized to consist of a facial hemangioma, buphthalmos, seizures, and radiographic evidence of intracranial calcification (*Table 24*).[28–30] Most patients, however, have a forme fruste rather than the entire syndrome. In contrast to most other systemic hamartomatoses, there is no recognizable hereditary pattern associated with SW syndrome.

CLINICAL PRESENTATION

The ocular findings associated with SW syndrome include eyelid involvement with the nevus flammeus, prominent epibulbar blood vessels, glaucoma, retinal vascular tortuosity, and diffuse choroidal hemangioma (*Table 24*).

The facial hemangioma can frequently involve the eyelids (**265**). Although it is usually nilateral, bilateral involvement occasionally occurs. Involvement of the upper eyelid has a high association with ipsilateral glaucoma. Prominent tortuous epibulbar blood vessels, in both the conjunctiva and episclera, are common findings (**266**). Glaucoma is more common in patients with SW syndrome than in the other ONCS. In one study, if the facial hemangioma involved both the first and second division of the trigeminal nerve, the incidence was 15%.[28] The glaucoma occurs unilaterally on the side of the facial hemangioma.

The only important abnormality of the uveal tract in patients with SW syndrome is the diffuse choroidal hemangioma. Patients with this tumor usually have a bright red pupillary reflex in the involved eye ('tomato catsup fundus') as compared to the normal contralateral eye.

Table 24 Clinical features of encephalofacial cavernous hemangiomatosis (SW syndrome)

Eye	
Eyelid	Nevus flammeus
Episclera	Dilated vessels
Angle	Glaucoma
Retina	Vascular tortuosity
Choroid	Diffuse hemangioma
Brain	
Meninges	Hemangioma with calcification
Cerebrum	Maldevelopment
Skin	
Face	Nevus flammeus

The diffuse choroidal hemangioma is usually diagnosed when the affected patient is young (median age 8 years), either because the associated facial hemangioma prompts a fundus examination or because visual impairment occurs from hyperopic amblyopia or from a secondary retinal detachment. The diffuse choroidal hemangioma appears as a red-orange thickening of the choroid, often with overlying subretinal fluid. The tumor is usually a few millimeters thicker than normal choroid.

The details of fluorescein angiography, indocyanine green angiography, and ultrasonography, which can be helpful in the diagnosis, are discussed elsewhere.[1,3]

Histopathologically the choroidal hemangioma is a diffuse thickening of the choroid consisting of variable sized venous channels separated by thin intervascular septa.[1,3,30] Overlying retinal edema with cystoid changes, and fibrous and osseous metaplasia of the RPE are sometimes found.

OTHER FEATURES

The typical CNS change associated with SW syndrome is a diffuse leptomeningeal hemangiomatosis that is ipsilateral to the facial hemangioma.[1,3] The adjacent cerebral cortex can show secondary linear calcification on computed tomography (CT), referred to as the 'railroad track' sign. Convulsions, which frequently occur, are characteristically localized to the side contralateral to the CNS involvement.

The classic skin lesion of SW syndrome is the facial hemangioma, often referred to as nevus flammeus or port wine stain. Although it usually occurs in the cutaneous distribution of the fifth cranial nerve, it can have many variations, ranging from minor involvement of the first division of the nerve to massive involvement of all three divisions. It sometimes crosses the midline in an irregular pattern and it is occasionally bilateral.

MANAGEMENT/TREATMENT

Management of the diffuse choroidal hemangioma can be difficult and it varies with the extent of the tumor. It may range from observation only to laser photocoagulation or retinal detachment surgery or irradiation, depending on the clinical circumstances.[3]

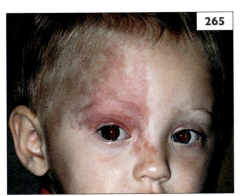

265 Sturge–Weber syndrome, with facial nevus flammeus.

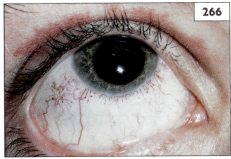

266 Conjunctival and episcleral dilated blood vessels in Sturge–Weber syndrome.

Oculoneurocutaneous cavernous hemangiomatosis

DEFINITION/OVERVIEW AND ETIOLOGY

There are several systemic syndromes that are characterized by multiple cavernous hemangiomas or other vascular malformations. This chapter includes only those with a combination of cavernous hemangiomas that involve the eye, skin, and CNS. Oculoneurocutaneous cavernous hemangiomatosis (ONCCH) is a syndrome characterized by cavernous hemangiomas that affect the retina, CNS, and skin (*Table 25*).[1,33–37] The retinal and skin tumors are frequently asymptomatic, but the CNS hamartomas can sometimes produce clinical symptoms. This syndrome appears to have an AD mode of inheritance.[33–37] A 7q locus has also been implicated in a large family with retinal cavernous hemangioma, choroidal cavernous hemangioma, and widespread CNS and cutaneous lesions.[35] Although the genetics is poorly understood, a mutation in the KRIT1 gene has been recognized in a family with retinal and CNS cavernous hemangiomas.[37]

CLINICAL PRESENTATION

The only ocular manifestation of this syndrome is the retinal cavernous hemangioma and the iris cavernous hemangioma, with the latter being extremely rare. The retinal lesions appear as a cluster of dark venous intraretinal aneurysms on ophthalmoscopic examination (**267**). There is no feeder artery and usually no yellow exudation, but white fibroglial tissue is characteristically present on the surface of the tumor. The main complication of retinal cavernous hemangioma is vitreous hemorrhage. Severe fibrogliosis and dragging of the retina can occur. During fluorescein angiography, the vascular channels comprising the lesion remain hypofluorescent until the late venous phase, when fluorescein begins slowly to enter the vascular spaces and produces the characteristic fluorescein–blood interface.

Table 25 Clinical features of retinal cavernous hemangiomatosis

Eye	
Retina	Cavernous hemangioma
Brain	
Cavernous hemangioma	
Skin	
Various vascular malformations	

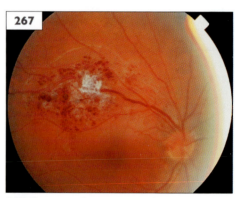

267 Cavernous hemangioma of the retina and CNS.

OTHER FEATURES

Vascular malformations in the CNS can lead to seizures, oculomotor palsies, and other neurologic symptoms. The hemangiomas of the skin in this syndrome are often subtle and are quite variable in their appearance and distribution on the body.

TREATMENT

Most patients require no treatment. Patients who experience recurrent vitreous hemorrhages may benefit from laser photocoagulation of the lesion.

Organoid nevus syndrome

DEFINITION/OVERVIEW AND ETIOLOGY

The organoid nevus syndrome (ONS) has recently been included with the ONCS.

CLINICAL PRESENTATION AND PROGNOSIS

ONS is characterized by the nevus sebaceous of Jadassohn, cerebral atrophy, epibulbar complex choristoma, posterior scleral cartilage, and occasionally other features (*Table 26*, overleaf).[38] The full syndrome is uncommon and the exact incidence is unknown. The two most important ophthalmologic features are the epibulbar complex choristoma and posterior scleral cartilage.

The epibulbar complex choristoma is a fleshy lesion of the conjunctiva that can extend onto the cornea (**268**). The posterior scleral cartilage produces a peculiar yellow-white discoloration of the fundus in the area of involvement. Since the cartilage produces a pattern similar to bone with ultrasonography and CT, it has sometimes been misinterpreted as a choroidal osteoma. The main dermatologic feature of the ONS is the nevus sebaceous of Jadassohn. It appears as a geographic yellow-brown lesion that often involves the preauricular region and extends onto the scalp, where it is associated with alopecia (**269**).

Patients with this syndrome can develop seizures, due mainly to enlarging subarachnoid cysts in the CNS. Rarely, the affected patient can have various cardiac and renal abnormalities.

TREATMENT

Most patients can be observed and do not require treatment. Larger or progressive lesions may require surgical excision.

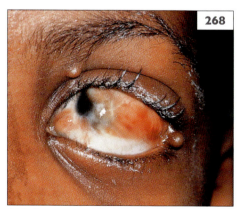

268 Organoid nevus syndrome: epibulbar complex choristoma.

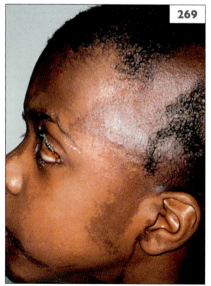

269 Nevus sebaceous of Jadassohn showing linear nevus sebaceous and alopecia in organoid nevus syndrome.

Introduction

Neurologic disorders affecting the eye and the visual pathways are an important potential cause for decreased vision and morbidity in the pediatric population. Identification of these disorders is important in order to prevent vision loss but also to identify other potentially lethal abnormalities of the nervous system.

Cortical visual impairment

DEFINITION/OVERVIEW AND ETIOLOGY

Cortical visual impairment (CVI) implies visual abnormalities secondary to damage to the posterior visual pathways, and mainly to the lateral geniculate body, the optic radiations, and the occipital cortex. The term 'cortical blindness' is old terminology which is no longer in favor. Blindness implies that the patient has no vision and no ability to recover. Both of those implications are incorrect. Cerebral visual impairment is synonymous with CVI and is preferred by some authors.

The most common cause of CVI is hypoxic ischemic injury. This is particularly the case in preterm infants. Their immature vascular system is prone to pressure fluctuations with resultant wound ischemia to the watershed area lying in the periventricular region. Within the periventricular area are the optic radiations. Also residing in this area is the germinal matrix, the area of the brain where all neurons originate. It is a very metabolically active area in the ventricular wall. The vasculature is friable and prone to hypoxic ischemic injury, leading to hemorrhage, termed germinal matrix hemorrhage. This hemorrhage can break through from the periventricular white matter into the ventricle leading to intra-ventricular hemorrhage, and possible subsequent hydrocephalus.

CLINICAL PRESENTATION

Patients with CVI display a wide range of visual disability ranging from no light perception to normal visual acuity but with visual field deficits. Cognitive visual disability is also considered a form of cortical impairment and includes difficulties navigating and route finding, difficulty finding objects in crowded scenes (making reading difficult), and difficulty recognizing people's faces.[1]

Other causes of CVI include hypoxia and ischemia unrelated to preterm delivery. Asphyxia and ischemia can occur in term infants. Congenital cerebral malformations, head trauma, metabolic and neurodegenerative disorders, meningitis and encephalitis, and hydrocephalus can all cause CVI.

DIAGNOSIS AND DIFFERENTIAL DIAGNOSIS

Diagnosis is made using the patient's history of brain injury and lack of visual attentiveness. Most patients have neurologic deficits that correspond to their vision loss. Vision loss very rarely occurs in isolation from any other neurologic problems or brain damage.[2] Examination reveals variable degrees of decreased vision or visual attentiveness, no nystagmus, normal pupillary reactivity, and a normal retina and optic nerve examination. Because the damage to the visual pathways is behind the lateral geniculate body, there will be no optic atrophy in most cases. Therefore, a normal eye exam with very poor vision is a classic presentation for CVI. Magnetic resonance imaging (MRI) is the best means of studying the occipital cortices and may be helpful in patients with suspected CVI.

Differential diagnosis includes any anterior pathway visual disturbance causing vision loss.

MANAGEMENT/TREATMENT

There is no treatment to improve vision. Treatment is aimed at providing low-vision services and supporting the vision available.

Migraine headache

DEFINITION/OVERVIEW AND ETIOLOGY

Migraine is not simply a headache but a constellation of abnormal neurologic events. It is often inherited and more often occurs in females than males; when children are analyzed separately, however, boys and girls under 7 years of age have an equal prevalence. Females predominate after that age. Children present differently from adults. Migraines typically begin at puberty and decrease in frequency at menopause. The median attack rate is 1.5 per month and the median duration is 24 hours, with a range of 4–72 hours, slightly less in children.

The neurologic events that lead to migraine all are poorly understood but felt to be secondary to hyperexcitable brainstem nuclei activating portions of the cortex. This increased activity leads to decreased blood flow and spreading cortical electrical depression, producing neurologic events such as visual aura. There is also dilation of the meningeal vessels with the release of inflammatory products leading to pain.

CLINICAL PRESENTATION

The migraine headache is often a throbbing hemicranial pain but can be anywhere on the head. It is also often accompanied by nausea and/or vomiting, photophobia, and phonophobia. Patients often sleep, and rest relieves the pain. Pediatric migraneurs often have a history of migraine equivalent which includes colic, recurrent abdominal pain, cyclic vomiting, or night terrors. Patients may experience irritability or lethargy. Triggering factors include menstruation, hunger, stress, chocolate and caffeine, sleep deprivation and, occasionally, visual triggers such as flickering lights or a computer screen. Approximately 4% of all pediatric headaches are migraine.

Transient visual disturbances occur more frequently in the pediatric age group, in some 18% of children with migraine. The stereotypical aura usually lasts 25–30 minutes. Since the visual aura is created by the brain, both eyes 'see' the image in the same hemifield. Some children can describe the classical scintillating scotoma which consists of a 'fog', or 'seeing through water', or an area of loss of vision in one hemifield, surrounded by a colored shimmery zigzag line, which moves across the visual field. The scintillating scotoma then regresses. The clinical presentation described above is classic migraine. It can occur prior to a headache. If it occurs in the absence of a headache it is termed acephalgic migraine. If the scintillating scotoma occurs in just one eye it is a retinal event and is termed retinal migraine.

Some patients present with cranial nerve palsies such as cranial nerve 3, 4, and 6. The paresis begins at the peak of the headache and last days to weeks after the headache resolves. These are very rare.

DIAGNOSIS AND DIFFERENTIAL DIAGNOSIS

The diagnosis of migraine is based on history. There is often a family history of migraine or sick headaches. Intracranial masses can also cause headache and vomiting, particularly in the morning on awakening.

MANAGEMENT/TREATMENT

Pharmacologic treatment for pediatric headache can be divided into abortive and prophylactic therapy. Most patients seek no treatment other than over-the-counter medications for symptomatic relief of their migraine headaches such as aspirin, acetaminophen, and ibuprofen. Medications can also include amitriptyline, propranolol, selective serotonin reuptake inhibitors, anticonvulsants, tricyclic antidepressants, calcium channel blockers, and 5-HT2 antagonists.

Congenital motor nystagmus

DEFINITION/OVERVIEW

Nystagmus is an involuntary rhythmic movement of the eyes. The beating of the eyes in usually in the horizontal direction and is present in all positions of gaze. The etiology is unknown but it may be heritable. It is theorized that there is an ocular motor circuitry problem.

CLINICAL PRESENTATION

Patients with congenital nystagmus present with nystagmus at 2–4 months of age. At the time of onset the vision is somewhat reduced when compared to the visual attentiveness of children without nystagmus, but the vision improves quickly and the parents usually report no reduction in vision after 6 months of age. The typical eye exam reveals good vision, and normal pupils, retinas, and optic nerves.

Over time the amplitude of the nystagmus lessens and it becomes less noticeable. Head shaking may accompany the nystagmus. In time patients may develop a head turn. This forces the eyes into an extreme gaze position and quietens the nystagmus, termed a null point. Another dampening mechanism is convergence, so patients will hold near material very close for best vision. Patients do not complain of oscillation of the environment, termed oscillopsia. The ultimate visual acuity of these patients is usually better than 20/60, and can be near normal.

DIAGNOSIS AND DIFFERENTIAL DIAGNOSIS

The diagnosis is often made clinically. The eye exam reveals no retinal or optic nerve pathology. An electoretinogram to rule out any retinal dystrophy can also be considered. Neuroimaging is usually not performed unless other neurologic abnormalities are present and the nystagmus is atypical.

Care should be taken to rule out sensory causes of nystagmus such as any abnormality of the retina or optic nerve that leads to vision loss. Poor vision from congenital retinal or optic nerve disease causes an early-onset nystagmus and poor vision, unlike the normal or near normal vision in patients with congenital motor nystagmus. Common congenital retina and optic nerve disorders that cause nystagmus are: albinism, Leber congenital amaurosis, cone–rod dystrophy, optic neve hypoplasia, retinal and/or optic nerve colobomas.

MANAGEMENT/TREATMENT

Drug therapy to dampen the nystagmus is not successful. Some advocate base-out prisms to induce convergence. Contact lenses may dampen the nystagmus. Surgery on the extraocular muscles can improve an abnormal head position that is adopted to dampen the nystagmus (null point). Surgery to improve visual function and dampen the amplitude of the nystagmus in some patients may be performed by detaching all four horizontal rectus muscles and then reattaching them at the same site.[3]

Spasmus nutans

DEFINITION/OVERVIEW AND ETIOLOGY

Spasmus nutans is a constellation of nystagmus, head nodding, and a torticollis. It is an acquired form of nystagmus that generally appears between 1 and 3 years of age. The etiology of typical spasmus nutans is unknown. However, rarely a suprasellar tumor such as a chiasmal glioma can cause clinical findings identical to those seen in spasmus nutans.[4]

CLINICAL PRESENTATION

Children present with a shimmering, small-amplitude, high-frequency nystagmus that is often asymmetric between the two eyes; in some cases the condition appears to be monocular. It is usually horizontal in direction but there can be a vertical component. Vision is good. A combination of head nodding and lateral shaking is also present and may be compensatory. A head tilt or turn is a variable finding and presents in less than half the cases. The nystagmus often remits a few years after onset.[5]

DIAGNOSIS AND DIFFERENTIAL DIAGNOSIS

Diagnosis is based on the clinical findings. A suprasellar tumor can rarely present with spasmus nutans. Some neurodegenerative diseases have also occasionally been known to cause nystagmus typical of spamus nutans, such as Pelizaeus–Merzbacher disease and Leigh disease.

MANAGEMENT/TREATMENT

There is no treatment for typical idiopathic spasmus nutans. Neuroimaging should be performed to rule out a suprasellar tumor.

Opsoclonus

DEFINITION/OVERVIEW AND ETIOLOGY

Opsoclonus is an acquired ocular movement abnormality that is characterized by involuntary chaotic bursts of multidirectional nystagmus. If the oscillations are purely horizontal, they are termed ocular flutter. Opsoclonus differs from nystagmus in that the oscillations are not rhythmic and are punctuated by silent periods.

The etiology of opsoclonus is secondary to neuroblastoma, due to a paraneoplastic phenomenon, and secondary to encephalitis affecting the cerebellum, and less often to exposure to toxins or drugs, meningitis, and intracranial tumors. It is felt that there is an inhibition of the pause cells of the cerebellum, allowing the burst cells to fire without interruption. In the case of neuroblastoma it has been hypothesized that a peptide produced by the tumor directly affects the cerebellum and causes the opsoclonus, or that the opsoclonus is due to an immunological cross-reactivity between the tumor and normal cerebellar neurons.

CLINICAL PRESENTATION

Patients present with a bizarre chaotic nystagmus, with the eyes moving in different directions, followed by periods of quiet. Young patients often complain of oscillopsia and have fairly good visual function in spite of the large-amplitude nystagmus. The eye exam is normal except for the movement abnormality. Patients with neuroblastoma may also exhibit myoclonus.

DIAGNOSIS AND DIFFERENTIAL DIAGNOSIS

After the diagnosis of opsoclonus is made, a work-up for neuroblastoma in the abdomen, chest or neck must be carried out with MR imaging. A toxin screen can be considered as well as neuroimaging of the brain. Because of its unique and remarkable appearance, no ocular movement abnormality can be confused with opsoclonus.

Horner's syndrome

DEFINITION/OVERVIEW AND ETIOLOGY

Any lesion along the oculosympathetic pathway can cause Horner's syndrome. There are three parts or orders to the oculosympathetic pathway. First-order sympathetic fibers arise from the hypothalamus and descend uncrossed through the brainstem and terminate/synapse in the spinal cord at the level of C8–T2. Second-order sympathetic fibers exit the spinal cord at the level of T1 and enter the sympathetic cervical chain, where they arch over the pulmonary apex and the subclavian artery and then ascend the common carotid artery to synapse in the superior cervical ganglion at the bifurcation of the carotid artery. Third-order fibers exit the superior cervical ganglion and ascend along the internal carotid artery, traveling into the cavernous sinus, and entering the orbit to innervate the iris dilator and Muller muscle, the eyelid retractor muscles.

First-order neuron lesions include Arnold–Chiari malformation, meningitis, cerebral vascular accident involving the brainstem, and demyelinating disorders. Second-order neuron lesions include tumor at the apex of the lung, brachial plexus injury from birth trauma, central venous catheterization, trauma or surgical injury (radical neck dissection, thyroid surgery, carotid angiography, cardiac surgery), chest tubes, lymphadenopathy,

lesions of the middle ear (acute otitis media), and neuroblastoma. Third-order lesions include internal carotid artery dissection, idiopathic inflammation of the orbit, carotid-cavernous fistula, herpes zoster, and migraine headaches.

CLINICAL PRESENTATION

When the sympathetic innervation to the eye is interrupted the retractor muscles of the eyelids are weakened, allowing the upper lid to droop and the lower lid to rise (this is called ptosis of the upper and lower lids) (**270**). The dilator muscle of the iris is weakened, allowing the pupil to become smaller. Vasomotor and sudomotor control of parts of the face may be impaired. This combination of ptosis, pupil miosis, and anhidrosis is called Horner's syndrome. If the Horner's syndrome is congenital it may cause a lighter colored iris on the involved side.

DIAGNOSIS AND DIFFERENTIAL DIAGNOSIS

The diagnosis can be made clinically with this constellation of features: mild (1–2 mm) ptosis of the upper and lower lids, smaller pupil on the involved side which responds well to light, with the pupil asymmetry between the two eyes greater in darkness than in light, and a pupil that dilates more slowly when the lights are extinguished (dilation lag). Depending on the location of the lesion on the sympathetic chain there may be loss of sweating and redness on the involved side of the face with exertion. A lighter colored iris supports the diagnosis of a congenital Horner's syndrome.

The diagnosis of Horner's syndrome can be further substantiated by pharmacologic testing with 4–10% cocaine solution. Cocaine blocks the reuptake of norepinephrine into the sympathetic nerve endings. In the normal eye the cocaine causes dilation of the pupil. However, if there is any lesion on the sympathetic chain an insufficient quantity of norepinephrine will accumulate and the involved pupil will not dilate as well as the normal one. Hydroxyamphetamine drops can be used to distinguish between first-/second-order neuron involvement and third-order neuron involvement.[6, 7]

The differential diagnosis would include physiologic anisocoria (natural variation in pupil size, not pathologic). Cranial third nerve palsy causes ptosis but also should display motility

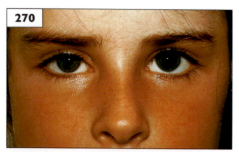

270 Right Horner's syndrome with slight ptosis, enophthalmos, pupillary constriction and decreased sweating. (From Strobel S *et al. Paediatrics and Child Health – The Great Ormond Street Colour Handbook*, Manson Publishing.)

disturbances, and the pupil should be large and nonreactive if the third nerve palsy involves the pupil. Iris sphincter muscle damage from trauma or intraocular inflammation can lead to a smaller pupil. Use of certain iris sphincter constricting eyedrops could lead to a smaller pupil.

MANAGEMENT/TREATMENT

As noted above it may be necessary to test with cocaine drops to confirm the diagnosis of Horner's syndrome. If the etiology is known, such as chest surgery, chest tubes, neck surgery, central venous catheterization, brachial plexus injury, or brainstem lesions on MRI, then no further work-up is indicated. If the etiology is unknown a work-up is indicated regardless of whether the onset of the Horner's syndrome is congenital or acquired. Work-up should include MRI of brain and orbits, neck, and upper chest to the level of the aortic arch. This ensures complete imaging of the oculosympathetic pathway. Many cases have no obvious etiology. The ptosis can be corrected with surgery but it is usually quite mild and not problematic. Mild dilating drops can enlarge the pupil but typically are not used by these patients. The vision in the involved eye is normal.

Congenital ocular motor apraxia

DEFINITION/OVERVIEW AND ETIOLOGY

Congenital ocular motor apraxia is characterized by impaired ability to generate quick (typically horizontal) eye movements on command. The eye movements can be elicited with horizontal head movements but not volitionally.[8] CNS abnormalities have been noted which include bilateral lesions of the frontoparietal cortex, agenesis of the corpus callosum, hydrocephalus, and cerebellar abnormalities. Frequently neuroimaging is normal.

CLINICAL PRESENTATION

Congenital ocular motor apraxia is characterized by an inability to generate normal voluntary horizontal saccades. The movement abnormality is noted in the first few months of life. The child may not appear to fixate and follow objects normally and can be erroneously diagnosed as being blind. Between the ages of 3 and 5 months the child will begin a characteristic head thrusting in order to move the eyes horizontally to fixate on targets. Vertical voluntary eye movements are typically normal. The head thrusts made by these patients reflect an adaptive strategy to change their eye position. In order to see an object the head will thrust toward the target and overshoot it. As the head is thrust the eyes deviate in the opposite direction and slowly come to rest on the target. Then the head slowly normalizes its position. The mechanism evoked is called the vestibulo-oculoreflex.

DIAGNOSIS AND DIFFERENTIAL DIAGNOSIS

The diagnosis of congenital ocular motor apraxia is made clinically. Lesions of the cerebral hemispheres can cause movement abnormalities. Blindness from anterior or posterior visual pathway disease can imitate congenital ocular motor apraxia.

MANAGEMENT/TREATMENT

There is no treatment for congenital ocular motor apraxia. The head thrusts may improve in later childhood.

Myasthenia gravis

DEFINITION/OVERVIEW AND ETIOLOGY

Myasthenia gravis is a disease of abnormal neuromuscular transmission characterized by variable muscle weakness and fatigability of affected skeletal muscles, particularly the extraocular muscles and eyelids. There is a reduction in the number of acetylcholine receptors available at the muscle endplate. The nerve terminal releases an adequate amount of acetylcholine but with fewer endplates and endplate potentials produced, the end result is inefficient neuromuscular transmission and a weak muscle. The decrease in number of postsynaptic acetylcholine receptors is believed to be due to an autoimmune process whereby acetylcholine receptor antibodies are produced and block the receptors. For unknown reasons the disease affects predominantly the extraocular muscles and eyelids.

CLINICAL PRESENTATION

The hallmark feature of myasthenia gravis is variability of strength of the affected muscles. Ptosis may occur as an isolated sign or in association with extraocular muscle involvement. It is usually fleeting and fluctuating, shifting from one eye to the other. The ptosis may be bilateral and usually is asymmetric. The ptosis may be absent on awakening but appear later in the day. Involvement of the extraocular muscles, like ptosis, is extremely common in patients with myasthenia gravis. In most cases eye alignment abnormalities are associated with ptosis. All degrees of ocular motor dysfunction may occur from a single isolated muscle involvement to complete ophthalmoplegia.[9]

The disease may be purely ocular but in the most severe form occurs as part of a major systemic disorder with other skeletal muscles involved. Other signs and symptoms include weakness in the muscles of mastication, extensors of the neck, trunk, and limbs, dysphasia, hoarseness, dysarthria, and dyspnea. Dysphasia and dyspnea can be life-threatening. The onset of myasthenia gravis may occur at any age but is uncommon in children. A transient neonatal form, caused by the placental transfer of acetylcholine receptor antibodies from mothers with myasthenia gravis, typically resolves quickly.

DIAGNOSIS AND DIFFERENTIAL DIAGNOSIS

The diagnosis of myasthenia gravis can be made clinically by identifying typical signs and symptoms. Roughly half of patients with ocular myasthenia will have elevated acetylcholine receptor antibodies on serologic testing. The diagnosis can also be made pharmacologically by overcoming the receptor block through the administration of acetylcholinesterase inhibitors such as edrophonium. Other office-based tests can be performed such as the sleep test or ice pack test. The sleep test is performed by having the patient take a 30-minute nap and upon awakening the ptosis or motility disturbance is reassessed. Improvement is highly suggestive of myasthenia gravis. The ice pack test is appropriate for patients with ptosis but not strabismus. An ice pack is placed on the closed eyelid for 2 minutes. If there is improvement in the ptosis on removal of the ice pack this is suggestive of myasthenia gravis.[10] Repetitive nerve stimulation shows a decremental response in many patients with systemic myasthenia gravis. Single fiber electromyography is most sensitive but is not widely available.

Differential diagnoses that should be considered are: botulism, chronic progressive external ophthalmoplegia (Kearns–Sayre syndrome), Lambert–Eaton myasthenic syndrome, drug-induced myasthenic-like syndrome, and congenital myasthenic syndromes.

MANAGEMENT/TREATMENT

Medical treatment for myasthenia gravis includes acetylcholinesterase inhibitors, corticosteroids, and other immunosuppressive agents. Thymectomy is the treatment of choice in patients with generalized myasthenia gravis with thymic enlargement. Purely ocular myasthenia gravis is usually not treated by thymectomy. The presence of a thymoma requires thymectomy.

Ocular tumors

Carol L. Shields, MD and Jerry A. Shields, MD

- **Introduction**

- **Clinical signs of childhood ocular tumors**
  Eyelid and conjunctiva
  Intraocular tumors
  Orbital tumors

- **Diagnostic approaches**
  Eyelid and conjunctiva
  Intraocular tumors
  Orbital tumors

- **Therapeutic approaches**
  Eyelid and conjunctiva
  Intraocular tumors
  Orbital tumors

- **Eyelid tumors**
  Capillary hemangioma
  Facial nevus flammeus
  Kaposi's sarcoma
  Basal cell carcinoma
  Melanocytic nevus
  Neurofibroma
  Neurilemoma (schwannoma)

- **Conjunctival tumors**
  Introduction
  Choristomatous conjunctival tumors
  Epithelial conjunctival tumors
  Melanocytic conjunctival tumors
  Vascular conjunctival tumors
  Xanthomatous conjunctival tumors
  Lymphoid/leukemic conjunctival tumors
  Non-neoplastic lesions that simulate conjunctival tumors
  Conclusions

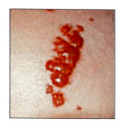 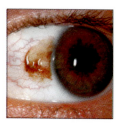 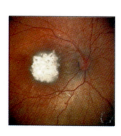 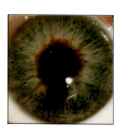

- **Intraocular tumors**
  Retinoblastoma
  Retinal capillary hemangioma
  Retinal cavernous hemangioma
  Retinal racemose hemangioma
  Astrocytic hamartoma of the retina
  Melanocytoma of the optic nerve
  Intraocular medulloepithelioma
  Choroidal hemangioma
  Choroidal osteoma
  Uveal nevus
  Uveal melanoma
  Congenital hypertrophy of retinal
  pigment epithelium
  Leukemia

- **Orbital tumors**
  Dermoid cyst
  Teratoma
  Capillary hemangioma
  Lymphangioma
  Juvenile pilocytic astrocytoma
  Rhabdomyosarcoma
  Granulocytic sarcoma ('chloroma')
  Lymphoma
  Langerhan's cell histiocytosis
  Metastatic neuroblastoma

Introduction

Several benign and malignant ocular tumors can occur in childhood. Tumors in the ocular region can lead to loss of vision, loss of the eye and, in the case of malignant neoplasms, to loss of life. Therefore, it is important for the clinician to recognize childhood ocular tumors and to refer affected patients for further diagnostic studies and appropriate management. Based on the authors' extensive clinical experience with ocular tumors during the last 35 years, some general concepts of childhood eye tumors are reviewed and the clinical manifestations of selected specific tumors of the eyelid, conjunctiva, intraocular structures and orbit in children are discussed.[1–5]

Clinical signs of childhood ocular tumors

The clinical characteristics of childhood ocular tumors vary as to whether the tumor is located in the eyelids, conjunctiva, intraocular tissues, or the orbit.

Eyelid and conjunctiva

Eyelid and conjunctival tumors are generally quite evident, prompting an early visit to a physician. Since most tumors in the ocular area have characteristic features, an accurate diagnosis of eyelid and conjunctival tumors can usually be made with inspection alone. Therefore, additional diagnostic studies are often unnecessary.

Intraocular tumors

Unlike tumors of the eyelids and conjunctiva, intraocular tumors are not readily visible. Infants and very young children do not complain of visual loss and their visual acuity is difficult to assess. However, there are several features that should alert the pediatrician to consider the possibility of an intraocular tumor and prompt a timely referral.

LEUKOCORIA

One of the more important signs of an intraocular tumor in children is leukocoria, or a white pupillary reflex (**271**). There are many causes of leukocoria in children.[2,4–7] The more common causes include congenital cataract, retinal detachment due to retinopathy of prematurity, persistent hyperplastic primary vitreous, and Coats' disease. Retinoblastoma is probably the most serious condition to cause leukocoria in children. Any child with leukocoria should be referred promptly to an ophthalmologist for further diagnostic evaluation.

STRABISMUS

Most children with strabismus do not have an intraocular tumor. However, about 30% of patients with retinoblastoma present initially with either esotropia or exotropia, due to the tumor location in the macular area which disrupts the child's fixation. It is important that a retinal examination using the indirect ophthalmoscope be performed on every child with strabismus to exclude an underlying tumor.

VISUAL IMPAIRMENT

An older child with an intraocular tumor may complain of visual impairment or may be found to have decreased vision on visual testing in school. This usually occurs from destruction of the central retina by the tumor or by the presence of vitreous hemorrhage, hyphema, or secondary cataract formation.

Orbital tumors

Unlike tumors of the eyelid and conjunctiva, orbital tumors cannot be directly visualized. Therefore, they often attain a relatively large size before becoming clinically evident. They generally present with proptosis or displacement of the eye. Pain, diplopia, and conjunctiva edema may also be early clinical features of an orbital tumor. Computed tomography (CT) and magnetic resonance imaging (MRI) have revolutionized the diagnosis and treatment of orbital tumors.[8] It is important to understand that CT in children could be associated with future cancer risk.[9]

Diagnostic approaches

Although some atypical tumors can defy clinical diagnosis, most ophthalmic tumors in children can be accurately diagnosed by a competent ophthalmologist or ocular oncologist.

Eyelid and conjunctiva

Most eyelid and conjunctival tumors are recognized by their typical clinical features, and special diagnostic studies are of little additional help. Smaller suspicious tumors in these tissues can be removed by excisional biopsy and the diagnosis established histopathologically. Larger tumors where the resulting defect cannot be repaired primarily, are best diagnosed by incisional biopsy and definitive treatment is withheld until a definite diagnosis has been established.

Intraocular tumors

Lesions of the iris can often be recognized with external ocular examination or slit-lamp biomicroscopy. Tumors of the retina and choroid can be visualized with ophthalmoscopy, which often reveals typical features depending on the type of tumor. Many small tumors are difficult to visualize and may only be detected by an experienced ophthalmologist using binocular indirect ophthalmoscopy. Ancillary studies such as fundus photography, autofluorescence, fluorescein angiography, indocyanine green angiography, ocular ultrasonography, and occasionally CT or MRI are of supplemental value in establishing the diagnosis. Optical coherence tomography (OCT) is a newer fundus scanning method using a rapid, noncontact technique with color-coded images in about 5 minutes. Children comfortably tolerate this technique.[10] OCT can provide *in vivo*, high-resolution information on the retina to the 10 μm level. Fine-needle aspiration biopsy (FNAB) has recently been employed in selected intraocular tumors of children.[11] Such procedures in children often require general anesthesia.

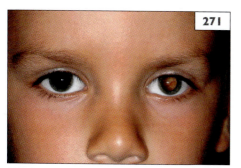

271

271 Leukocoria secondary to retinoblastoma.

Orbital tumors

Some orbital tumors occur in an anterior location and can be recognized by their extension into the conjunctiva and eyelid area. This is particularly true of childhood vascular tumors such as capillary hemangioma and lymphangioma. Other tumors reside in the deeper orbital tissues and are less accessible to inspection, palpation, and biopsy. Orbital ultrasonography can be performed quickly in many ophthalmologists' offices and can sometimes provide useful diagnostic information in cases of anterior orbital tumors. As mentioned earlier, CT and MRI have revolutionized orbital tumor diagnosis in children and have greatly improved the management of such cases.

Therapeutic approaches

The treatment of an ocular tumor in a child also depends on the location of the tumor and the size of the lesion.

Eyelid and conjunctiva

True neoplasms of the eyelid and conjunctiva can be removed surgically by a qualified ophthalmologist or ocular oncologist. Inflammatory lesions that simulate neoplasia can be managed by antibiotics or corticosteroids, depending on the diagnosis. Some malignant neoplasms such as leukemias and lymphomas are best managed with a limited diagnostic biopsy followed by irradiation and/or chemotherapy.

Intraocular tumors

The management of intraocular tumors is more complex. Certain benign intraocular tumors that are asymptomatic are usually managed by serial observation. Some symptomatic benign tumors can be treated with laser or cryotherapy depending on the mechanism of visual impairment. Malignant tumors, such as retinoblastoma, sometimes require enucleation of the eye. In recent years, however, there has been a trend away from enucleation for retinoblastoma, with the increasing use of more conservative methods of management, such as chemoreduction, thermotherapy, cryotherapy, and plaque radiotherapy.[2,4,12,13] Over the past 15 years, there has been a strong trend toward using chemoreduction to reduce the tumor(s) to a small size so that enucleation and irradiation can be avoided.[13]

Orbital tumors

The treatment of an orbital tumor varies greatly with the clinical or histopathologic diagnosis. Benign vascular tumors, such as capillary hemangioma and lymphangioma, can be managed by serial observation or patching treatment of the opposite eye to decrease the severity of associated amblyopia. Circumscribed tumors in the anterior orbit may be managed by excisional biopsy. Many malignant tumors, such as rhabdomyosarcoma and orbital leukemia, may require limited biopsy to establish the diagnosis, followed by irradiation or chemotherapy.[3,5]

Eyelid tumors

There are many pediatric cutaneous tumors that can affect the skin of the eyelids.[3,14] Only the more important tumors will be considered here.

Capillary hemangioma

The capillary hemangioma or strawberry hemangioma can occur on the skin in 10% of infants and is recognized to be more common in premature infants and twins (**272–275**). Capillary hemangioma of the eyelids can be a reddish, diffuse or circumscribed mass.[15] It usually has clinical onset at birth, or shortly thereafter, tends to enlarge for a few months, and then slowly regresses. The main complications of this benign tumor are strabismus and amblyopia. In recent years the most frequently used treatment has been refraction, glasses for refractive error, patching of the opposite eye, and close follow-up. More recently, there has been a trend toward corticosteroids or complete surgical excision of those lesions that are relatively small and localized. Intralesional or oral corticosteroids may hasten regression of the tumor in some cases (**274, 275**). Radiotherapy is almost never used today. Newer therapy using beta-blocker medications, both topical timoptic and oral propanolol, has been successful in treating capillary hemangioma. More research is being conducted in the use of these medications for this condition.

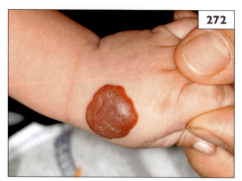

272 Cutaneous hemangioma in twin #2 on the hand.

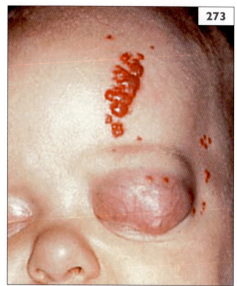

273 Extensive capillary hemangioma of the eyelid, facial skin, and orbit before treatment with systemic corticosteroids.

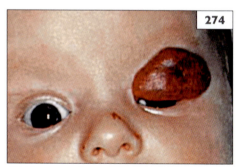

274 Large capillary hemangioma of the eyelid obstructing vision, before treatment.

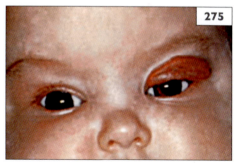

275 The capillary hemangioma in **264** after 2 months of oral corticosteroids. Note the tumor reduction and facial weight gain.

Facial nevus flammeus

Facial nevus flammeus is a congenital cutaneous vascular lesion that occurs in the distribution of the fifth cranial nerve (**276**). It may be an isolated entity or it may occur with variations of the SW syndrome. Infants with this lesion have a higher incidence of ipsilateral glaucoma, diffuse choroidal hemangioma, and secondary retinal detachment. Affected infants should be referred to an ophthalmologist as early as possible in order to diagnosis and treat these serious ocular conditions. Management of the cutaneous lesion includes observation, cosmetic make-up, or laser treatment.

Kaposi's sarcoma

Opportunistic neoplasms such as Kaposi's sarcoma can be found in immunosuppressed children, particularly those with acquired immune deficiency syndrome (AIDS). Although the affected patient can display red cutaneous lesions elsewhere, the eyelid can occasionally be the initial site of involvement. The lesion appears as a reddish-blue subcutaneous mass near the eyelid margin. It generally responds best to chemotherapy and radiotherapy.

Basal cell carcinoma

Although basal cell carcinoma is primarily a disease of adults, it is occasionally seen in younger patients, particularly if there is a family history of the basal cell carcinoma syndrome. It generally occurs on the lower eyelid as a slowly progressive mass that frequently develops a central ulcer (rodent ulcer). Lesions near the eyelid margin often develop loss of eyelashes in the area of involvement. Treatment is local excision using frozen section control and eyelid reconstruction.

Taylor *et al.* reviewed 39 patients with basal cell carcinoma syndrome (Gorlin–Goltz syndrome) and found the age of presentation to be between 5 and 72 years.[16] The presenting clinical features included odontogenic keratocyst (n=17 patients), basal cell carcinoma (n=13), and congenital malformations (n=2). Seventeen of the 39 patients confirmed a family history of the syndrome in a parent. Basal cell carcinoma developed in 18 of 28 (64%) patients before the age of 30 years. Thus this syndrome should be explored in any child with basal cell carcinoma.

Melanocytic nevus

A melanocytic nevus is a tumor composed of benign melanocytes. It can occur on the eyelid as a variably-pigmented well-circumscribed lesion, identical to those that occur elsewhere on the skin. It does not usually cause loss of cilia. In some instances, the nevus is congenital and large and involves both the upper and lower eyelids and is termed 'kissing nevus' or 'divided nevus'. There is some evidence that early intervention with curettage of the lesion within the first 3–4 weeks after birth can successfully remove the lesion without the need for extensive grafting. The nevus at an early stage is superficial and can be scraped off the superficial skin, whereas its involvement deepens into the subcutaneous tissue over time, making surgical removal more difficult. Following curettage, the affected infant is treated with topical antibiotic ointment and the skin heals by granulation.

The blue nevus is often apparent at birth, whereas the junctional or compound nevus may not become clinically apparent until puberty. Transformation into malignant melanoma is rare and usually occurs later in life. Although most eyelid nevi in children can be safely observed, they are occasionally excised because of cosmetic considerations or because of fear of malignant transformation.

Neurofibroma

A neurofibroma can occur on the eyelid as a diffuse or plexiform lesion that is often associated with von Recklinghausen's neurofibromatosis. In the earliest stages the lesion produces a characteristic S-shaped curve to the upper lid. Larger lesions produce thickening of the eyelid with secondary blepharoptosis (**277**). Since these diffuse tumors are often difficult or impossible to completely excise, they should be managed by periodic observation or surgical debulking if they cause a major cosmetic problem.[17]

Neurilemoma (schwannoma)

Neurilemoma is a benign peripheral nerve sheath tumor that is composed purely of Schwann cells of peripheral nerves. It more commonly occurs in the orbit of young adults, but it can appear as a solitary eyelid lesion in children.[18] It often occurs as a circumscribed solitary lesion (**278**) unassociated with neurofibromatosis. It is a benign tumor that can be excised surgically.

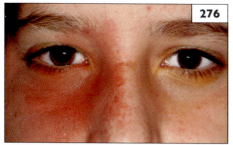

276 Nevus flammeus of the face in a child with Sturge–Weber syndrome.

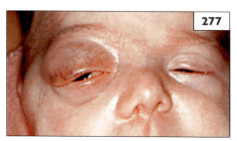

277 Neurofibroma of the eyelid and orbit in an infant.

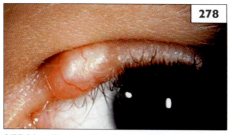

278 Neurilemoma in a 9-year-old boy.

Conjunctival tumors

Introduction

Tumors of the conjunctiva and epibulbar tissues involve a large spectrum of conditions ranging from benign lesions such as limbal dermoid, myxoma, and scleral melanocytosis to aggressive, life-threatening malignancies such as melanoma, Kaposi's sarcoma, and sebaceous carcinoma.[1,3,19–22] The clinical differentiation of the various tumors is based primarily on the clinical features of the tumor as well as the patient's history. The clinical features as well as the management of each tumor are discussed in detail elsewhere, based on the authors' personal experience with over 1600 patients with conjunctival tumors over a 30-year period.[22]

Several previously published surveys[20–22] have reported on the incidence of conjunctival lesions in adults. However, the epidemiologic features, anatomic characteristics, and malignant potential of such lesions differ in the pediatric age group. There have been only three large series of conjunctival tumors in children, two using a pathologic approach,[23,24] and one from clinical data[1] (*Tables 27, 28, overleaf*).

In a clinical series of 262 children referred to an oncology service with a conjunctival tumor, the most common lesions were of melanocytic (67%), choristomatous (10%), vascular (9%), and benign epithelial (2%) origin[1] (*Table 27*). Ten percent of cases were non-neoplastic lesions simulating a tumor such as epithelial inclusion cyst, nonspecific inflammation/infection, episcleritis, scleritis, and foreign body.

The following tumors are classified based on tissues of origin including choristomatous, epithelial, melanocytic, vascular, fibrous, xanthomatous, and lymphoid/leukemic origin.

Choristomatous conjunctival tumors

A variety of tumors can be present at birth or become clinically apparent shortly after birth. Most of the lesions are choristomas, consisting of displaced tissue elements not normally found in these areas. A simple choristoma is comprised of one tissue element such as epithelium, whereas a complex choristoma represents variable combinations of ectopic tissues such as bone, cartilage, and lacrimal gland.

Table 27 Clinical diagnostic categories of conjunctival tumors in 262 children[1]

Classification of tumors	Number of patients (~%)	Classification of tumors	Number of patients (~%)
Choristomatous	26 (10)	Myxomatous	0 (0)
Benign epithelial	5 (2)	Lipomatous	0 (0)
Premalignant and malignant epithelial	1 (<1)	Lacrimal gland	0 (0)
		Lymphoid	4 (2)
Melanocytic	175 (67)	Leukemic	0 (0)
Vascular	23 (9)	Metastatic	0 (0)
Fibrous	2 (<1)	Secondary	0 (0)
Neural	0 (0)	Non-neoplastic lesions simulating a tumor	25 (10)
Xanthomatous	1 (<1)		

Data from the Oncology Service at Wills Eye Institute

Table 28 Comparison of data from three series of conjunctival lesions in young patients

Classification of tumors	% tumors	% tumors	% tumors
Data source	Clinical series Shields, Shields (2007)[1] n = 262	Pathology series Cunha et al. (1987)[24] n = 282	Pathology series Elsas, Green (1975)[23] n = 302
Choristomatous	10	22	33
Benign epithelial (papilloma)	2	10	7
Premalignant and malignant epithelial	<1	0	1
Melanocytic	67	23	29
Vascular	9	6	2
Fibrous	<1	na	<1
Neural	0	1	na
Xanthomatous	<1	na	na
Myxomatous	0	na	na
Lipomatous	0	4	2
Lacrimal gland	0	na	na
Lymphoid	2	3	na
Leukemic	0	na	na
Metastatic	0	na	na
Secondary	0	na	na
Non-neoplastic lesions simulating a tumor*	10	30*	23

*Includes epithelial inclusion cyst, inflammatory lesions, vernal conjunctivitis, pyogenic granuloma, nonspecific granuloma, foreign body, scar tissue, keloid, and others.

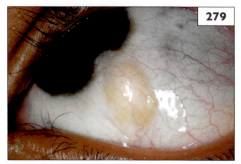
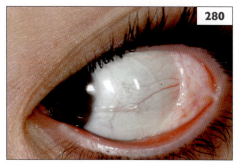

279, 280 Congenital choristomas. **279:** Conjunctival dermoid; **280:** conjunctival lipodermoid.

DERMOID

Conjunctival dermoid is a congenital well-circumscribed yellow-white solid mass that involves the bulbar or limbal conjunctiva.[25,26] It characteristically occurs inferotemporally and often this tumor has fine white hairs (**279**). In rare cases, it can extend to the central cornea or be located in other quadrants on the bulbar surface. Most often dermoid straddles the limbus, but in rare instances it can be extensive and involve the full thickness of the cornea, anterior chamber, and iris stroma. The more severe dermoids occur earlier in embryogenesis.

Conjunctival dermoid can occur as a solitary lesion or can be associated with Goldenhar's syndrome. The patient should be evaluated for ipsilateral or bilateral preauricular skin appendages, hearing loss, eyelid coloboma, orbitoconjunctival dermolipoma, and cervical vertebral anomalies. Histopathologically, the conjunctival dermoid is a simple choristomatous malformation that consists of dense fibrous tissue lined by conjunctival epithelium with deeper dermal elements including hair follicles and sebaceous glands.

The management of an epibulbar dermoid includes observation if the lesion is small and visually asymptomatic. It is possible to excise the lesion for cosmetic reasons, but the remaining corneal scar can be cosmetically unacceptable. Larger or symptomatic dermoids can produce visual loss from astigmatism. These can be approached by lamellar keratosclerectomy with primary closure of overlying tissue if the defect is superficial, or closure using corneal graft if the defect is deep or full thickness. The cosmetic appearance might improve, but the refractive and astigmatic errors and visual acuity might not change. When the lesion involves the central cornea, a lamellar or penetrating keratoplasty is necessary and long-term amblyopia should be anticipated.

DERMOLIPOMA

Dermolipoma is believed to be congenital, but it classically remains asymptomatic for years and might not be detected until adulthood. It typically occurs in the conjunctival fornix superotemporally and appears as a yellow, soft, fluctuant mass with fine white hairs on its surface (**280**). It can extend into the orbital fat and onto the bulbar conjunctiva, sometimes reaching the limbus.

Dermolipoma has features similar to orbital fat on CT and MRI. Histopathologically, it is lined by conjunctival epithelium on its surface and the subepithelial tissue has variable quantities of collagenous connective tissue and adipose tissue. Pilosebaceous units and lacrimal gland tissue might be present. The majority of dermolipomas require no treatment, but larger ones or those that are cosmetically unappealing can be managed by excision of the entire orbitoconjunctival lesion through a conjunctival forniceal approach, or by removing the anterior portion of the lesion in a manner similar to that used to remove prolapsed orbital fat.

EPIBULBAR OSSEOUS CHORISTOMA

Epibulbar osseous choristoma is a firm deposit of bone, usually located in the bulbar conjunctiva superotemporally (**281**).[3] It is believed to be congenital and typically remains undetected until palpated by the older patient. On ultrasonography or CT the mass demonstrates a calcium component. This tumor is usually managed by observation. Occasionally a foreign body sensation necessitates excision of the mass using a conjunctival forniceal incision followed by dissection of the tumor to bare sclera.

LACRIMAL GLAND CHORISTOMA

Lacrimal gland choristoma is a congenital lesion, discovered in young children as an asymptomatic pink stromal mass, typically in the superotemporal or temporal portion of the conjunctiva. It is speculated that this lesion represents small sequestrations of the embryonic evagination of the lacrimal gland from the conjunctiva. The lacrimal gland choristoma can masquerade as a focus of inflammation due to its pink color. Rarely, this mass can be cystic due to ongoing secretions if there is no connection to the conjunctival surface. Excisional biopsy is usually performed to confirm the diagnosis.

COMPLEX CHORISTOMA

The conjunctival dermoid and epibulbar osseous choristoma are simple choristomas as they contain one tissue type such as skin or bone. A complex choristoma contains a greater variety of tissue derived from two germ layers such as lacrimal tissue and cartilage. It is variable in its clinical appearance and can cover much of the epibulbar surface or it may form a circumferential growth pattern around the limbus. The complex choristoma has an association with the linear nevus sebaceous of Jadassohn (**282**).[25] The nevus sebaceous of Jadassohn includes cutaneous features with nevus sebaceous in the facial region and neurologic features including seizures, mental retardation, arachnoidal cyst, and cerebral atrophy. The ophthalmic features of this syndrome include epibulbar complex choristoma and posterior scleral cartilage. The management of complex choristoma depends upon the extent of the lesion. Observation and wide local excision followed by mucous membrane graft reconstruction are options.

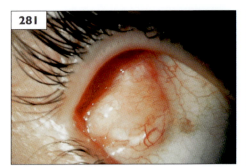

281 Congenital choristomas: conjunctival osseous choristoma.

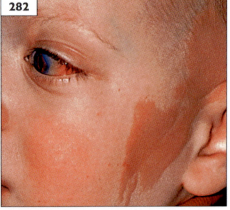

282 Complex conjunctival choristoma in a child with nevus sebaceous of Jadassohn and organoid nevus syndrome.

Epithelial conjunctival tumors

There are several benign and malignant tumors that can arise from the squamous epithelium of the conjunctiva.

PAPILLOMA

Squamous papilloma is a benign tumor, documented to be associated with human papillomavirus (subtypes 6, 11, 16, and 18) infection of the conjunctiva.[27,28] This tumor can occur in both children and adults. It is speculated that the virus is acquired through transfer from the mother's vagina to the newborn's conjunctiva as the child passes through the mother's birth canal. Papillomas appear as a pink fibrovascular frond of tissue arranged in a sessile or pedunculated configuration (**283**). The numerous fine vascular channels ramify through the stroma beneath the epithelial surface of the lesion. In children, the lesion is usually small, multiple, and located in the inferior fornix. Histopathologically, the lesion shows numerous vascularized papillary fronds lined by acanthotic epithelium.

There are several treatment options for small sessile papillomas in a child. Sometimes, periodic observation allows for slow spontaneous resolution of the viral-produced tumor. Larger or more pedunculated lesions with foreign body sensation, chronic mucous production, hemorrhagic tears, incomplete eyelid closure, and poor cosmetic appearance probably require surgical excision. Complete removal of the mass without direction manipulation of the tumor (no touch technique) is advisable to avoid spreading of the virus.[29,30] Double freeze–thaw cryotherapy is applied to the remaining conjunctiva around the excised lesion in order to prevent tumor recurrence. In some instances, the pedunculated tumor is frozen alone and then excised while frozen or allowed to slough off the conjunctival surface later. Topical interferon and mitomycin C have been employed for resistant or multiply recurrent conjunctival papillomas.[31,32] For difficult recurrent lesions, oral cimetidine for several months following surgical resection can minimize recurrence by boosting the patient's immune system and suppressing the virally-stimulated mass.[33]

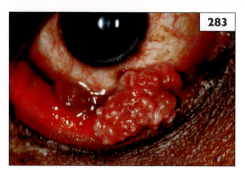

283 Conjunctival papilloma.

HEREDITARY BENIGN INTRAEPITHELIAL DYSKERATOSIS

Hereditary benign intraepithelial dyskeratosis (HBID) is a rare benign condition seen in an inbred isolate of Caucasian, African-American, and American Indians (Haliwa Indians). This group resided initially in North Carolina. It is an autosomal dominant (AD) disorder characterized by bilateral elevated fleshy plaques on the nasal or temporal perilimbal conjunctiva and on the buccal mucosa. It can remain asymptomatic or can cause redness and foreign body sensation. It is characterized histopathologically by acanthosis, dyskeratosis on the epithelial surface and deep within the epithelium, and prominent chronic inflammatory cells. HBID does not usually require aggressive treatment. Smaller, less symptomatic lesions can be treated with ocular lubricants and topical corticosteroids. Larger symptomatic lesions can be managed by local resection with mucous membrane grafting if necessary.

SQUAMOUS CELL CARCINOMA/ CONJUNCTIVAL INTRAEPITHELIAL NEOPLASIA

Squamous cell carcinoma and conjunctival intraepithelial neoplasia (CIN) are malignancies of the surface epithelial cells. Intraepithelial neoplasia displays anaplastic cells within the epithelium, whereas squamous cell carcinoma displays extension of anaplastic cells through the basement membrane into the conjunctival stroma. Clinically, invasive squamous cell carcinoma is usually larger and more elevated

Table 29 Differential diagnosis of pigmented epibulbar lesions[1]

Condition	Anatomic location	Color	Depth	Margins	Laterality	Other features	Progression
Nevus	Inter-palpebral limbus usually	Brown or yellow	Stroma	Well defined	Unilateral	Cysts	<1% progress to conjunctival melanoma
Racial melanosis	Limbus > bulbar > palpebral conjunctiva	Brown	Epithelium	Ill defined	Bilateral	Flat, no cysts	Very rare progression to conjunctival melanoma
Ocular melanocytosis	Bulbar conjunctiva	Gray	Episclera	Ill defined	Unilateral more so than bilateral	Congenital, usually 2 mm from limbus, often with periocular skin pigmentation	<1% progress to uveal melanoma
Primary acquired melanosis (PAM)	Anywhere, but usually bulbar conjunctiva	Brown	Epithelium	Ill defined	Unilateral	Flat, no cysts	Progresses to conjunctival melanoma in up to nearly 50% of cases that show cellular atypia
Malignant melanoma	Anywhere	Brown or pink	Stroma	Well defined	Unilateral	Vascular nodule, dilated feeder vessels, may be nonpigmented	32% develop metastasis by 15 years

than CIN. Leukoplakia can be seen with either condition.

Patients who are medically immunosuppressed for organ transplantation, those with human immunodeficiency virus (HIV), or those with underlying deoxyribonucleic acid (DNA) repair abnormalities like xeroderma pigmentosum are at particular risk of developing conjunctival squamous cell carcinoma and malignant melanoma. In these cases, the risk of life-threatening metastatic disease is greater.

The management of squamous cell carcinoma of the conjunctiva varies with the extent of the lesion. Tumors in the limbal area require alcohol epitheliectomy for the corneal component and partial lamellar scleroconjunctivectomy with wide margins for the conjunctival component, followed by freeze–thaw cryotherapy to the remaining adjacent bulbar conjunctiva. Extensive tumors or those tumors that are recurrent, especially with an extensive corneal component, are treated with adjuvant topical mitomycin C, 5-fluorouracil, or interferon.[31,32,34,35]

Melanocytic conjunctival tumors

There are several lesions that arise from the melanocytes of the conjunctiva and episclera. The most important ones include nevus, racial melanosis, primary acquired melanosis, and malignant melanoma (*Table 29*). Ocular melanocytosis should be included in this section as its scleral pigmentation can masquerade as conjunctival pigmentation.

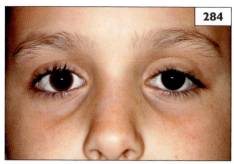

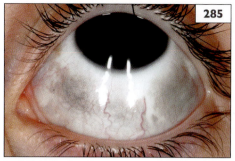

284 Ocular melanocytosis. Heterochromia with light brown right iris and dark brown left iris.

285 Episcleral melanocytosis.

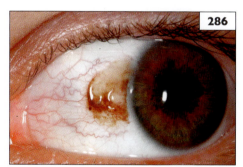

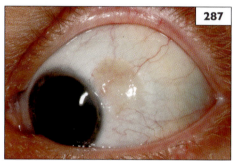

286, 287 Melanocytic conjunctival lesions. **286:** Partially pigmented conjunctival nevus with cysts; **287:** nonpigmented conjunctival nevus.

OCULAR MELANOCYTOSIS

Ocular melanocytosis is a congenital pigmentary condition of the periocular skin, sclera, orbit, meninges, and soft palate. Typically, there is no conjunctival pigment. However, this condition is clinically confused with primary acquired melanosis (*Table 29*). In ocular melanocytosis, flat, gray pigment scattered posterior to the limbus on the sclera is visualized through the thin overlying conjunctival tissue (**284, 285**). The entire uvea can also be affected by similar increased pigment. This condition imparts a 1 in 400 risk for the development of uveal melanoma and not conjunctival melanoma.[36] Affected patients should be followed once or twice yearly for the development of uveal, orbital, or meningeal melanoma.

NEVUS

The conjunctival nevus is the most common melanocytic tumor. It becomes clinically apparent in the first or second decade of life as a discrete, variably pigmented, slightly elevated lesion that contains fine clear cysts in 65% of cases.[37,38] Conjunctival nevi can manifest as a darkly pigmented (65%), lightly pigmented (19%), and completely nonpigmented (16%) mass (**286, 287**).[38] It is typically located in the interpalpebral bulbar conjunctiva near the limbus and remains stationary throughout life, with less than a 1% risk for transformation into malignant melanoma.[37,38] Over time, a nevus can become more or less pigmented in 5% of cases and show evidence of enlargement in 7%.[38]

Histopathologically the conjunctival nevus is composed of nests of benign melanocytes in the stroma near the basal layers of the epithelium. Like cutaneous nevus, it can be junctional, compound, or deep. The management is usually periodic observation with photographic comparison. If growth is documented, then local excision of the lesion should be considered. In some cases, excision for cosmetic reasons is desired. At the time of excision, the entire mass is removed using the no touch technique, and if it is adherent to the globe, then a thin lamella of underlying sclera is removed intact with the tumor. Standard double freeze–thaw cryotherapy is applied to the remaining conjunctival margins. These precautions are employed to prevent recurrence of the nevus and also to prevent recurrence should the lesion prove to be a melanoma.

RACIAL MELANOSIS

Racial melanosis is an acquired pigmentation of the conjunctiva usually detected in darkly pigmented individuals and occasionally in children. This pigment is most often present at the limbus and less on the limbal cornea and bulbar conjunctiva. This pigmentation can occasionally be patchy in appearance and rarely does melanoma arise from this condition. Histopathologically, the pigmented cells are benign melanocytes located in the basal layer of the epithelium. The recommended management is observation.

PRIMARY ACQUIRED MELANOSIS

Primary acquired melanosis (PAM) is an important benign conjunctival pigmentary condition that can give rise to conjunctival melanoma. In contrast to conjunctival nevus, it is acquired in middle age and rarely in children. It appears diffuse, patchy, flat, and noncystic. In contrast to ocular melanocytosis, the pigment is acquired, located within the conjunctiva, and appears brown, not gray, in color (**288**).[39,40] In contrast to racial melanosis, PAM generally is found in fair-skinned individuals as a unilateral patchy condition.

Histopathologically, PAM is characterized by the presence of abnormal melanocytes near the basal layer of the epithelium. Pathologists should attempt to classify the melanocytes as having atypia or no atypia based on nuclear features and growth pattern. PAM with atypia carries a 13–46% risk for ultimate evolution into malignant melanoma, whereas PAM without atypia carries a nearly 0% risk for melanoma development.[39,40]

The management of PAM depends on the extent of involvement and the association with melanoma. If there is only a small region of PAM, occupying less than 3 'clock hours' of the conjunctiva, then periodic observation or complete excisional biopsy and cryotherapy are options. If the PAM occupies more than three clock hours, then incisional map biopsy of all four quadrants is warranted, followed by double freeze–thaw cryotherapy to all affected pigmented sites. If the patient has a history of melanoma or if there are areas of nodularity or vascularity suspicious for melanoma, then a more aggressive approach is warranted with complete excisional biopsy of the suspicious areas using the no touch technique.[29,30] Topical mitomycin C can also be beneficial, especially if there is recurrent corneal PAM. This medication should be used with extreme caution in children due to its toxicities.[41]

MALIGNANT MELANOMA

Malignant melanoma of the conjunctiva most often arises from PAM, but can also arise from a pre-existing nevus or *de novo*.[42–44] It typically arises in middle-aged to older adults, but rare cases of conjunctival melanoma in children have been recognized (**289**). In the authors' practice, 1% of all conjunctival melanoma occur in children. Conjunctival melanoma shows considerable clinical variability, as it can be pigmented or nonpigmented, pink, yellow, or brown in color, and involve the limbal, bulbar, forniceal, or palpebral conjunctiva.

Vascular conjunctival tumors

There are severeal vascular tumors of the conjunctiva including capillary hemangioma, lymphangioma, pyogenic granuloma, cavernous hemangioma, racemose hemangioma, varix, hemangiopericytoma, and Kaposi's sarcoma. The first three conditions are typically found in children or young adults.

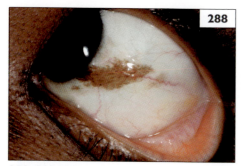
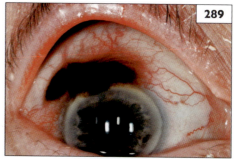

288, 289 Melanocytic conjunctival lesions. **288:** Primary acquired melanosis; **289:** conjunctival melanoma.

CAPILLARY HEMANGIOMA

Capillary hemangioma of the conjunctiva generally presents in infancy several weeks following birth, as a red stromal mass, sometimes associated with a cutaneous or orbital component. Similar to its cutaneous counterpart, the conjunctival mass might enlarge over several months and then spontaneously involute. Management includes observation most commonly, but surgical resection or local or systemic prednisone can be employed.

LYMPHANGIOMA

Conjunctival lymphangioma can occur as an isolated conjunctival lesion or it can represent a superficial component of a deeper diffuse orbital lymphangioma. It usually becomes clinically apparent in the first decade of life and appears as a multiloculated mass containing variable-sized clear dilated cystic channels. In most instances, blood is visible in many of the cystic spaces. These have been called 'chocolate cysts'. The treatment of conjunctival lymphangioma is often difficult because surgical resection or radiotherapy cannot completely eradicate the mass.

PYOGENIC GRANULOMA

Pyogenic granuloma is a proliferative fibrovascular response to prior tissue insult by inflammation, surgery, or nonsurgical trauma. It is sometimes classified as a polypoid form of acquired capillary hemangioma. It appears clinically as an elevated red mass, often with a prominent blood supply. Microscopically, it is composed of granulation tissue with chronic inflammatory cells and numerous small-caliber blood vessels. Since the lesion is rarely pyogenic nor granulomatous, the term 'pyogenic granuloma' may be a misnomer. Pyogenic granuloma will sometimes respond to topical corticosteroids but many cases ultimately require surgical excision.

Xanthomatous conjunctival tumors

Xanthomatous conjunctival tumors include juvenile xanthogranuloma, found in children, and xanthoma and reticulohistiocytoma, typically found in adults.

JUVENILE XANTHOGRANULOMA

Juvenile xanthogranuloma is a cutaneous condition that presents as painless, pink skin papules with spontaneous resolution, generally in children under the age of 2 years. Rarely, conjunctival, orbital, and intraocular involvement is noted. In the conjunctiva, the mass appears as an orange-pink stromal mass, typically in teenagers or young adults. If the classic skin lesions are noted, the diagnosis is established clinically and treatment with observation or topical steroid ointment is provided. Otherwise, biopsy is suggested and recognition of the typical histopathologic features of histiocytes admixed with Touton's giant cells confirms the diagnosis.

Lymphoid/leukemic conjunctival tumors

Lymphoid and leukemic tumors of the conjunctiva can appear as an orange-pink stromal mass. Systemic evaluation for underlying malignancy is important.

LYMPHOID TUMORS

Lymphoid tumors can occur in the conjunctiva as isolated lesions or they can be a manifestation of systemic lymphoma.[45–47] This condition is most often found in older adults and rarely in children. Clinically, the lesion appears as a diffuse, slightly elevated pink mass located in the stroma or deep to Tenon's fascia, most commonly in the forniceal region. This appearance is similar to that of smoked salmon; hence it is termed the 'salmon patch'. It is not possible to differentiate clinically between a benign and malignant lymphoid tumor. Therefore, biopsy is necessary to establish the diagnosis and a systemic evaluation should be done in all affected patients to exclude the presence of systemic lymphoma. The lymphoid tumors found in children are most often hyperplasia and not lymphoma and generally not associated with systemic lymphoma. Treatment of the conjunctival lesion should include chemotherapy or rituximab if the patient has systemic lymphoma or external beam irradiation (2000–4000 cGy) if the lesion is localized to the conjunctiva. Other options include excisional biopsy and cryotherapy, local interferon injections, or observation. There is new information that some lymphoid tumors are related to *Helicobacter pylori* or *Chlamydia psittaci* infection, and treatment with appropriate antibiotics could be beneficial.

LEUKEMIA

Leukemia generally manifests in the ocular region as hemorrhages from associated anemia and thrombocytopenia rather than leukemic infiltration. In the rare instance of leukemic infiltration of the conjunctiva, the mass appears pink and smooth within the conjunctival stroma at either the limbus or the fornix, similar to a lymphoid tumor. Biopsy reveals sheets of large leukemic cells. Treatment of the systemic condition is advised with secondary resolution of the conjunctival infiltration.

Non-neoplastic lesions that simulate conjunctival tumors

A number of non-neoplastic conditions can simulate neoplasms. These include epithelial inclusion cyst, inflammatory lesions, vernal conjunctivitis, pyogenic granuloma, nonspecific granuloma, foreign body, scar tissue, keloid, and others. In most instances, the history and clinical findings should allow for the diagnosis; however, excision of the mass might be necessary in order to exclude a neoplasm.

Conclusions

Most conjunctival tumors in children are benign. The majority of conjunctival tumors in children are pigmented or nonpigmented nevi. Conjunctival nevi often manifest intralesional cysts. Conjunctival nevi rarely evolve into melanoma (<1%). Episcleral melanocytosis is a sign of possible uveal melanocytosis and all affected eyes should be dilated once or twice a year for examination as there is a small risk for uveal melanoma. Conjunctival papillomas can be treated with observation, cryotherapy, topical chemotherapy, or interferon, and oral cimetidine.

Intraocular tumors

Retinoblastoma

Retinoblastoma represents approximately 4% of all pediatric malignancies and is the most common intraocular malignancy in children.[2,4,48] It is estimated that 250–300 new cases of retinoblastoma are diagnosed in the US each year and 5,000 cases are found worldwide. Large countries like India and China individually estimate approximately 1,000 new cases of retinoblastoma per year. Most (>95%) children with retinoblastoma in the US and other medically developed nations survive their malignancy, whereas approximately 50% survive worldwide. The reason for the poor survival in undeveloped nations relates to late detection of advanced retinoblastoma, often presenting with orbital invasion or metastatic disease. In Brazil, the mean age at presentation for retinoblastoma is approximately 25 months, compared to 18 months or less in the US.[49] The average Brazilian family delays seeking medical care for a mean of 6 months. The delay is longer if the only symptom is strabismus in an eye with retinoblastoma (lagtime is 9 months) compared to children with symptoms of leukocoria (lagtime is 6 months) or tumor mass (lagtime is 2 months).

SYSTEMIC CONCERNS WITH RETINOBLASTOMA

Retinoblastoma can be grouped in four different ways: sporadic or familial, unilateral or bilateral, nonheritable or heritable, and somatic or germline mutation. About two-thirds of all cases are unilateral and one-third of cases are bilateral. Genetically, it is simpler to discuss retinoblastoma with the latter classification of somatic or germline mutation. Germline mutation implies that the mutation is present in all cells of the body whereas somatic mutation means that only the tissue of concern, the retinoblastoma, has the mutation. All patients are offered genetic testing for retinoblastoma. The testing is performed on the tumor specimen (when available) and a blood sample. Mutations for retinoblastoma have been found predominantly on chromosome 13 long arm.[50]

Patients with germline mutation have mutation in both the tumor and the peripheral blood, whereas those with somatic mutation show only mutation in the tumor and not the blood. This implies that all cells might be affected with the mutation in germline cases so these patients could be at risk for other cancers (second cancers and pinealoblastoma). Patients with bilateral and familial retinoblastoma have presumed germline mutation because they have multifocal or heritable disease. Patients with unilateral sporadic retinoblastoma usually carry a somatic mutation, but approximately 7–15% of these patients will show a germline mutation. Multistep clinical molecular screening of 180 unrelated individuals with retinoblastoma found germline RB1 mutations in 77 out of 85 bilateral retinoblastoma patients (91%), 7 out of 10 familial unilateral patients (70%), and 6 out of 85 unilateral sporadic patients (7%). Mutations included 36 novel alterations spanning the entire RB1 gene.[50] Thus it is important to have children with retinoblastoma tested for genetic mutations, particularly those with unilateral sporadic retinoblastoma.

Children with retinoblastoma are at risk for three important, life-threatening problems: metastasis from retinoblastoma, intracranial neuroblastic malignancy (trilateral retinoblastoma/pinealoblastoma), and second primary cancers.

Retinoblastoma metastasis typically develops within 1 year of the diagnosis of the intraocular tumor. Those at greatest risk for metastasis show histopathologic features of retinoblastoma invasion beyond the lamina cribrosa in the optic nerve, in the choroid, sclera, orbit, or anterior chamber.[51–53] It is critical that a qualified ophthalmic pathologist examines the eye for the high-risk features. Optic nerve invasion has been found in approximately 30% of eyes that come to enucleation and choroidal invasion in approximately 30% of eyes.[51–53] So this feature is not uncommon and could be life-threatening to the patient. Patients with postlaminar optic nerve invasion or gross (>2 mm) choroidal invasion or a combination of any optic nerve or choroidal invasion should be treated with chemotherapy. The chemotherapy generally involves vincristine, etoposide, and carboplatin for 4–6 months to prevent metastastic disease.[53]

Pinealoblastoma or related brain tumors typically occur in the first 5 years of life, most often within 1 year of diagnosis of the retinoblastoma.[54,55] This has been termed

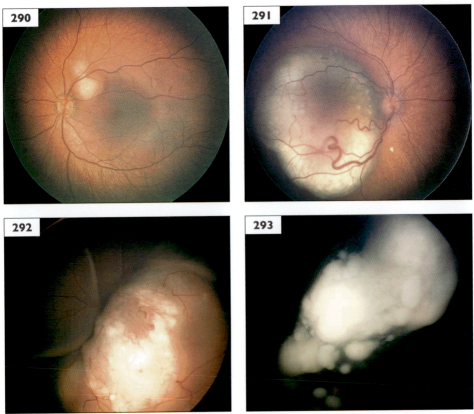

290–293 Clinical appearance of retinoblastoma. **290:** Small-sized intraretinal retinoblastomas; **291:** medium-sized intraretinal retinoblastoma with surrounding subretinal fluid; **292:** large-sized exophytic retinoblastoma with subretinal fluid; **293:** endophytic retinoblastoma.

'trilateral' retinoblastoma and overall is found in about 3% of all children with retinoblastoma, but those with germline mutation manifest this tumor in up to 10% of cases.[55] Unfortunately, pinealoblastoma is usually fatal with only a few survivors. Systemic chemotherapy, particularly the chemoreduction protocol currently used for retinoblastoma, might prevent trilateral retinoblastoma.[56] This remarkable observation indicates that neoadjuvant chemotherapy could be beneficial. Longer follow-up in our series of over 300 children with retinoblastoma treated with chemoreduction continues to show the same trend, with very few cases of pinealoblastoma. It should be noted that benign pineal cyst can simulate pinealoblastoma and can best

be differentiated using high-resolution MRI.[57] Pineal cysts are not uncommon in the pediatric population and are most often coincidentally found on MRI. With MRI, the cyst shows gadolinium enhancement of the wall but not the center cavity, whereas pinealoblastoma are typically larger than cysts and show full enhancement. Pineal cysts require no treatment.

Second cancers occur in survivors of bilateral or heritable (germline mutation) retinoblastoma.[58–60] Patients with hereditary retinoblastoma have approximately a 4% chance of developing a second cancer during the first 10 years of follow-up, 18% during the first 20 years, and 26% within 30 years.[58] Second cancers most often include osteogenic sarcoma,

Table 30 International Classification of Retinoblastoma

Group	Quick reference	Specific features
A	Small tumor	Rb ≤3 mm*
B	Larger tumor	Rb >3 mm* or
	Macula	• macular Rb location [≤3 mm to foveola]
	Juxtapapillary	• juxtapapillary Rb location [≤1.5 mm to disc]
	Subretinal fluid	• Rb with subretinal fluid
C	Focal seeds	Rb with
		• subretinal seeds ≤3 mm from Rb and/or
		• vitreous seeds ≤3 mm from Rb
D	Diffuse seeds	Rb with
		• subretinal seeds >3 mm from Rb and/or
		• vitreous seeds >3 mm from Rb
E	Extensive Rb	Extensive Rb nearly filling globe or
		• neovascular glaucoma
		• opaque media from intraocular hemorrhage
		• invasion into optic nerve, choroid, sclera, orbit, anterior chamber

Rb: retinoblastoma

* refers to 3 mm in basal dimension or thickness

spindle cell sarcoma, chondrosarcoma, rhabdomyosarcoma, neuroblastoma, glioma, leukemia, sebaceous cell carcinoma, squamous cell carcinoma, and malignant melanoma. Therapeutic radiotherapy previously delivered for the retinoblastoma can further increase the rate of second cancers. Hereditary retinoblastoma patients who received ocular radiation carried a 29% chance of developing a periocular second cancer compared with only a 6% risk in hereditary retinoblastoma patients treated without radiotherapy.[58] Less than 50% of patients survive their second cancer and they are at risk of developing a third nonocular cancer (22% by 10 years) at a mean interval of 6 years.[60] Survivors continue to be at risk for fourth and fifth nonocular cancers. There is some concern that patients treated with chemoreduction, particularly etoposide, might be at risk for secondary acute myelogenous leukemia.[61]

DIAGNOSIS AND MANAGEMENT/TREATMENT

The clinical manifestations of retinoblastoma vary with the stage of the disease.[2,4,12,48] A small retinoblastoma less than 2 mm in diameter appears transparent or slightly translucent in the sensory retina. Larger tumors stimulate dilated retinal blood vessels feeding the tumor, foci of intrinsic calcification, and can produce subretinal fluid (exophytic pattern), subretinal seeding, and vitreous seeding (endophytic pattern) (290–293). Retinoblastoma of any size can produce leukocoria, but this is most often seen with large tumors. Several classifications of retinoblastoma have been developed including the Reese Ellsworth classfication and the more recent International Classification of Retinoblastoma (ICRB) (*Table 30*).[48,62] The ICRB is simple to remember and is useful for the prediction of chemoreduction success.[63] Based on the ICRB,

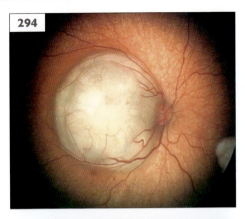

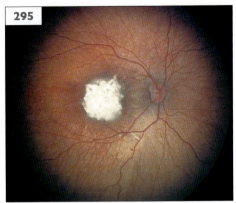

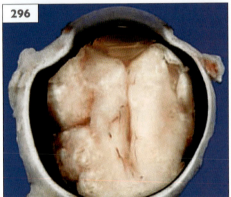

294–296 Clinical appearance of retinoblastoma. **294:** Macular retinoblastoma before chemoreduction; **295:** macular retinoblastoma (same as in **294**) following chemoreduction and thermotherapy; **296:** large retinoblastoma managed with enucleation.

chemoreduction success is achieved in 100% of group A, 93% of group B, 90% of group C, and 47% of group D eyes (**294, 295**).[63]

Management of retinoblastoma is tailored to each individual case and based on the overall situation, including the threat of metastatic disease, risks for second cancers, systemic status, laterality of the disease, size and location of the tumor(s), and estimated visual prognosis. The currently available treatment methods comprise intravenous chemoreduction (carboplatin, etoposide, and vincristine), subconjunctival carboplatin boost, thermotherapy, cryotherapy, laser photocoagulation, plaque radiotherapy, external beam radiotherapy, and enucleation (**296**) (*Table 31*).[12,13]

For unilateral retinoblastoma, enucleation is necessary in approximately 75% of cases and conservative treatment (nonenucleation methods) is possible in 25%.[13] The reason for the high rate of enucleation is that unilateral

sporadic retinoblastoma is typically detected when the disease is advanced. For children with less advanced unilateral disease, chemoreduction plus focal consolidation of each tumor with thermotherapy or cryotherapy, or the use of plaque radiotherapy, is beneficial. For bilateral retinoblastoma, chemoreduction plus thermotherapy or cryotherapy is necessary in most cases and about 60% of patients require enucleation of one eye for dangerously advanced tumor.[13] Enucleation of both eyes is only necessary in 1% of cases.[13]

Chemoreduction for retinoblastoma has now been used for 15 years.[64–67] Many observations on the success and limitations of this technique have been published. Chemoreduction will reduce retinoblastoma by approximately 35% in tumor base and nearly 50% in tumor thickness. Subretinal fluid will completely resolve in approximately 75% of eyes that present with total retinal detachment. Subsequently, several

Table 31 Treatment strategy based on laterality and retinoblastoma grouping

International Classification of Retinoblastoma	Unilateral	Bilateral*
A	Laser or cryotherapy	Laser or cryotherapy
B	VC or plaque	VC
C	VEC or plaque	VEC
D	Enucleation or VEC	VEC+SCC
E	Enucleation	Enucleation but if both eyes equally advanced then VEC+SCC+planned low-dose EBRT

* Treatment in bilateral cases is usually based on the most advanced eye.

EBRT: External beam radiotherapy; Laser: laser photocoagulation; Plaque: plaque radiotherapy; SCC: subconjunctival carboplatin; VC: vincristine, carboplatin plus thermotherapy or cryotherapy; VEC: vincristin, etoposide, carboplatin plus thermotherapy or cryotherapy.

reports elaborated on the response of vitreous and subretinal seeds to chemoreduction. In spite of these successes, vitreous and subretinal seeds pose the greatest problem with potential for recurrence, often remote from the main tumor. In a report on 158 eyes with retinoblastoma treated using vincristine, etoposide, and carboplatin for 6 cycles, all retinoblastomas, subretinal seeds, and vitreous seeds showed initial regression.[65] However, approximately 50% of the eyes with vitreous seeds showed at least one vitreous seed recurrence at 5 years and 62% of the eyes with subretinal seeds showed at least one subretinal seed recurrence at 5 years.[65] Of the 158 eyes, recurrence of at least one retinal tumor per eye was found in 51% of eyes by 5 years. A more recent analysis of 457 consecutive retinoblastomas focused on individual tumor control with chemoreduction and focal tumor consolidation.[67] Tumors treated with chemoreduction alone showed recurrence in 45% by 7 years' follow-up, whereas those treated with chemoreduction plus thermotherapy, cryotherapy, or both showed recurrence in 18% by 7 years.

Following chemoreduction, tumor consolidation with thermotherapy or cryotherapy is important for tumor control. Macular retinoblastoma represents a specially difficult situation regarding therapy. Consolidation with thermotherapy in the foveal region could lead to immediate visual loss so controversy exists regarding the need for, or benefit of, adjuvant focal thermotherapy following chemoreduction. In an analysis of 68 macular retinoblastomas, 35% of those treated with chemoreduction alone showed recurrence by 4 years compared to 17% of those treated with chemoreduction plus extrafoveal thermotherapy.[68] Surprisingly, small retinoblastomas were most likely to show tumor recurrence. This is believed to be related to the reduced chemotherapy dose received from small feeder vessels or to the more well-differentiated features of small retinoblastomas with less responsiveness to chemotherapy.

Plaque radiotherapy is a method of brachytherapy in which a radioactive implant is placed on the sclera over the base of a retinoblastoma to irradiate the tumor transclerally. It is limited to tumors less than 16 mm in base and 8 mm in thickness and complete treatment can be achieved in approximately 4 days. Plaque radiotherapy provides long-term tumor control in 90% of eyes when used as a primary treatment.[2,4,69] In those eyes that need plaque radiotherapy for tumor recurrence after chemoreduction, complete control of the tumor is achieved in 96% of cases.[69] Plaque radiotherapy can be used for extensive recurrent subretinal seeds or vitreous seeds but there is a higher failure rate. All eyes treated with plaque radiotherapy should be monitored for radiation maculopathy and papillopathy.

Enucleation is an important and powerful method for managing retinoblastoma.[2,4,70] Enucleation is employed for advanced tumor with no hope for useful vision in the affected eye, or if there is a concern for invasion of the tumor into the optic nerve, choroid, or orbit. Eyes with unilateral group D or E are usually managed with primary enucleation. Eyes with bilateral group D or E generally need secondary enucleation in one eye following chemoreduction.

A number of ocular disorders in infants and children can resemble retinoblastoma. The most common pseudoretinoblastomas include Coats' disease, persistent hyperplastic primary vitreous (PHPV), also known as persistent fetal vasculature (PFV), and ocular inflammation such as toxocariasis.[2,4,6] Retinoblastoma should be considered in any child with retinal detachment, vitreous hemorrhage, or intraocular mass. It is important that the diagnosis of retinoblastoma be confidently excluded before treatment of a pseudoretinoblastoma. Vitrectomy or retinal detachment repair should be withheld in a child until the diagnosis of retinoblastoma is reliably excluded.[71] Any child with unexplained, atraumatic hyphema or vitreous hemorrhage should be evaluated for retinoblastoma using clinical examination, ultrasonography, and possibly even CT or MRI. Consultation with an ocular oncologist experienced with retinoblastoma could be helpful in confirming the clinical diagnosis and directing therapy.

Retinal capillary hemangioma

Retinal capillary hemangioma is a reddish-pink retinal mass that can occur in the peripheral fundus or adjacent to the optic disc.[72] The tumor often has prominent dilated retinal blood vessels that supply and drain the lesion (**297**). Untreated lesions can cause intraretinal exudation and retinal detachment. Fluorescein angiography shows rapid filling of the tumor with dye and intense late staining of the mass. Patients with retinal capillary hemangioma should be evaluated for the von Hippel–Lindau syndrome (VHL), an AD condition characterized by cerebellar hemangioblastoma, pheochromocytoma, hypernephroma, and other visceral tumors and cysts. If the tumor produces macular exudation or retinal detachment, it can be treated with methods of laser photocoagulation, cryotherapy, photodynamic therapy, plaque radiotherapy, or external beam radiotherapy. The gene responsible for this syndrome has been localized to the short arm of chromosome 3.

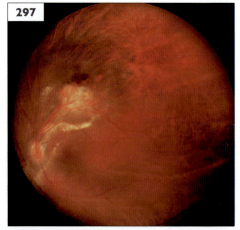

297 Retinal capillary hemangioma with subretinal fluid and exudation in a child with von Hippel–Lindau syndrome.

Retinal cavernous hemangioma

The retinal cavernous hemangioma typically appears as a globular or sessile intraretinal lesion that is composed of multiple vascular channels that have a reddish-blue color.[2,4] It may show patches of gray-white fibrous tissue on the surface, but it does not cause the exudation that characterizes the retinal capillary hemangioma. Cavernous hemangioma is a congenital retinal vascular hamartoma that is probably present at birth. This tumor can be associated with similar intracranial and cutaneous vascular hamartomas, but the syndrome does not have the visceral tumors that characterize the VHL syndrome. As a general rule, retinal cavernous hemangioma requires no active treatment. If vitreous hemorrhage should occur, laser or cryotherapy to the tumor can be attempted. If vitreous blood does not resolve, removal by vitrectomy may be necessary.

Retinal racemose hemangioma

The retinal racemose hemangioma is not a true neoplasm but rather a simple or complex arteriovenous communication.[2,4] It is characterized by a large dilated tortuous retinal artery that passes from the optic disc for a variable distance into the fundus where it then communicates directly with a similarly dilated retinal vein that passes back to the optic disc (298, 299). It can occur as a solitary unilateral lesion or it can be part of the Wyburn-Mason syndrome, which is characterized by other similar lesions in the midbrain and sometimes the orbit, mandible, and maxilla. It does not appear to have a hereditary tendency.

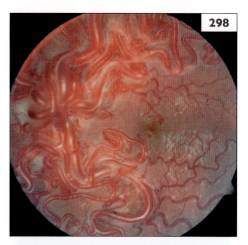

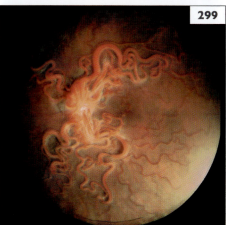

298, 299 Retinal racemose hemangioma. **298:** Macular image showing the tortuous, dilated vessels; **299:** wide-angle image showing the entire extent of the hemangioma.

Astrocytic hamartoma of the retina

Astrocytic hamartoma of the retina is a yellow-white intraretinal lesion that can also occur in the peripheral fundus or in the optic disc region. The lesion can be homogeneous or it may contain glistening foci of calcification (**300**). Unlike retinal capillary hemangioma, it does not generally produce significant exudation or retinal detachment. Patients with astrocytic hamartoma of the retina should be evaluated for tuberous sclerosis, characterized by intracranial astrocytoma, cardiac rhabdomyoma, renal angiomyolipoma, pleural cysts, and other tumors and cysts. Growing astrocytic hamartoma can be treated with photodynamic therapy.[73]

Melanocytoma of the optic nerve

Melanocytoma of the optic nerve is a deeply pigmented congenital tumor that overlies a portion of the optic disc (**301**).[2,74] Unlike uveal melanoma, which occurs predominantly in Caucasians, melanocytoma occurs with equal frequency in all races. It must be differentiated from malignant melanoma.

Intraocular medulloepithelioma

Medulloepithelioma is an embryonal tumor that arises from the primitive medullary epithelium or the inner layer of the optic cup.[2,4,75] It generally becomes clinically apparent in the first decade of life and appears as a fleshy, often cystic mass in the ciliary body (**302, 303**). Cataract and secondary glaucoma are frequent complications. Although approximately 60–90% are cytologically malignant, intraocular medulloepithelioma tends to be only locally invasive and distant metastasis is exceedingly rare. Larger tumors generally require enucleation of the affected eye. It is possible that some smaller tumors can be resected locally without enucleation.[75]

Choroidal hemangioma

Choroidal hemangioma is a benign vascular tumor that can occur as a circumscribed lesion in adults or as a diffuse tumor in children.[2,4,76] The diffuse choroidal hemangioma usually occurs in association with ipsilateral facial nevus flammeus or variations of the Sturge–Weber syndrome. Ipsilateral congenital glaucoma is a frequent association. Secondary retinal detachment frequently occurs. Affected children often develop amblyopia in the involved eye. If vision loss from retinal detachment is found, then treatment of circumscribed hemangioma involves photodynamic therapy, whereas diffuse hemangioma is treated with external beam radiotherapy.

Choroidal osteoma

Choroidal osteoma is a benign choroidal tumor that is probably congenital. Although it has been recognized in infancy, it may not be diagnosed clinically until young adulthood.[2,4,77] It is more common in females. It consists of a plaque of mature bone that generally occurs adjacent to the optic disc (**304**). It generally shows slow enlargement and choroidal neovascularization, with subretinal hemorrhage a frequent complication. The pathogenesis is unknown. Serum calcium and phosphorus levels are normal.

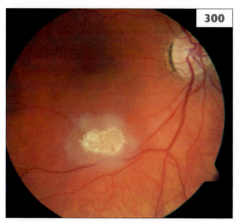

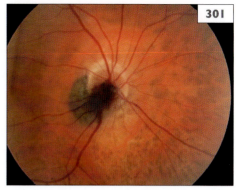

301 Optic disc melanocytoma with choroidal component.

300 Retinal astrocytic hamartoma with glistening calcification.

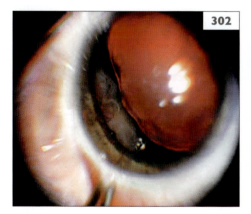

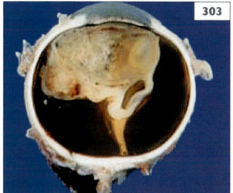

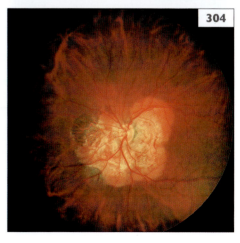

302, 303 Medulloepithelioma of the ciliary body. **302:** Mass is visible peripheral to the lens on scleral depression; **303:** following enucleation in another case, the mass is seen in the ciliary body with total retinal detachment.

304 Choroidal osteoma surrounding the optic disc.

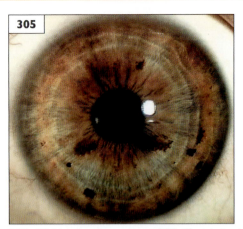
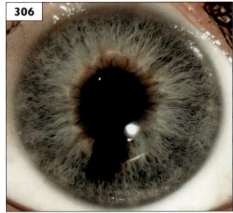

305, 306 Iris freckles and nevi. **305:** Flat iris freckles on iris surface; **306:** slightly thickened iris nevus distorting the iris stroma and causing corectopia.

Uveal nevus

Uveal nevus is a flat or minimally elevated, variably pigmented tumor that may occur in the iris (**305, 306**) or in the choroid (**307–309**). Although it is most likely to be congenital it is usually asymptomatic and not usually recognized until later in life. Although most uveal nevi are stationary and nonprogressive, malignant transformation into melanoma can occur in rare instances.[78,79] Factors that predict risk of transformation into melanoma are listed in *Table 32*.

An important variant of iris nevus is the presence of bilateral multiple slightly elevated melanocytic lesions of the iris, known as Lisch nodules. These lesions become clinically apparent at about age 5 years and are often the first sign of von Recklinghausen's neuro-fibromatosis.

Uveal melanoma

Although uveal melanoma is generally a disease of adulthood, it is occasionally diagnosed in children.[80] It is a variably pigmented elevated mass that shows slow progression (**310**). If it is not treated early, it has a tendency to metastasize to liver, lung, and other distant sites. Most advanced tumors are treated by enucleation. Radiotherapy or local tumor resection can be employed for less advanced tumors.

Table 32 Clinical features predictive of growth of small choroidal melanoma (≤3 mm thickness)[79]

TFSOM (mnemomic for *To Find Small Ocular Melanoma*)

T = Thickness >2 mm
F = Fluid subretinal
S = Symptoms
O = Orange pigment
M= Margin within 3 mm of optic disc

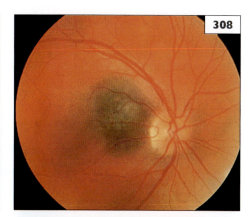

307–309 Choroidal freckles and nevi.
307: Flat macular choroidal freckle;
308: slightly thickened suspicious choroidal nevus in macular region; **309:** very suspicious choroidal nevus versus small melanoma with orange pigment and subretinal fluid.

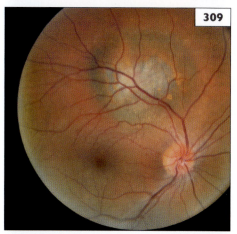

310 Choroidal melanoma with shallow subretinal fluid and documented growth in a 16-year-old boy.

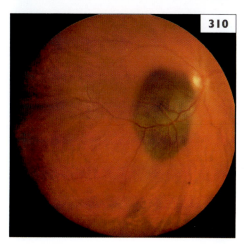

Congenital hypertrophy of retinal pigment epithelium

Congenital hypertrophy of the retinal pigment epithelium (CHRPE) is a well-circumscribed, flat, pigmented lesion that can occur anywhere in the fundus.[81] It often shows depigmented lacunae within the lesion and a surrounding pale halo. It can occur as a solitary lesion or it can be multiple as part of a congenital grouped pigmentation lesion (**311, 312**). Similar but distinct multifocal pigmented lesions may be a marker for familial adenomatous polyposis and Gardner's syndrome, in which patients have a high likelihood of developing colonic cancer.

Leukemia

Childhood leukemias can occasionally exhibit tumor infiltration in the retina, optic disc, and uveal tract. Infiltration is characterized by a swollen optic disc and thickening of the retina and choroid, often with hemorrhage and secondary retinal detachment. Intraocular leukemic infiltrates are generally responsive to irradiation and chemotherapy, but they generally portend a poor systemic prognosis.

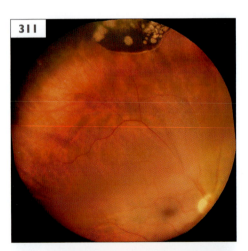

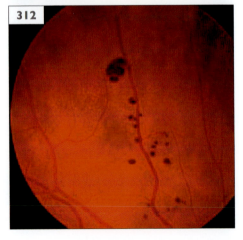

311, 312 Congenital hypertrophy of the retinal pigment epithelium. **311:** Solitary type with lacunae and halo; **312:** multifocal type.

Orbital tumors

A variety of neoplasms and related space-occupying lesions can affect the orbit.[3,5,82] Orbital cellulitis secondary to sinusitis and inflammatory pseudotumors are more common than true neoplasms. Only about 5% of orbital lesions in children that come to biopsy prove to be malignant.[82,83] Cystic lesions are the most common group and vascular lesions are the second most common. This section covers orbital tumors and cysts but does not discuss orbital inflammatory or infectious conditions.

Dermoid cyst

Dermoid cyst is the most common noninflammatory space-occupying orbital mass in children.[84,85] It usually appears in the first decade of life as a fairly firm, fixed, subcutaneous mass at the superotemporal orbital rim near the zygomaticofrontal suture (**313, 314**). Occasionally, a dermoid cyst may occur deeper in the orbit unattached to bone. Although it is sometimes stationary, it does have a tendency to enlarge slowly. It can occasionally rupture, inciting an intense inflammatory reaction. Management is either serial observation or surgical removal of the mass.

Teratoma

A teratoma is a cystic mass that contains elements of all three embryonic germ layers.[3,5] An orbital teratoma causes proptosis that is generally quite apparent at birth. The diagnosis should be confirmed by imaging studies. Larger orbital teratomas can destroy the eye. Smaller teratomas can be removed intact without sacrificing the eye, but larger ones that have caused blindness may require orbital exenteration.

Capillary hemangioma

Capillary hemangioma is the most common orbital vascular tumor of childhood.[3,5,15] It usually is clinically apparent at birth or within the first few weeks after birth. It tends to cause progressive proptosis during the first few months of life and then it becomes stable and slowly regresses. Orbital imaging studies show a diffuse, poorly circumscribed, orbital mass that enhances with contrast material. The best management is refraction and treatment of induced amblyopia with patching of the opposite eye. Local injection of corticosteroids or oral corticosteroids can hasten regression of the mass and minimize complications. Occasionally, surgical resection of circum-scribed tumors is performed.

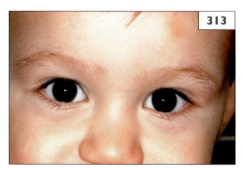

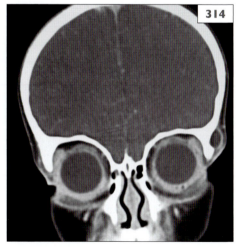

313, 314 Dermoid cyst near the lateral orbital rim, barely visible clinically. **313:** Slight elevation of lateral orbital skin is shown; **314:** coronal CT showing the cystic mass.

Lymphangioma

Lymphangioma is an important vascular tumor of the orbit in children.[3,5,86,87] It tends to become clinically apparent during the first decade of life. It can cause abrupt proptosis following orbital trauma, secondary to hemorrhage into the lymphatic channels within the lesion (**315–317**). Such spontaneous hemorrhages, called chocolate cysts, can require aspiration or surgical evacuation to prevent visual loss from compression of the eye. Occasionally surgical resection or debulking of the mass is necessary. More recently, aspiration of large cysts followed by injection of tissue glue has been performed to assist in identification of the tumor margins[88] and even to avoid major surgery as the glue often clots the tumor and leads to shrinkage.

Juvenile pilocytic astrocytoma

Juvenile pilocytic astrocytoma ('optic nerve glioma') is the most common orbital neural tumor of childhood.[3,5] It is a cytologically benign hamartoma that is generally stationary or very slowly progressive. The affected child develops ipsilateral visual loss and slowly progressive axial proptosis (**318**). Orbital imaging studies show an elongated or oval shaped mass which is well-circumscribed because of the overlying dura mater. There is greater incidence of this tumor in patients with neurofibromatosis. Since surgical excision necessitates blindness, the best management is periodic observation and surgical removal if there is blindness and cosmetically unacceptable proptosis. In cases that extend to the optic chiasm and are surgically unresectable, radiotherapy may be necessary.

Rhabdomyosarcoma

Rhabdomyosarcoma is the most important primary orbital malignant tumor of childhood.[3,5,89,90] It usually occurs in the first decade of life with a mean age of 8 years at the time of diagnosis. It causes fairly rapid proptosis and displacement of the globe, usually without pain or major inflammatory signs (**319**). Imaging studies show an irregular but fairly well-circumscribed mass usually in the extraconal anterior orbit (**320**). Although orbital exenteration was often employed in the past, more recent experience has suggested that the best cure is obtained by performing a biopsy to confirm the diagnosis, and treating with combined irradiation and chemotherapy, using vincristine, cytoxan, and adriamycin.

Granulocytic sarcoma ('chloroma')

Granulocytic sarcoma is soft tissue infiltration by myelogenous leukemia.[5,91,92] Although leukemia usually appears first in the blood and bone marrow, the orbit soft tissues may be the first site to become clinically apparent. The child presents with a fairly rapid onset of proptosis and displacement of the globe. Confirmation of the orbital lesion can be made by biopsy and the condition treated by chemotherapy or low-dose irradiation.

Lymphoma

The most important lymphoma to affect the orbit of children is Burkitt's lymphoma. Although this tumor was originally recognized exclusively in African tribes, it is being recognized more often in patients with the autoimmune deficiency syndrome (AIDS) and as an American form in otherwise healthy children.[3,5]

Langerhan's cell histiocytosis

Eosinophilic granuloma can affect the orbital bones as an intraosseous bone-destructive inflammatory lesion.[3,5] Although it can occur anywhere in the orbit, it most often occurs in the anterior portion of the frontal and zygomatic bones. Recent ultrastructural studies have suggested that the stem cell in eosinophilic granuloma and certain other tumors in the histiocytic X group is the Langerhan's cell. Hence, the term Langerhan's cell histiocytosis is becoming preferable.

Metastatic neuroblastoma

Although orbital metastasis in children can occur secondary to Wilm's and Ewing's tumors, metastatic neuroblastoma is the most common metastatic orbital tumor of childhood.[3,5] The majority of children with orbital metastasis of neuroblastoma have a previously diagnosed primary neoplasm in the adrenal gland. However, the orbital metastasis can be diagnosed before the adrenal primary in about 3% of cases.

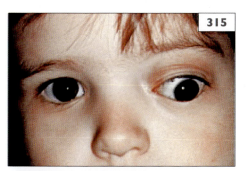

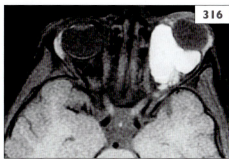

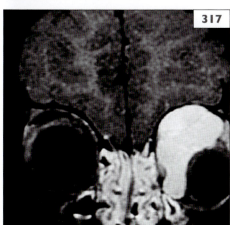

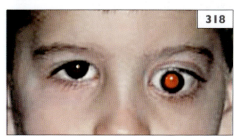

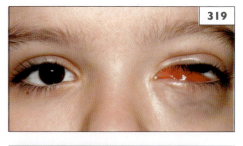

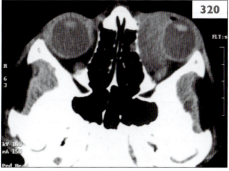

315–317 Orbital lymphangioma producing rapid proptosis in a young child.
315: Downward displacement of the globe;
316: axial MRI showing bright signal in the blood-filled cyst; 317: coronal MRI showing the mass displacing the globe.

318 Juvenile pilocytic astrocytoma of optic nerve causing proptosis.

319, 320 Orbital rhabdomyosarcoma.
319: Proptosis and tumor involving the inferior fornix; 320: axial CT showing mass in medial orbit.

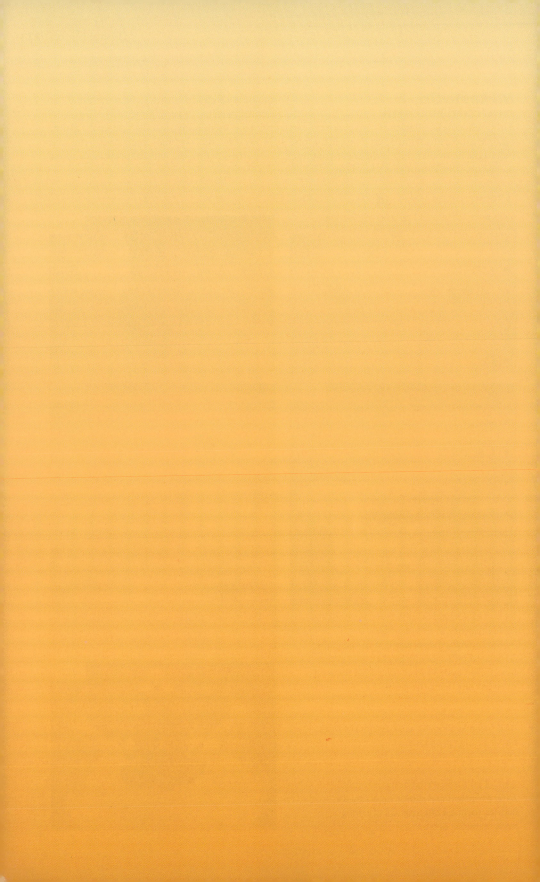

Ocular trauma

Denise Hug, MD

- **Introduction**

- **Eyelid**

- **Open globe**

- **Ocular surface injury**

- **Intraocular trauma**

- **Iridodialysis**

- **Cataract**

- **Retina**

- **Optic nerve injury**

- **Orbital fracture**

- **Other orbital injury**

- **Child abuse**
  Shaking injury

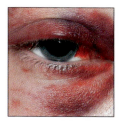
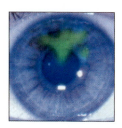
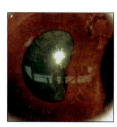
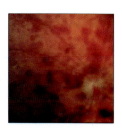

Introduction

Trauma to the eye and surrounding structures (adnexa) can come from different sources and can vary in intensity from minimal to sight-threatening. This chapter will review some of the most common etiologies of ocular trauma and its management.

Eyelid

Eyelid trauma is a common issue in the pediatric population. The injury can occur from simple blunt trauma, or a laceration can occur from a sharp object. Tissue avulsion of the eyelid may occur in more complicated trauma, such as from a dog bite. Blunt trauma to the eyelid can result in ecchymosis and edema (**321**). These are self-limiting and can be treated with iced compresses and analgesics. Blunt trauma may also be associated with injuries to the eye and orbit, so careful inspection of the surrounding structures is neccessary.

Eyelid foreign bodies are relatively uncommon but must be removed in an effort to minimize injury to the eye (**322**). Small, superficial foreign bodies under the upper eyelid can cause linear, vertical abrasions of the cornea (seen with fluorescein). The upper eyelid should be everted and the foreign body removed with a moist cotton swab.

Eyelid lacerations may vary from simple to complex (**323, 324**). When evaluating an eyelid laceration examination details should include: depth of the laceration, its location, and if there is involvement of the canaliculus. Most superficial eyelid lacerations may be closed by the primary caregiver, but if the laceration is deep, it should be evaluated by an ophthalmologist. The levator muscle is responsible for elevation of the eyelid and runs deep to the obicularis oculi muscle. If the levator muscle is compromised and not recognized at initial repair, ptosis will occur. If orbital fat is visible in the laceration, the laceration has compromised the skin, obicularis oculi, levator, and orbital septum and must be meticulously repaired to avoid ptosis. Eyelid margin involvement (**325**) also requires careful repair to avoid notch formation. A residual notch can lead to ocular surface problems in the future, resulting in corneal scarring and loss of vision.

Trauma involving the canaliculus (**326**) will require repair with intubation of the naso-lacrimal duct to avoid future problems with tearing. Canalicular involvement may be subtle, so consideration must be given if there is a laceration medially or if the mechanism is that of avulsion. Finally, with any eyelid injury, the eye must be carefully inspected for damage. For example, it is fairly common in dog-bite trauma for injuries involving the eye, scalp, and extremities to be present for which the child must be examined (**327**).

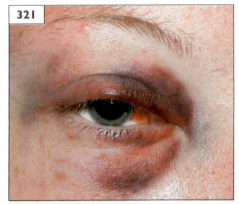

321 Ecchymosis.

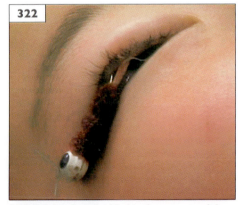

322 Fish hook embedded in the upper eyelid.

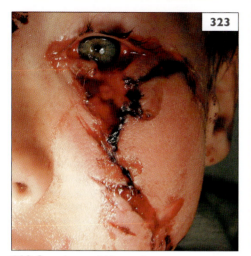

323 Complex eyelid laceration.

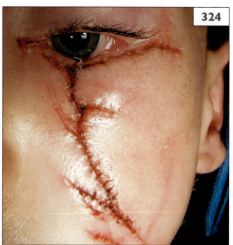

324 Postoperative repair of a complex eyelid laceration.

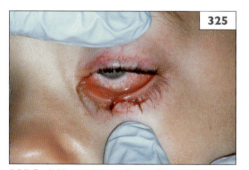

325 Eyelid laceration on lower lid margin.

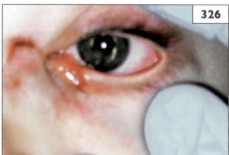

326 Canalicular laceration.

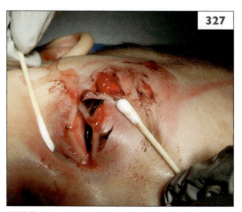

327 Dog bite with eyelid and scalp injuries.

Open globe

A penetrating, perforating, or blunt injury resulting in compromise of the cornea or sclera of the eye is one of the most sight-threatening injuries that can be sustained. This is known as an open globe. A penetrating injury extends only partially through the tissue of reference while a perforation extends through the full thickness of the tissue. An open globe is a true ophthalmologic emergency which requires prompt, careful evaluation and repair to minimize vision loss. Vision loss can result from corneal scarring, loss of intraocular contents, or infection. Evaluation involves careful history including time and mechanism of the injury, as well as visual acuity and inspection of the eye. A full-thickness corneal (**328**) wound will often present with prolapse of iris tissue through the wound. If this is not immediately evident, a peaked or irregular pupil may be seen (**329**). Scleral compromise may be more difficult to identify because of overlying structures. The thinnest part of the sclera is at the corneoscleral junction (the limbus) and just posterior to the insertion of the rectus muscles. When an open globe is caused by blunt force injury, these are the two areas most likely involved. The overlying conjunctiva may not be compromised but a subconjunctival hemorrhage may be present, obscuring the view. In these cases, a shallow anterior chamber, low intraocular pressure (IOP), or pigment within the involved area should be identified. If the patient has been diagnosed with an open globe, the examination should be stopped, an eye shield should be placed immediately (**330, 331**), and the ophthalmologist contacted.

The presence of an intraocular foreign body (**332–334**) should be suspected in cases of open globe secondary to a high-velocity projectile, such as a BB (pellet). Intraocular foreign bodies must always be surgically removed.

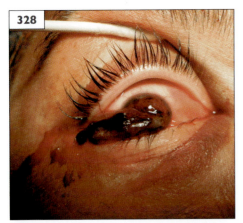

328 Full-thickness laceration with prolapse of intraocular contents.

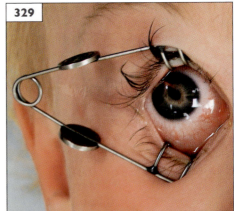

329 Peaked pupil from iris prolapse, secondary to full-thickness corneal laceration.

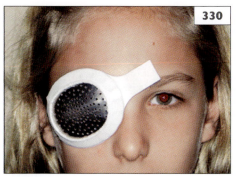

330 Metal shield placed for protection.

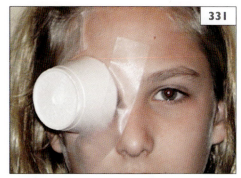

331 Styrofoam cup placed for protection.

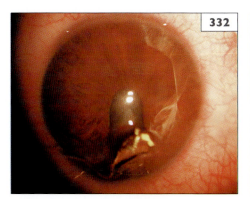

332 Intraocular metallic fragment.

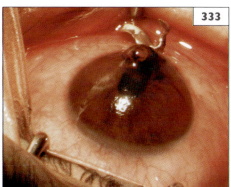

333 Removed metallic fragment.

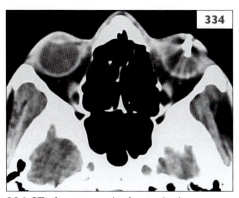

334 CT of an intraocular foreign body.

Ocular surface injury

The conjunctiva is the thin, connective tissue that covers the sclera. A common injury to the pediatric eye is a subconjunctival hemorrhage (**335**). This is most often caused by blunt injury or Valsalva maneuver. Subconjunctival hemorrhages are usually painless and self-limiting, and require no treatment. The mechanism of injury is important to rule out additional complications, such as scleral laceration. A conjunctival laceration (**336**) may occur without involving the underlying sclera. Treatment of conjunctival laceration is dependent on its extent. Most lacerations will heal without surgical intervention, but extensive or complex lacerations may require suturing. Nonsurgical repair involves lubrication with antibiotic or antibiotic–steroid ophthalmic ointment until closure occurs.

The cornea is composed of five layers with the epithelium being the most superficial layer. When all or part of the epithelium is lost secondary to a trauma, it is called a corneal abrasion. Evaluation includes history, visual acuity, and inspection. The abrasion can readily be identified with the instillation of fluorescein and observation with blue light (**337–339**). Treatment involves analgesics and cycloplegic agent with frequent instillation of an antibiotic ophthalmic ointment. Patching of the eye was once considered standard practice but has not been shown to improve healing time or increase comfort. A corneal abrasion in a contact lens wearer should not be patched as this may increase the risk for *Pseudomonas* infection. The abrasion should be re-evaluated in 1–2 days to ensure healing and that no infection has occurred.

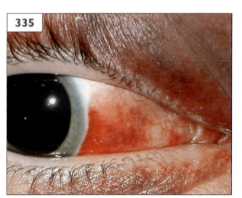

335 Subconjunctival hemorrhage.

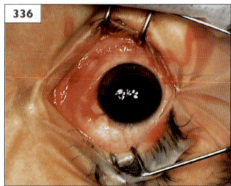

336 Conjunctival laceration.

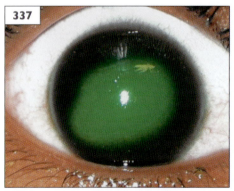

337 Corneal abrasion with fluorescein staining.

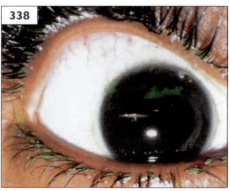

338 Corneal abrasion with fluorescein staining.

Corneal foreign bodies are another source of pediatric ocular trauma, and may be organic or nonorganic (**340**). All corneal foreign bodies must be removed to minimize risk of infection, inflammation, and scarring. A superficial, peripheral foreign body may be removed in the office in a cooperative child. After removal, the treatment is the same as that of an abrasion. Deep or central foreign bodies may need to be removed in the controlled environment of the operating room to minimize corneal scarring. Metallic foreign bodies are more complicated because the iron in the foreign body often oxidizes and may cause rust to be deposited in the cornea. The rust must be removed to ensure proper healing. Therefore, it is best to have the metallic foreign body and rust removed by an ophthalmologist.

Chemical injuries to the ocular surface may be sight-threatening and should be considered an ophthalmic emergency. It is important to identify the substance to which the eye was exposed. Acidic chemicals tend to precipitate in the ocular tissues. Bases tend to coagulate the ocular tissues and will penetrate deeper into the eye. Upon arrival, the child with a chemical exposure should receive *immediate* irrigation with saline for 10 minutes. The pH of the ocular surface should then be checked and irrigation continued until neutrality. If significant exposure has occurred, the patient should be seen promptly by an ophthalmologist to initiate further treatment. The goal of treatment is to minimize vision-threatening sequelae such as conjunctival scarring, corneal scarring/opacification, glaucoma, cataract, vision loss, and phthisis (**341**).

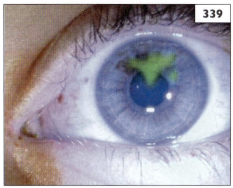

339 Corneal abrasion with fluorescein staining.

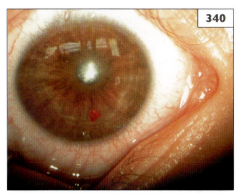

340 Corneal foreign body.

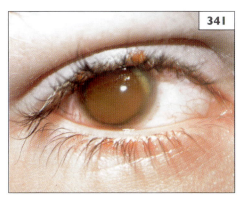

341 Early phthisis.

Intraocular trauma

Traumatic iritis occurs after blunt trauma to the eye. The symptoms include eye pain, photophobia, tearing, and blurred vision. The symptoms usually present within 3 days of injury. Iritis is the presence of intraocular inflammation demonstrated by conjunctival injection and the presence of white cells in the anterior chamber. Traumatic iritis is treated with a cycloplegic agent to immobilize the iris, which in turn improves comfort. Many practitioners also recommend topical steroid treatment to reduce inflammation.

Hyphema can be caused by blunt or penetrating injury to the eye and represents a vision-threatening situation. Blunt force to the eye causes posterior displacement of the lens–iris diaphragm, which results in tearing of structures, including vessels, in the iris root. When these vessels tear, blood is released into the anterior chamber, causing a hyphema (**342, 343**). The IOP acts as a tamponade to stop the bleeding and allow the formation of fibrin clot. Symptoms of a hyphema include immediate decrease in vision and pain. Hyphema is diagnosed by observing blood in the anterior chamber. If a view of posterior structures is obscured, ultrasonography may be useful to rule out retinal detachment or intraocular foreign body. Treatment of hyphema involves efforts to minimize the vision-threatening sequelae such as rebleeding, glaucoma, and corneal blood staining (**344**). A shield is placed on the affected eye, and a cycloplegic agent is used to immobilize the iris. Additionally, topical steroids are used to minimize intraocular inflammation and antiemetics should be considered if the patient is experiencing nausea. All nonsteroidal anti-inflammatories and asprin must be avoided. Frequent visits are required to check IOP and for new bleeding. If IOP is elevated, topical and systemic pressure-lowering medications are used. If the pressure is not controlled by such measures then surgical intervention may be required to minimize the risk of permanent vision loss. Patients with sickle cell disease present an additional concern in managing hyphema. Because of the shape and relative rigidity of the red blood cells in these patients, their clearance through the normal outflow pathways can be limited. This creates a higher risk for developing increased IOP. Additionally, the sickle cell patient's optic nerve is more predisposed to damage from ischemia, and so these patients can sustain permanent vision loss at a lower IOP than expected.

Iridodialysis

Iridodialysis occurs secondary to blunt trauma when the iris root becomes disinserted from the sclera. Hyphema is often present and should be treated if present. If the iridodialysis is small and the patient is asymptomatic (**345**), then treatment may not be needed. If the iridodialysis is large, it may cover the pupil or form a secondary pupil which may cause monocular diplopia or reduced vision (**346**). If this occurs then surgical intervention may be required.

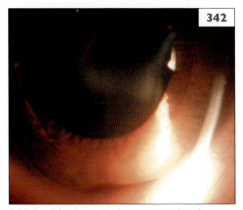

342 Small hyphema in the anterior chamber.

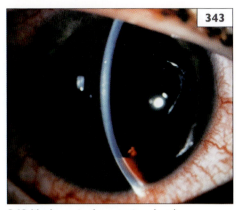

343 Hyphema in the anterior chamber.

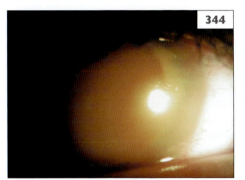

344 Corneal blood staining secondary to hyphema.

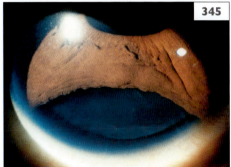

345 Asymptomatic iridodialysis.

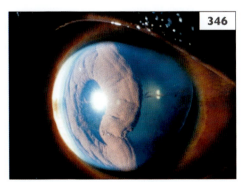

346 Large, symptomatic iridodialysis.

Cataract

A traumatic cataract may develop secondary to a penetrating, perforating, or blunt trauma and may be an immediate, early, or late sequela to ocular trauma. Penetrating and perforating injuries may cause cataract formation from direct injury to the lens, specifically, the lens capsule. Once the integrity of the lens capsule is compromised, the aqueous fluid and inflammatory mediators enter the lens, causing swelling and opacification. In addition, lens proteins may then leak into the anterior chamber, causing significant inflammation and glaucoma. Cataract secondary to blunt injury (**347**) is not always immediately evident. If the opacity is small and in the peripheral lens, no intervention may be needed. When the cataract interferes with vision then surgical intervention offers a chance for visual rehabilitation (**348**). Once the cataractous lens has been surgically removed, its optical power must be replaced by that of an intraocular lens implant, contact lens, or glasses. In children with visual immaturity, occlusion therapy may be required to maximize their vision after surgery, and prevent the development of amblyopia.

Lens dislocation can be caused by blunt trauma and may be partial or complete. It occurs when a blunt force causes rapid anterior–posterior shortening of the eye accompanied by equatorial expansion. This, in turn, causes stretching and disruption of the lens zonules. The lens dislocates in the direction of the intact zonules. When the center of the lens no longer resides in the center of the pupil, a large refractive shift and optical distortion occurs. If the effect is large enough, vision may be affected and surgical intervention may be required.

Retina

The choroid is responsible for nutrition of the external retina. In blunt force trauma, a rupture in the choroid may occur. This is often accompanied by subretinal hemorrhage (**349**). The hemorrhage may resolve without further issue but the choroidal break is permanent. Choroidal rupture can lead to subretinal neovascularization, which in turn may lead to retinal detachment and permanent vision loss. Children who have suffered this type of injury must be monitored by an ophthalmologist over their lifetime.

The retina may also be injured by blunt force trauma, resulting in edema of the neural cells of the retina. When this occurs, it is termed commotio retinae (**350**). This does not require treatment and is usually self-limiting. When the edema involves the macula, it may lead to permanent vision loss if there is disruption of the retinal pigmented epithelium after resolution of the edema.

Retinal detachment may occur secondary to blunt or penetrating injury (**351**). It may occur at the time of injury or may present later, usually within the first month after injury. Treatment of retinal detachment is always surgical.

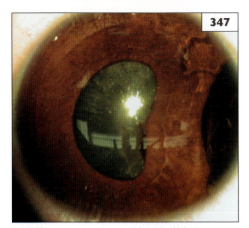

347 Traumatic cataract with iridodialysis.

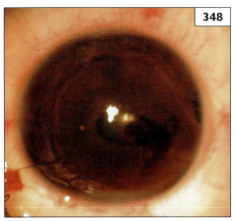

348 After repair of iridodialysis, cataract extraction and placement of intraocular lens.

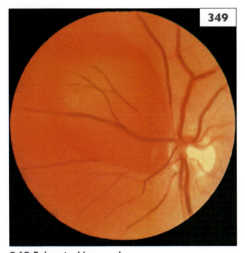

349 Subretinal hemorrhage.

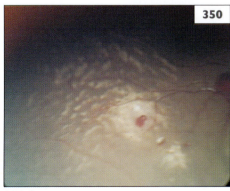

350 Commotio retinae.

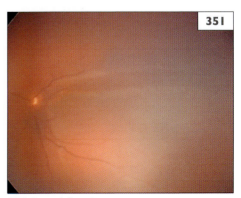

351 Retinal detachment.

Optic nerve injury

The optic nerve may be injured in both penetrating and blunt trauma. The injury may occur at any point between the globe and the chiasm. Traumatic injury to the optic nerve, regardless of cause or location, causes a reduction in vision and a pupillary defect. Direct trauma to the intraorbital optic nerve may cause transection, partial transection, or optic nerve sheath hemorrhage. Optic nerve sheath hemorrhage will lead to axonal compression and vascular compromise. Fractures involving the skull base may cause injury to the intracranial portions of the optic nerve. Treatment decisions are difficult because there are no universally accepted guidelines and the prognosis for good visual outcome is often poor. Medical management involves observation and the use of high-dose corticosteroids. Because many of these patients have multiple injuries, care must be taken to rule out contraindications of corticosteroid use prior to initiating treatment. Finally, the use of corticosteroids as treatment for traumatic optic neuropathy has not been proven in a prospective, randomized, double-blind, placebo-controlled study to improve visual outcomes. Surgical intervention involves optic nerve sheath decompression for nerve sheath hemorrhages. Decompression of the optic canal may be performed if there is compression of the optic nerve by bone fragment. Optic canal decompression is very controversial in the absence of direct bone compression. If compression of the optic nerve is secondary to orbital hemorrhage, prompt lateral canthotomy and cantholysis should be performed to relieve intraorbital pressure.

Orbital fracture

The orbit is the bony structure surrounding the eye. Any of these bones may fracture in a traumatic incident. The superior and lateral walls are the least common fracture sites, but the superior orbital fracture is the most significant because of the potential for intracranial injury (**352, 353**). The medial wall of the orbit is very susceptible to fracture because of the thin nature of the lamina papyracea. Perhaps the most common site of fracture from blunt trauma is the orbital floor (**354**). This is often referred to as a blow-out fracture. The mechanism for a blow-out fracture proposes that a blunt force compresses the globe, which then has equatorial expansion creating increased intraorbital pressure. In turn, the weakest part of the orbital floor fractures. At times, the fracture may act as a trapdoor, entrapping orbital contents within the fracture site. The patient often presents with a recent history of periocular trauma and pain. Diplopia, eyelid swelling, eye movement restriction, and hypesthesia may or may not be present. A complete ophthalmic exam including history of injury, visual acuity, pupil exam, ocular alignment and motility exam, anterior segment exam, and fundus exam is required. There are often accompanying ocular injuries. The diagnosis of fracture is suspected if eye misalignment, eye movement restriction, or enophthalmos (sunken eye) is present. The diagnosis is verified by orbital computed tomography (CT) scan. Medical management includes ice compressed to the orbit for the first 24–48 hours and elevation of the head of the bed. Broad-spectrum antibiotics are sometimes recommended for 14 days because of the exposure of the orbital contents to the sinus cavity. Instructions not to blow their nose is vital in patients with medial wall fractures in order to avoid orbital emphysema and possible optic nerve compression.

Neurosurgical consultation is recommended for orbital roof fractures. Indications for surgical repair of orbital fractures are diplopia in primary or downgaze that persists 2 weeks, and enophthalmos or fracture of the orbital floor involving greater that than one-half of the floor. Most surgeons prefer to repair the fracture 1–2 weeks after injury because of the improvement in acute orbital edema. If extraocular muscle entrapment is present, most surgeons will operate in the acute phase. These patients have significant pain, nausea, and vomiting that is difficult to control. Rarely, extraocular muscle entrapment can cause activation of the oculocardiac reflex, requiring urgent fracture repair.

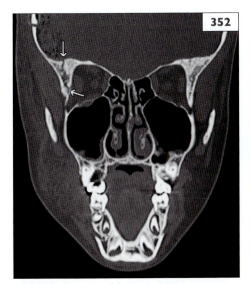

352 Right lateral wall fracture.

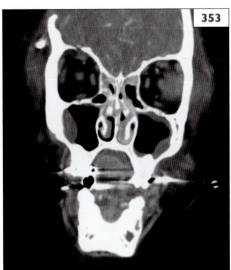

353 Right roof fracture.

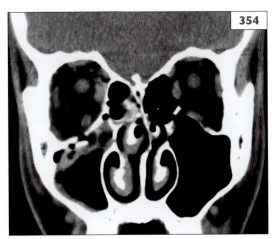

354 Right orbital floor fracture.

Other orbital injury

Intraorbital foreign bodies are relatively uncommon but must be considered whenever a laceration or puncture wound involves the brow or eyelids. Clinical presentation is variable, ranging from asymptomatic to pain, decreased vision, and diplopia. A complete ophthalmic exam is required to rule out other ocular trauma. A head and orbital CT scan should be performed if intraorbital foreign body is suspected (**355**). The medial wall and orbital roof are thin and objects may penetrate into the paranasal sinuses or anterior cranial fossa. Not all intraorbital foreign bodies must be removed. Indications for surgery include: organic or copper material, signs of infection, signs of optic nerve compression, fistula formation, large foreign body, sharp foreign body, and compromise of extraocular muscles or nerves.

Traumatic retrobulbar hemorrhage occurs after blunt trauma to the orbit in which a blood vessel breaks and blood extravasates into the confined space of the orbit. This hemorrhage can cause significant loss of vision from optic nerve compression or acute glaucoma. The patient often presents with pain, acute loss of vision, history of recent trauma, proptosis, and subconjunctival hemorrhage or conjunctival injection. Examination includes visual acuity, pupil examination, color vision, measurement of IOP and evaluation of the central retinal artery. If elevated IOP, decreased vision, or abnormal pupil exam is present, then lateral canthotomy and cantholysis should be performed to minimize the risk of permanent vision loss.

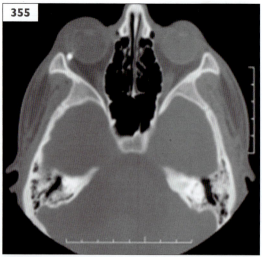

355 BB (pellet) within the right lateral rectus capsule, adjacent to the globe.

Child abuse

The ocular manifestations of child abuse may be from direct injury or indirect injury, such as shaking. Periocular contusions, eyelid abrasions, lacerations, conjuctival hemorrhages, corneal injuries, hyphema, cataract, lens dislocation, and retinal and vitreous hemorrhages have all been described in child abuse cases. When child abuse is suspected the ophthalmologist may play an integral role in the diagnosis.

Shaking injury

Young children who have suffered a shaking or shaking/impact injury often do not present until respiratory depression or seizure activity occurs. During the evaluation of the child, neuroimaging almost always demonstrates subdural hematoma and often also involves subarachnoid hemorrhage. The most common ocular manifestation of shaking injury is retinal hemorrhage. These hemorrhages involve multiple layers: preretinal, nerve fiber layer, deep retinal, and subretinal (**356, 357**). Vitreous hemorrhage may also be present. Traumatic retinoschisis occurs when the retinal hemorrhage is accompanied by retinal disruption. The retina splits and the resulting cavity fills with blood. Because of retinal anatomy and vitreoretinal adhesions, the cavities usually occur in the macular region.

The retinal hemorrhages usually resolve over weeks to months without sequelae. If subretinal hemorrhages are present in the macular region, retinal pigment epithelial disruption may occur, which can cause permanent vision loss. Traumatic retinoschisis cavities may take a significantly longer time to resolve and visual prognosis in these children is not as good. If vitreous hemorrhage is present, a vitrectomy may be warranted to remove the blood. These children are at risk for developing amblyopia. Visual prognosis may be difficult to determine because visual recovery is also dependent on the accompanying intracranial injuries.

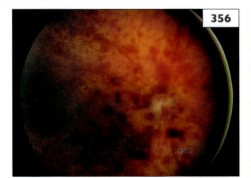

356 Retinal hemorrhages in shaken baby syndrome.

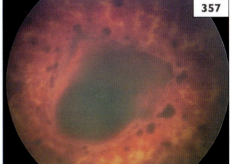

357 Retinal hemorrhages with macular schisis cavity.

References and bibliography

CHAPTER 1
References

1 Warwich R (1977). *Eugene Wolff's Anatomy of the eye and orbit*, 7th edn. Saunders, Philadelphia.
2 Milder B (1987). The lacrimal apparatus. In: *Adler's Physiology of the eye*, 8th edn. RA Moses, WM Hart (eds). Mosby, St. Louis, pp. 15–35.
3 Nelson LB, Catalano RA (1989). *Atlas of Ocular Motility*. Saunders, Philadelphia.
4 Demer JL (2007). Mechanics of the orbita. *Dev Ophthalmol* **40**:132–157.
5 Narasimhan A, Tychsen L, Poukens V, *et al*. (2008). Horizontal rectus muscles anatomy in naturally and artificially strabismic monkeys. *Invest Ophthalmol Vis Sci* **48**:2576–2588.
6 Lagreze WA, Zobor G (2007). A method for noncontact measurement of corneal diameter in children. *Am J Ophthalmol* **144**:141–142.
7 Ronneburer A, Basarab J, Howland HC (2006). Growth of the cornea from infancy to adolescence. *Ophthalmol Physiol Opt* **26**:80–87.
8 Dada T, Sihota R, Gadia R, *et al*. (2007). Comparison of anterior segment optical coherence tomography and ultrasound biomicroscopy for assessment of the anterior segment. *J Cataract Refract Surg* **33**:837–840.
9 Friberg TR, Lace JW (1988). A comparison of the elastic properties of human choroid and sclera. *Exp Eye Res* **47**:429–436.
10 Boubriak OA, Urban JPG, Bron AJ (2005). Differential effects of aging on transport properties of anterior and posterior human sclera. *Exp Eye Res* **76**:701–703.
11 Knop E, Knop N (2005). The role of eye-associated lymphoid tissue in corneal immune protection. *J Anat* **206**:271–285.
12 Dartt DA (2002). Regulation of mucin and fluid secretion by conjunctival epithelial cells. *Prog Retin Eye Res* **21**:555–576.
13 Ohashi Y, Dogru M, Tsubota K (2006). Laboratory findings in tear fluid analysis. *Clinica Chimica Acta* **369**:17–28.
14 Konstantopoulos A, Hossain P, Anderson DF (2007). Recent advances in ophthalmic anterior segment imaging: a new era for ophthalmic diagnosis? *Br J Ophthalmol* **91**:551–557.
15 Jakobiec FA, Ozanics V (1990). General topographic anatomy of the eye. In: *Biomedical Foundation of Ophthalmology*. TD Duane, EA Jaeger (eds). Lippincott, Philadelphia.
16 Snell R, Lemp MA (1971). *Clinical Anatomy of the Eye*. Blackwell Scientific, Boston.
17 Hogan MJ, Alvarado JA, Weddell JE (1971). *Histology of the Human Eye*. Saunders, Philadelphia.
18 Straatsma BR, Hall MO, Allen RA, Crescitelli F (eds) (1969). *The Retina: Morphology, Function, and Clinical Characteristics*. University of California Press, Berkeley.

CHAPTER 2
References

1 American Academy of Pediatrics Red Reflex Subcommittee Policy statement (2002). Red reflex examination in infants. *Pediatrics* **109**(5):980–981.
2 Nelson LB, Rubin SE, Wagner RS, *et al*. (1984). Developmental aspects in the assessment of visual function in young children. *Pediatrics* **73**:375–384.
3 Wagner RS (1998). Pediatric eye examination. In: *Harley's Pediatric Ophthalmology*. LB Nelson (ed). Saunders, Philadelphia, ch 3 p. 82.
4 Simons K (1996). Preschool vision screening: rationale, methodology and outcome. *Surv Ophthalmol* **41**:3–30.
5 Committee on Practice and Ambulatory Medicine and Section on Ophthalmology (2003). Eye examination in infants, children and young adults by pediatricians. *Pediatrics* **111**(4):902–907.
6 Von Noorden GK (1990). *Binocular Vision and Ocular Motility: Theory and Management of Strabismus*, 4th edn. Mosby, St. Louis, p. 163.
7 Parks MM (1969). The monofixational syndrome. *Trans Am Ophthalmol Soc* **67**:609–657.
8 Committee on Practice and Ambulatory Medicine and Section on Ophthalmology (2002). Use of photoscreening for children's vision screening. *Pediatrics* **109**(3):524–525.

9 Freedman HL, Preston KL (1992). Polaroid photoscreening for amblyogenic factors: an improved methodology. *Ophthalmology* **99**:1785–1795.

10 Friendly DS, Weiss LP, Barnet AB, *et al*. (1986). Pattern-reversal visual evoked potentials in the diagnosis of amblyopia in children. *Am J Ophthalmol* **102**:329–339.

CHAPTER 3
References

1 Gilbert C, Foster A (2001). Childhood blindness in the context of VISION 2020 – the right to sight. *Bull World Health Organ* **79**(3):227–232.
2 Terry TL (1942). Extreme prematurity and fibroblastic overgrowth of persistent vascular sheath behind each crystalline lens. I. Preliminary report. *Am J Ophthalmol* **25**:203–204.
3 Hess JH (1934). Oxygen unit for premature and very young infants. *Am J Dis Child* **7**:916–917.
4 Silverman WA (1980). *Retrolental fibroplasia. A Modern Parable*. Grune & Stratton, New York.
5 Campbell K (1951). Intensive oxygen therapy as a possible cause of retrolental fibroplasia: a clinical approach. *Med J Aust* **2**:48–50.
6 Patz A, Hoech LE, DeLaCruz E (1952). Studies on the effect of high oxygen administration in retrolental fibroplasia. I. Nursery observations. *Am J Ophthalmol* **35**:1248–1253.
7 Kinsey VE, Jacobus JT, Hemphill FM (1956). Retrolental fibroplasia. Cooperative study of retrolental fibroplasia and the use of oxygen. *Arch Ophthalmol* **56**:481–547.
8 Patz A (1953). Oxygen studies in retrolental fibroplasia. II. The production of the microscopic changes of retrolental fibroplasia in experimental animals. *Am J Ophthalmol* **136**:1511–1522.
9 Ashton N, Ward B, Serpell G (1954). Effect of oxygen on developing retinal vessels with particular reference to the problem of retrolental fibroplasia. *Br J Ophthalmol* **38**(7):397–432.
10 Dollery CT, Bulpitt CJ, Kohner EM (1969). Oxygen supply to the retina from the retinal and choroidal circulations at normal and increased arterial oxygen tensions. *Invest Ophthalmol* **8**(6):588–594.
11 Chan-Ling T, Tout S, Hollander H, *et al*. (1992). Vascular changes and their mechanisms in the feline model of retinopathy of prematurity. *Invest Ophthalmol Vis Sci* **33**(7):2128–2147.
12 Katz ML, Robison WG Jr (1988). Autoxidative damage to the retina: potential role in retinopathy of prematurity. *Birth Defects Orig Artic Ser* **24**(1):237–248.
13 Pierce EA, Foley ED, Smith LE (1996). Regulation of vascular endothelial growth factor by oxygen in a model of retinopathy of prematurity. *Arch Ophthalmol* **114**(10):1219–1228.

14 Hellstrom A, Engstrom E, Hard AL, *et al*. (2003). Postnatal serum insulin-like growth factor I deficiency is associated with retinopathy of prematurity and other complications of premature birth. *Pediatrics* **112**(5):1016–1020.
15 Avery ME (1960). Recent increase in mortality from hyaline membrane disease. *J Pediatr* **57**:553–559.
16 Hatfield EM (1972). Blindness in infants and young children. *Sight Sav Rev* **42**(2):69–89.
17 Cross KW (1973). Cost of preventing retrolental fibroplasia? *Lancet* **2**(7835):954–956.
18 Nelson KB, Grether JK (1999). Causes of cerebral palsy. *Curr Opin Pediatr* **11**(6):487–491.
19 Patz A (1970). The need for further research in retrolental fibroplasia. *Sight Sav Rev* **40**(1):7–11.
20 Coats DK (2005). Retinopathy of prematurity: involution, factors predisposing to retinal detachment, and expected utility of preemptive surgical reintervention. *Trans Am Ophthalmol Soc* **103**:281–312.
21 Lala-Gitteau E, Majzoub S, Saliba E, *et al*. (2007). [Epidemiology for retinopathy of prematurity: risk factors in the Tours hospital (France)]. *J Fr Ophtalmol* **30**(4):366–373.
22 Valcamonico A, Accorsi P, Sanzeni C, *et al*. (2007). Mid- and long-term outcome of extremely low birth weight (ELBW) infants: an analysis of prognostic factors. *J Matern Fetal Neonatal Med* **20**(6):465–471.
23 Wright KW, Sami D, Thompson L, *et al*. (2006). A physiologic reduced oxygen protocol decreases the incidence of threshold retinopathy of prematurity. *Trans Am Ophthalmol Soc* **104**:78–84.
24 Chen J, Smith LE (2007). Retinopathy of prematurity. *Angiogenesis* **10**(2):133–140.
25 Wallace DK, Veness-Meehan KA, Miller WC (2007). Incidence of severe retinopathy of prematurity before and after a modest reduction in target oxygen saturation levels. *J AAPOS* **11**(2):170–174.
26 Liu PM, Fang PC, Huang CB, *et al*. (2005). Risk factors of retinopathy of prematurity in premature infants weighing less than 1600 g. *Am J Perinatol* **22**(2):115–120.
27 Kim TI, Sohn J, Pi SY, *et al*. (2004). Postnatal risk factors of retinopathy of prematurity. *Paediatr Perinat Epidemiol* **18**(2):130–134.
28 Shah VA, Yeo CL, Ling YL, *et al*. (2005). Incidence & risk factors of retinopathy of prematurity among very low birth weight infants in Singapore. *Ann Acad Med Singapore* **34**(2):169–178.
29 Noyola DE, Bohra L, Paysse EA, *et al*. (2002). Association of candidemia and retinopathy of prematurity in very low birthweight infants. *Ophthalmology* **109**(1):80–84.
30 Mittal M, Dhanireddy R, Higgins RD (1998). *Candida* sepsis and association with retinopathy of prematurity. *Pediatrics* **101**(4 Pt 1):654–657.

31 Manzoni P, Maestri A, Leonessa M, *et al*. (2006). Fungal and bacterial sepsis and threshold ROP in preterm very low birth weight neonates. *J Perinatol* **26**(1):23–30.

32 Englert JA, Saunders RA, Purohit D, *et al*. (2001). The effect of anemia on retinopathy of prematurity in extremely low birth weight infants. *J Perinatol* **21**(1):21–26.

33 Gaynon MW (2006). Rethinking STOP-ROP: is it worthwhile trying to modulate excessive VEGF levels in prethreshold ROP eyes by systemic intervention? A review of the role of oxygen, light adaptation state, and anemia in prethreshold ROP. *Retina* **6**(7 Suppl):S18–S23.

34 Modanlou HD, Gharraee Z, Hasan J, *et al*. (2006). Ontogeny of VEGF, IGF-I, and GH in neonatal rat serum, vitreous fluid, and retina from birth to weaning. *Invest Ophthalmol Vis Sci* **7**(2):738–744.

35 Villegas Becerril E, Fernandez Molina F, Gonzalez R, *et al*. (2005). [Serum IGF-I levels in retinopathy of prematurity. New indications for ROP screening.] *Arch Soc Esp Oftalmol* **80**(4):233–238.

36 Villegas Becerril E, Gonzalez Fernandez R, Fernandez Molina F, *et al*. (2005). Growth factor levels and ROP. *Ophthalmology* **112**(12):2238.

37 Villegas-Becerril E, Gonzalez-Fernandez R, Perula-Torres L, *et al*. (2006). [IGF-I, VEGF and bFGF as predictive factors for the onset of retinopathy of prematurity (ROP).] *Arch Soc Esp Oftalmol* **81**(11):641–646.

38 The Committee for the Classification of Retinopathy of Prematurity (1984). An international classification of retinopathy of prematurity. *Arch Ophthalmol* **102**(8):1130–1134.

39 The International Committee for the Classification of the Late Stages of Retinopathy of Prematurity (1987). An international classification of retinopathy of prematurity. II. The classification of retinal detachment. *Arch Ophthalmol* **105**(7):906–912.

40 International Committee for the Classification of Retinopathy of Prematurity (2005). The International Classification of Retinopathy of Prematurity revisited. *Arch Ophthalmol* **123**(7):991–999.

41 Palmer EA, Flynn JT, Hardy RJ, *et al*. for the Cryotherapy for Retinopathy of Prematurity Cooperative Group (1991). Incidence and early course of retinopathy of prematurity. *Ophthalmology* **98**(11):1628–1640.

42 Jones JG, MacKinnon B, Good WV, *et al*. (2005). The early treatment for ROP (ETROP) randomized trial: study results and nursing care adaptations. *Insight* **30**(2):7–13.

43 Good WV (2004). Final results of the Early Treatment for Retinopathy of Prematurity (ETROP) randomized trial. *Trans Am Ophthalmol Soc* **102**:233–248; discussion 248–250.

44 Repka MX, Palmer EA, Tung B, for the Cryotherapy for Retinopathy of Prematurity Cooperative Group (2000). Involution of retinopathy of prematurity. *Arch Ophthalmol* **118**(5):645–649.

45 Flynn JT, Bancalari E, Bachynski BN, *et al*. (1987). Retinopathy of prematurity. Diagnosis, severity, and natural history. *Ophthalmology* **94**(6):620–629.

46 Mintz-Hittner HA, Kretzer FL (1990). The rationale for cryotherapy with a prophylactic scleral buckle for Zone I threshold retinopathy of prematurity. *Doc Ophthalmol* **74**(3):263–268.

47 Kretzer FL, Hittner HM (2000). Pathogenesis and antioxidant suppression of retinopathy of prematurity. In: *Handbook of Free Radicals and Antioxidants in Biomedicine*. JQA Miquel, H Weber (eds). CRC Press Inc, Boca Raton, Florida.

48 Coats DK, Miller AM, Hussein MA, *et al*. (2005). Involution of retinopathy of prematurity after laser treatment: factors associated with development of retinal detachment. *Am J Ophthalmol* **140**(2):214–222.

49 (2006). Erratum. *Pediatrics* **118**(3):1324. Original article: American Academy of Pediatrics Section on Ophthalmology (2006). Screening examination of premature infants for retinopathy of prematurity. *Pediatrics* **117**(2):572–576.

50 Aprahamian AD, Coats DK, Paysse EA, *et al*. (2000). Compliance with outpatient follow-up recommendations for infants at risk for retinopathy of prematurity. *J AAPOS* **4**(5):282–286.

51 Wallace DK, Coats DK, Paysse EA (1998). Retinopathy of prematurity survey results. *J AAPOS* **2**(2):65–66.

52 O'Neil JW, Hutchinson AK, Saunders RA, *et al*. (1998). Acquired cataracts after argon laser photocoagulation for retinopathy of prematurity. *J AAPOS* **2**(1):48–51.

53 Paysse EA, Miller A, Brady McCreery KM, *et al*. (2002). Acquired cataracts after diode laser photocoagulation for threshold retinopathy of prematurity. *Ophthalmology* **109**(9):1662–1665.

54 Fuchino Y, Hayashi H, Kono T, *et al*. (1995). Long-term follow up of visual acuity in eyes with stage 5 retinopathy of prematurity after closed vitrectomy. *Am J Ophthalmol* **120**(3):308–316.

55 Capone A Jr, Trese MT (2001). Lens-sparing vitreous surgery for tractional stage 4A retinopathy of prematurity retinal detachments. *Ophthalmology* **108**(11):2068–2070.

56 Prenner JL, Capone A Jr, Trese MT (2004). Visual outcomes after lens-sparing vitrectomy for stage 4A retinopathy of prematurity. *Ophthalmology* **111**(12):2271–2273.

57 Paysse EA, Coats DK, Hussein MA, *et al*. (2006). Long-term outcomes of photorefractive keratectomy for anisometropic amblyopia in children. *Ophthalmology* **113**(2):169–176.

58 Cryotherapy for Retinopathy of Prematurity Cooperative Group (2001). Multicenter Trial of Cryotherapy for Retinopathy of Prematurity: ophthalmological outcomes at 10 years. *Arch Ophthalmol* **119**(8):1110–1118.

59 Cryotherapy for Retinopathy of Prematurity Cooperative Group (2001). Contrast sensitivity at age 10 years in children who had threshold retinopathy of prematurity. *Arch Ophthalmol* **119**(8):1129–1133.

60 VanderVeen DK, Coats DK, Dobson V, *et al.* (2006). Prevalence and course of strabismus in the first year of life for infants with prethreshold retinopathy of prematurity: findings from the Early Treatment for Retinopathy of Prematurity study. *Arch Ophthalmol* **124**(6):766–773.

61 Finer NN, Schindler RF, Grant G, *et al.* (1982). Effect of intramuscular vitamin E on frequency and severity of retrolental fibroplasia. A controlled trial. *Lancet* **1**(8281):1087–1091.

62 Hittner HM, Godio LB, Rudolph AJ, *et al.* (1981). Retrolental fibroplasia: efficacy of vitamin E in a double-blind clinical study of preterm infants. *New Engl J Med* **305**(23):1365–1371.

63 Johnson L, Schaffer D, Boggs TR Jr (1974). The premature infant, vitamin E deficiency and retrolental fibroplasia. *Am J Clin Nutr* **27**(10):1158–1173.

64 Ozkan H, Duman N, Kumral A, *et al.* (2006). Inhibition of vascular endothelial growth factor-induced retinal neovascularization by retinoic acid in experimental retinopathy of prematurity. *Physiol Res* **55**(3):267–275.

65 DiBiasie A (2006). Evidence-based review of retinopathy of prematurity prevention in VLBW and ELBW infants. *Neonatal Netw* **25**(6):393–403.

66 (No Authors listed) (2000). Supplemental Therapeutic Oxygen for Prethreshold Retinopathy Of Prematurity (STOP-ROP): a randomized, controlled trial. I: primary outcomes. *Pediatrics* **105**(2):295–310.

67 Abman S (2002). Monitoring cardiovascular function in infants with chronic lung disease of prematurity. *Arch Dis Child Fetal Neonatal Ed* **87**:F15.

68 Askie LM, Henderson-Smart DJ, Irwig L, *et al.* (2003). Oxygen-saturation targets and outcomes in extremely preterm infants. *New Engl J Med* **349**(10):959–967.

69 Hay WW Jr, Bell EF (2000). Oxygen therapy, oxygen toxicity, and the STOP-ROP trial. *Pediatrics* **105**(2):424–425.

70 Mills MD (2000). STOP-ROP results suggest selective use of supplemental oxygen for prethreshold ROP. *Arch Ophthalmol* **118**(8):1121–1122.

71 Rota R, Riccioni T, Zaccarini M, *et al.* (2005). Marked inhibition of retinal neovascularization in rats following soluble-flt-1 gene transfer. *J Gene Med* **6**(9):992–1002.

72 Demorest BH (1996). Retinopathy of prematurity requires diligent follow-up care. *Surv Ophthalmol* **41**(2):175–178.

73 Steinkuller PG, Du L, Gilbert C, *et al.* (1999). Childhood blindness. *J AAPOS* **3**(1):26–32.

CHAPTER 4
References

1 Noorden GK (1997). Mechanisms of amblyopia. *Adv Ophthalmol* **34**:93–115.

2 Thompson JR, Woodruff G, Hiscox FA, *et al.* (1991). The incidence and prevalence of amblyopia detected in childhood. *Public Health* **105**:455–462.

3 Preslan MW, Novak A (1996). Baltimore Vision Screening Project. *Ophthalmology* **103**:105–109.

4 Preslan MW, Novak A (1998). Baltimore Vision Screening Project. Phase 2. *Ophthalmology* **105**:150–153.

5 Rahi JS, Sripathi S, Gilbert CE, *et al.* (1995). Childhood blindness in India: causes in 1318 blind school students in nine states. *Eye* **9**(Pt 5):545–550.

6 National Eye Institute Office of Biometry and Epidemiology (1984). *Report on the National Eye Institute Visual Acuity Impairment Survey Pilot Study*. National Eye Institute, Bethesda, Maryland, pp. 81–84.

7 Woodruff G, Hiscox F, Thompson JR, *et al.* (1994). The presentation of children with amblyopia. *Eye* **8**(Pt 6):623–626.

8 Sjostrand J, Abrahamsson M (1995). Risk factors in amblyopia. *Eye* **4**(Pt 6):787–793.

9 Keech RV, Kutschke PJ (1995). Upper age limit for the development of amblyopia. *J Pediatr Ophthalmol Strabismus* **32**:89–93.

10 Williams C, Harrad RA, Harvey I, *et al.* for the ALSPAC Study Team (Avon Longitudinal Study of Pregnancy and Childhood) (2001). Screening for amblyopia in preschool children: results of a population-based, randomised controlled trial. *Ophthalmic Epidemiol* **8**:279–295.

11 Rahi J, Logan S, Timms C, *et al.* (2002). Risk, causes, and outcomes of visual impairment after loss of vision in the non-amblyopic eye: a population-based study. *Lancet* **360**:597–602.

12 Tommila V, Tarkkanen A (1981). Incidence of loss of vision in the healthy eye in amblyopia. *Br J Ophthalmol* **65**:575–577.

13 Van Leeuwen R, Eijkemans MJ, Vingerling JR, *et al.* (2007). Risk of bilateral visual impairment in individuals with amblyopia: the Rotterdam study. *Br J Ophthalmol* **91**:1450–1451.

14 Webber AL, Wood JM, Gole GA, *et al.* (2008). Effect of amblyopia on self-esteem in children. *Optom Vis Sci* **85**:1074–1081.

15 Koklanis K, Abel LA, Aroni R (2006). Psychosocial impact of amblyopia and its treatment: a multidisciplinary study. *Clin Experiment Ophthalmol* **34**:743–750.

16 Packwood EA, Cruz OA, Rychwalski PJ, *et al.* (1999). The psychosocial effects of amblyopia study. *J AAPOS* **3**:15–17.

17 Beauchamp GR, Bane MC, Stager DR, *et al.* (1999). A value analysis model applied to the management of amblyopia. *Trans Am Ophthalmol Soc* **97**:349–367; discussion 367–372.

18 Headon MP, Powell TP (1973). Cellular changes in the lateral geniculate nucleus of infant monkeys after suture of the eyelids. *J Anat* **116**:135–145.

19 Magramm I (1992). Amblyopia: etiology, detection, and treatment. *Pediatr Rev* **13**:7–14.

20 Vaegan, Taylor D (1979). Critical period for deprivation amblyopia in children. *Trans Ophthalmol Soc UK* **99**:432–439.

21 Lam GC, Repka MX, Guyton DL (1993). Timing of amblyopia therapy relative to strabismus surgery. *Ophthalmology* **100**:1751–1756.

22 Kushner BJ (1984). Functional amblyopia associated with abnormalities of the optic nerve. *Arch Ophthalmol* **102**:683–685.

23 Hubel DH, Wiesel TN (1963). Receptive fields of cells in striate cortex of very young, visually inexperienced kittens. *J Neurophysiol* **26**:994–1002.

24 Hubel DH, Wiesel TN, LeVay S (1977). Plasticity of ocular dominance columns in monkey striate cortex. *Philos Trans R Soc (Lond) B Biol Sci* **278**:377–409.

25 Wiesel TN (1982). Postnatal development of the visual cortex and the influence of environment. *Nature* **299**:583–591.

26 Shao LG, Zhang YH, Zhang DG (1994). [Experimental studies on the changes of immunocytochemistry of gamma-aminobutyric acidergic neurons in the lateral geniculate nuclei of amblyopic kittens.] *Zhonghua Yan Ke Za Zhi* **30**:437–440.

27 Graf MH, Becker R, Kaufmann H (2000). Lea symbols: visual acuity assessment and detection of amblyopia. *Graefes Arch Clin Exp Ophthalmol* **238**:53–58.

28 Vision in Preschoolers Study Group (2005). Preschool vision screening tests administered by nurse screeners compared with lay screeners in the vision in preschoolers study. *Invest Ophthalmol Vis Sci* **46**:2639–2648.

29 Clarke MP, Wright CM, Hrisos S, *et al.* (2003). Randomised controlled trial of treatment of unilateral visual impairment detected at preschool vision screening. *BMJ* **327**:1251.

30 Moseley MJ, Neufeld M, McCarry B, *et al.* (2002). Remediation of refractive amblyopia by optical correction alone. *Ophthalmic Physiol Opt* **22**:296–299.

31 Steele AL, Bradfield YS, Kushner BJ, *et al.* (2006). Successful treatment of anisometropic amblyopia with spectacles alone. *J AAPOS* **10**:37–43.

32 France TD, France LW (1999). Optical penalization can improve vision after occlusion treatment. *J AAPOS* **3**:341–343.

33 Pediatric Eye Disease Investigator Group (2003). The course of moderate amblyopia treated with atropine in children: experience of the amblyopia treatment study. *Am J Ophthalmol* **136**:630–639.

34 Scheiman MM, Hertle RW, Beck RW, *et al.* (2005). Randomized trial of treatment of amblyopia in children aged 7 to 17 years. *Arch Ophthalmol* **123**:437–447.

CHAPTER 5
Bibliography

Coats DK, Olitsky SE (2007). *Strabismus Surgery and Its Complications*. Springer, Berlin.

Olitsky SE, Nelson LB (2005). Strabismus disorders. In: *Harley's Pediatric Ophthalmology*, 5th edn. LB Nelson, SE Olitsky (eds). Lippincott, Williams & Wilkins, Baltimore.

CHAPTER 6
References

1 Kikkawa DO (2002). Ophthalmic facial anatomy and physiology. In: *Adlers's Physiology of the Eye*. P Kaufman, A Alm (eds). Saunders, Philadelphia, pp. 23–25.

2 Lawton A (1998). Structure and function of the eyelids and conjunctiva. In: *The Cornea*. Kaufman H, Barron B, McDonald M (eds). Butterworth-Heinemann, Boston.

3 Morrow GL, Abbott RL (1998). Conjunctivitis. *Am Family Phys* **57**:735–746.

4 Gigliotti F, Williams FT, Hayden FG, *et al.* (1981). Etiology of acute conjunctivitis in children. *J Pediatr* **98**:531–536.

5 Friedlaender MH (1995). A review of the causes and treatment of bacterial and allergic conjunctivitis. *Clin Therap* **17**:800–810.

6 Jackson WB (1993). Differentiating conjunctivitis of diverse origins. *Surv Ophthalmol* **38**(Supplement):91–104.

7 Lichtenstein SJ, Granet D, Gold R, *et al.* (2004). Acute conjunctivitis. *J Pediatr Ophthalmol Strabismus* **41**:134–138.

8 American Academy of Pediatrics (2006). School health. In: *Red Book: 2006 Report of the Committee on Infectious Diseases*, 27th edn, LK Pickering, CJ Baker, SS Long, *et al.* (eds). American Academy of Pediatrics, Elk Grove Village, Illinois, pp. 148–150.

9 Centers for Disease Control (2002). Outbreak of bacterial conjunctivitis at a College – New Hampshire, January–March, 2002. *Morb Mortal Wkly Rep* **51**(10):205–207 (www.cdc.gov/mmwr/preview/mmwrhtml/m m5204a2.htm).

10 Centers for Disease Control (2003). Pneumococcal conjunctivitis at an Elementary School – Maine, January 31, 2003. *Morb Mortal Wkly Rep* **52**(4):64–66 (www.cdc.gov/mmwr/preview/mmwrhtml/mm5110a1.htm).

11 Weiss A, Brinser JH, Nazar-Stewart V (1993). Acute conjunctivitis in childhood. *J Pediatr* **122**A(1):10–14.

12 Isenberg SJ, Apt L, Valenton M, *et al.* (2002). A controlled trial of povidone-iodine to treat infectious conjunctivitis in children. *Am J Ophthalmol* **134**:681–688.

13 Patel PB, Diaz MCG, Bennett JE, *et al.* (2007). Clinical features of bacterial conjunctivitis in children. *Acad Emerg Med* **14**(1):1–5.

14 Bodor FF (1982). Conjunctivitis–otitis media syndrome: more than meets the eye. *Pediatrics* **69**(6):695–698.

15 Bodor FF, Marchant CD, Shurin PA, *et al.* (1985). Bacterial etiology of conjunctivitis–otitis media syndrome. *Pediatrics* **76**(1):26–28.

16 Block SL, Hedrick J, Tyler R, *et al.* (2000). Increasing bacterial resistance in pediatric acute conjunctivitis (1997–1998). *Antimicrob Agents Chemotherap* **44**:1650–1654.

17 Lichtenstein SJ (October 2006). Corneal ulcer. In: *Pediatric Ophthalmic Conditions, Case Studies – a supplement to Month Prescribing Reference (MPR)*.

18 Lichtenstein SJ, Wagner RS (2007). Speed of bacterial kill with a fluoroquinolone compared with nonfluoroquinolones: clinical implications and a review of kinetics of kill. *Adv Therap* **24**(5):1098–1111.

19 Hwang D (2000). Antibiotic update. *Ocular Surg News* **10–11**.

20 McDermott PF, Zhao S, Wagner DD, *et al.* (2002). The food safety perspective of antibiotic resistance. *Animal Biotech* **13**:71–84.

21 Goldstein MH, Kowalski RP, Gordon YJ (1999). Emerging fluoroquinolone resistance in bacterial keratitis: a 5-year review. *Ophthalmology* **106**(7):1313–1318.

22 Marangon FB, Miller D, Muallem MS, *et al.* (2004). Ciprofloxacin and levofloxacin resistance among methicillin-sensitive *Staphylococcus aureus* isolates from keratitis and conjunctivitis. *Am J Ophthalmol* **137**(3):453–458.

23 Chalita MR, Hofling-Lima AL, Paranhos A Jr, *et al.* (2004). Shifting trends in *in vitro* antibiotic susceptibilities for common ocular isolates during a period of 15 years. *Am J Ophthalmol* **137**(1):43–51.

24 Yamada M, Yoshida J, Hatou S, *et al.* (2008). Mutations in the quinolone resistance determining region in *Staphylococcus epidermidis* recovered from conjunctiva and their association with susceptibility to various fluoroquinolones. *Br J Ophthalmol* **92**(6):848–851 (published online first, 6th May 2008: http://bjo.bmj.com/cgi/content/abstract/bjo.2007.129858v1).

25 Ohnsman CM (2007). Exclusion of students with conjunctivitis from school: policies of State Departments of Health. *J Pediatr Ophthalmol Strabismus* **44**:101–105.

26 Teoh DL, Reynolds S (2003). Diagnosis and management of pediatric conjunctivitis. *Pediatr Emerg Care* **19**:48–55.

27 Friedlander MH (1993). Conjunctivitis of allergic origin: clinical presentation and differential diagnosis. *Surv Ophthalmol* **38**(Supplement):105–114.

28 Ehlers WH, Donshik PC (1992). Allergic ocular disorders: a spectrum of diseases. *Contact Lens Assoc Ophthalmol J* **18**(2):117–124.

29 Abelson MB, George MA, Garofalo C (1993). Differential diagnosis of ocular allergic disorders. *Ann Allergy, Asthma, Immunol* **70**(2):95–107.

30 Dart JK, Buckley RJ, Monnickendan M, *et al.* (1985). Perennial allergic conjunctivitis: definition, clinical characteristics and prevalence. A comparison with seasonal allergic conjunctivitis. *Trans Ophthalmol Soc UK* **105** (Pt 5):513–520.

31 Ono SJ, Abelson MB (2005). Allergic conjunctivitis: update on pathophysiology and prospects for future treatment. *J Allergy Clin Immunol* **115**(1):118–122.

32 Ghaffar A (2002). Hypersensitivity reactions, medical microbiology . In: *Immunology*, 6th edn. Roitt, Brostoff, and Male (eds). Mosby, St Louis, ch 17.

33 Scoper SV, Berdy GJ, Lichtenstein SJ, *et al.* (2007). Perception and quality of life associated with the use of olopatadine 0.2% (Pataday™) in patients with active allergic conjunctivitis. *Adv Therap* **24**(6):1221–1232.

34 Anderson HR, Poloniecki JD, Strachan DP, *et al.* (2001). ISAAC Phase 1 Study Group. Immunization and symptoms of atopic disease in children: results from the International Study of Asthma and Allergies in Childhood. *Am J Pub Health* **91**(7):1126–1129.

35 Maggi E, Biswas P, Del Prete G, *et al.* (1991). Accumulation of Th-2 like helper T cells in the conjunctiva of patients with vernal conjunctivitis. *J Immunol* **146**:1169–1174.

36 Allansmith MR, Baird RS, Greiner JV (1979). Vernal conjunctivitis and contact lens associated papillary conjunctivitis compared and contrasted. *Am J Ophthalmol* **87**:544–555.

37 Buckley RJ (1980). Long-term experience with sodium cromoglycate in the management of vernal keratoconjunctivitis. In: *The Mast Cell.* J Pepys, AM Edward (eds). Pitman Medical, London.

38 Cameron JA (1995). Shield ulcers and plaques of the cornea in vernal keratoconjunctivitis. *Ophthalmology* **6**:985–993.

39 Dunn SP, Heidemann DG (1997). Giant papillary conjunctivitis. In: *Cornea–cornea and external disease: clinical diagnosis and management*. JH Krachmer, MJ Mannis (eds). Mosby, St. Louis, pp. 819–825.

40 Cullom RD, Chang B (1994). Cornea: phlyctenulosis. In: *The Wills Eye Manual: Office and Emergency Room Diagnosis and Treatment of Eye Disease*. RD Cullom, B Chang (eds). Lippincott, Philadelphia, pp. 64–65.

CHAPTER 7
References

1 Mann I (1957). *Developmental Abnormalities of the Eye*, 2nd edn. JB Lippincott , Philadelphia.

2 Peters A (1906). Ueber angeborene defektbildung der descemetschen membran. *Klin Monatsbl Augenheilkd* **44**:27–40.

3 Rezende RA, Uchoa UB, Uchoa R, *et al*. (2004). Congenital corneal opacities in a cornea referral practice. *Cornea* **23**(6):565–570.

4 Tripathi BJ, Tripathi RC (1989). Neural crest origin of human trabecular meshwork and its implications for the pathogenesis of glaucoma. *Am J Ophthalmol* **107**(6):583–590.

5 Bahn CF, Falls HF, Varley GA, *et al*. (1984). Classification of corneal endothelial disorders based on neural crest origin. *Ophthalmology* **91**(6):558–563.

6 Kivlin JD, Fineman RM, Crandall AS, *et al*. (1986). Peters' anomaly as a consequence of genetic and nongenetic syndromes. *Arch Ophthalmol* **104**(1):61–64.

7 Ciralsky J, Colby K (2007). Congenital corneal opacities: a review with a focus on genetics. *Semin Ophthalmol* **22**(4):241–246.

8 Holmstrom GE, Reardon WP, Baraitser M, *et al*. (1991). Heterogeneity in dominant anterior segment malformations. *Br J Ophthalmol* **75**(10):591–597.

9 Reese AB, Ellsworth RM (1966). The anterior chamber cleavage syndrome. *Arch Ophthalmol* **75**:307–318.

10 Waring GO III, Rodrigues MM, Laibson PR (1975). Anterior chamber cleavage syndrome. A stepladder classification. *Surv Ophthalmol* **20**(1):3–27.

11 Yang LL, Lambert SR (2001). Peters' anomaly. A synopsis of surgical management and visual outcome. *Ophthalmol Clin North Am* **14**(3):467–477.

12 Zaidman GW, Flanagan JK, Furey CC (2007). Long-term visual prognosis in children after corneal transplant surgery for Peters' anomaly type I. *Am J Ophthalmol* **144**(1):104–108.

13 Kupfer C, Kuwabara T, Kaiser-Kupfer M (1975). The histopathology of pigmentary dispersion syndrome with glaucoma. *Am J Ophthalmol* **80**(5):857–862.

14 Traboulski EI, Maumenee IH (1992). Peters' anomaly and associated congenital malformations. *Arch Ophthalmol* **110**(12):1739–1742.

15 Yang LL, Lambert SR, Lynn MJ, *et al*. (1999). Long-term results of corneal graft survival in infants and children with Peters' anomaly. *Ophthalmology* **106**(4):833–848.

16 Dana MR, Schaumberg DA, Moyes AL, *et al*. (1997). Corneal transplantation in children with Peters' anomaly and mesenchymal dysgenesis. Multicenter Pediatric Keratoplasty Study. *Ophthalmology* **104**(10):1580–1586.

17 Elliott JH, Feman SS, O'Day DM, *et al*. (1985). Hereditary sclerocornea. *Arch Ophthalmol* **103**(5):676–679.

18 Happle R, Daniels O, Koopman RJ (1993). MIDAS syndrome (microphthalmia, dermal aplasia, and sclerocornea): an X-linked phenotype distinct from Goltz syndrome. *Am J Med Genet* **47**(5):710–713.

19 Cape CJ, Zaidman GW, Beck AD, *et al*. (2004). Phenotypic variation in ophthalmic manifestations of MIDAS syndrome (microphthalmia, dermal aplasia, and sclerocornea). *Arch Ophthalmol* **122**(7):1070–1074.

20 Kenyon KR (1975). Mesenchymal dysgenesis in Peters' anomaly, sclerocornea and congenital endothelial dystrophy. *Exp Eye Res* **21**(2):125–142.

21 Howard RO, Abrahams IW (1971). Sclerocornea. *Am J Ophthalmol* **71**(6):1254–1258.

22 Kim T, Cohen EJ, Schnall BM, *et al*. (1998). Ultrasound biomicroscopy and histopathology of sclerocornea. *Cornea* **17**(4):443–445.

23 Sharma A, Sukhija J, Das A, *et al*. (2004). Large pedunculated congenital corneal dermoid in association with eyelid coloboma. *J Pediatr Ophthalmol Strabismus* **41**(1):53–55.

24 Sommer F, Pillunat LE (2004). [Epibulbar dermoids – clinical features and therapeutic methods.] *Klin Monatsbl Augenheilkd* **221**(10):872–877.

25 Dar P, Javed AA, Ben-Yishay M, *et al*. (2001). Potential mapping of corneal dermoids to Xq24-qter. *J Med Genet* **38**(10):719–723.

26 Xia K, Wu L, Xi X, *et al*. (2004). Mutation in PITX2 is associated with ring dermoid of the cornea. *J Med Genet* **41**(12): e129.

27 Henkind P, Marinoff G, Manas A, *et al*. (1973). Bilateral corneal dermoids. *Am J Ophthalmol* **76**(6): 972–977.

28 Renata A, Rezende EJ, Uchoandro C, *et al*. (2005). Congenital corneal opacities. In: *Cornea*. MJ Jay, H Krachmer, EJ Holland (eds). Elsevier Mosby, Philadelphia, pp. 311–338.

29 Stein RM, Cohen EJ, Calhoun JH, *et al*. (1987). Corneal birth trauma managed with a contact lens. *Am J Ophthalmol* **103**(4): 596–598.

30 Angell LK, Robb RM, Berson FG (1981). Visual prognosis in patients with ruptures in Descemet's membrane due to forceps injuries. *Arch Ophthalmol* **99**(12):2137–2139.

31 Gnanaraj L, Rao VJ (2000). Corneal birth trauma: a cause for sensory exotropia. *Eye* **14**(5):791–792.

32 Chadha V, Taguri AH, Devlin HC (2006). Pseudophakic bullous keratopathy in a case of corneal birth trauma. *Eye* **20**(12):1428–1429.

33 Maumenee AE (1960). Congenital hereditary corneal dystrophy. *Am J Ophthalmol* **50**:1114–1124.

34 Callaghan M, Hand CK, Kennedy SM, *et al.* (1999). Homozygosity mapping and linkage analysis demonstrate that autosomal recessive congenital hereditary corneal dystrophy (CHED) and autosomal dominant CHED are genetically distinct. *Br J Ophthalmol* **83**(1):115–119.

35 Toma NM, Ebenezer ND, Inglehearn CF, *et al.* (1995). Linkage of congenital hereditary endothelial dystrophy to chromosome 20. *Hum Mol Genet* **4**(12):2395–2398.

36 Vithana EN, Morgan P, Sundaresan P, *et al.* (2006). Mutations in sodium-borate cotransporter SLC4A11 cause recessive congenital hereditary endothelial dystrophy (CHED2). *Nat Genet* **38**(7):755–777.

37 Aldave AJ, Yellore VS, Bourla N, *et al.* (2007). Autosomal recessive CHED associated with novel compound heterozygous mutations in SLC4A11. *Cornea* **26**(7):896–900.

38 Kirkness CM, McCartney A, Rice NS, *et al.* (1987). Congenital hereditary corneal oedema of Maumenee: its clinical features, management, and pathology. *Br J Ophthalmol* **71**(2):130–144.

39 Judisch GF, Maumenee IH (1978). Clinical differentiation of recessive congenital hereditary endothelial dystrophy and dominant hereditary endothelial dystrophy. *Am J Ophthalmol* **85**(5Pt 1):606–612.

40 Al-Ghamdi A, Al-Rajhi A, Wagoner MD (2007). Primary pediatric keratoplasty: indications, graft survival, and visual outcome. *J AAPOS* **11**(1):41–47.

41 Al-Rajhi AA, Wagoner MD (1997). Penetrating keratoplasty in congenital hereditary endothelial dystrophy. *Ophthalmology* **104**(6):956–961.

42 Bredrup C, Knappskog PM, Majewski J, *et al.* (2005). Congenital stromal dystrophy of the cornea caused by a mutation in the decorin gene. *Invest Ophthalmol Vis Sci* **46**(2):420–426.

43 Witschel H, Fine BS, Grützner P, *et al.* (1978). Congenital hereditary stromal dystrophy of the cornea. *Arch Ophthalmol* **96**(6):1043–1051.

44 Héon E, Mathers WD, Alward WL, *et al.* (1995). Linkage of posterior polymorphous corneal dystrophy to 20q11. *Hum Mol Genet* **4**(3):485–488.

45 Krafchak CM, Pawar H, Moroi SE, *et al.* (2005). Mutations in TCF8 cause posterior polymorphous corneal dystrophy and ectopic expression of COL4A3 by corneal endothelial cells. *Am J Hum Genet* **77**(5):694–708.

46 Biswas S, Munier FL, Yardley J, *et al.* (2001). Missense mutations in COL8A2, the gene encoding the alpha2 chain of type VIII collagen, cause two forms of corneal endothelial dystrophy. *Hum Mol Genet* **10**(21):2415–2423.

47 Levy SG, Moss J, Noble BA, *et al.* (1996). Early-onset posterior polymorphous dystrophy. *Arch Ophthalmol* **114**(10):1265–1268.

48 Krachmer JH (1985). Posterior polymorphous corneal dystrophy: a disease characterized by epithelial-like endothelial cells which influence management and prognosis. *Trans Am Ophthalmol Soc* **83**:413–475.

49 McCartney AC, Kirkness CM (1998). Comparison between posterior polymorphous dystrophy and congenital hereditary endothelial dystrophy of the cornea. *Eye* **2**(Pt 1):63–70.

50 Kao WW, Liu CY (2002). Roles of lumican and keratocan on corneal transparency. *Glycoconj J* **19**(4–5):275–285.

51 Michelacci YM (2003). Collagens and proteoglycans of the corneal extracellular matrix. *Braz J Med Biol Res* **36**(8):1037–1046.

52 Hobbs JR, Hugh-Jones K, Barrett AJ, *et al.* (1981). Reversal of clinical features of Hurler's disease and biochemical improvement after treatment by bone-marrow transplantation. *Lancet* **2**(8249):709–712.

53 Pitz S, Ogun O, Bajbouj M, *et al.* (2007). Ocular changes in patients with mucopolysaccharidosis I receiving enzyme replacement therapy: a 4-year experience. *Arch Ophthalmol* **125**(10):1353–1356.

54 Herati RS, Knox VW, O'Donnell P, *et al.* (2008). Radiographic evaluation of bones and joints in mucopolysaccharidosis I and VII dogs after neonatal gene therapy. *Mol Genet Metab* **95**(3):142–151.

55 Moore D, Connock MJ, Wraith E, *et al.* (2008). The prevalence of and survival in Mucopolysaccharidosis I: Hurler, Hurler–Scheie and Scheie syndromes in the UK. *Orphanet J Rare Dis* **3**:24.

56 Summers CG, Whitley CB, Holland EJ, *et al.* (1994). Dense peripheral corneal clouding in Scheie syndrome. *Cornea* **13**(3):277–279.

57 Constantopoulos G, Dekabian AS, Scheie HG (1971). Heterogeneity of disorders in patients with corneal clouding, normal intellect, and mucopolysaccharidosis. *Am J Ophthalmol* **72**(6):1106–1117.

58 McDonnell JM, Green WR, Maumenee IH (1985). Ocular histopathology of systemic mucopolysaccharidosis, type II-A (Hunter syndrome, severe). *Ophthalmology* **92**(12):1772–1779.

59 Iwamoto M, Nawa Y, Maumenee IH, *et al*. (1990). Ocular histopathology and ultrastructure of Morquio syndrome (systemic mucopolysaccharidosis IV A). *Graefes Arch Clin Exp Ophthalmol* **228**(4):342–349.

60 Kenyon KR, Topping TM, Green WR, *et al*. (1972). Ocular pathology of the Maroteaux–Lamy syndrome (systemic mucopolysaccharidosis type VI). Histologic and ultrastructural report of two cases. *Am J Ophthalmol* **73**(5):718–741.

61 Cantor LB, Disseler JA, Wilson FM II (1989). Glaucoma in the Maroteaux–Lamy syndrome. *Am J Ophthalmol* **108**(4):426–430.

62 Sly WS, Quinton BA, McAlister WH, *et al*. (1973). Beta glucuronidase deficiency: report of clinical, radiologic, and biochemical features of a new mucopolysaccharidosis. *J Pediatr* **82**(2):249–257.

63 Rodrigues MM, Calhoun J, Harley RD (1975). Corneal clouding with increased acid mucopolysaccharide accumulation in Bowman's membrane. *Am J Ophthalmol* **79**(6):916–924.

64 Matalon RK (1996). Mucolipidoses. In: *Nelson Textbook of Pediatrics*. EB Richard, RM Kliegman, AM Arvin (eds). Saunders, Philadelphia, pp. 404–405.

65 Sphranger J, Gehler J, Cantz M (1977). Mucolipidosis I– a sialidosis. *Am J Med Genet* **1**(1):21–29.

66 Cibis GW, Harris DJ, Chapman AL, *et al*. (1983). Mucolipidosis I. *Arch Ophthalmol* **101**(6):933–939.

67 Libert J, Van Hoof F, Farriaux JP, *et al*. (1977). Ocular findings in I-cell disease (mucolipidosis type II). *Am J Ophthalmol* **83**(5):617–628.

68 Traboulsi EI, Maumenee IH (1986). Ophthalmologic findings in mucolipidosis III (pseudo-Hurler polydystrophy). *Am J Ophthalmol* **102**(5):592–597.

69 Berman ER, Livni N, Shapira E, *et al*. (1974). Congenital corneal clouding with abnormal systemic storage bodies: a new variant of mucolipidosis. *J Pediatr* **84**(4):519–526.

70 Schiffmann R, Dwyer NK, Lubensky IA, *et al*. (1998). Constitutive achlorhydria in mucolipidosis type IV. *Proc Natl Acad Sci USA* **95**(3):1207–1212.

71 Newman NJ, Starck T, Kenyon KR, *et al*. (1990). Corneal surface irregularities and episodic pain in a patient with mucolipidosis IV. *Arch Ophthalmol* **108**(2):251–254.

72 Dangel ME, Bremer DL, Rogers DL (1985). Treatment of corneal opacification in mucolipidosis IV with conjunctival transplantation. *Am J Ophthalmol* **99**(2):137–141.

73 Fabry H (2002). Angiokeratoma corporis diffusum – Fabry disease: historical review from the original description to the introduction of enzyme replacement therapy. *Acta Paediatr Suppl* **91**(439):3–5.

74 Sodi A, Ioannidis AS, Mehta A, *et al*. (2007). Ocular manifestations of Fabry's disease: data from the Fabry Outcome Survey. *Br J Ophthalmol* **91**(2):210–214.

75 Zarate YA, Hopkin RJ (2008). Fabry's disease. *Lancet* **372**(9647):1427–1435.

76 Tsilou E, Zhou M, Gahl W, *et al*. (2007). Ophthalmic manifestations and histopathology of infantile nephropathic cystinosis: report of a case and review of the literature. *Surv Ophthalmol* **52**(1):97–105.

77 Gahl WA, Thoene JG, Schneider JA (2002). Cystinosis. *New Engl J Med* **347**(2):111–121.

78 Melles RB, Schneider JA, Rao NA, *et al*. (1987). Spatial and temporal sequence of corneal crystal deposition in nephropathic cystinosis. *Am J Ophthalmol* **104**(6):598–604.

79 Kaiser-Kupfer MI, Gazzo MA, Datiles MB, *et al*. (1990). A randomized placebo-controlled trial of cysteamine eye drops in nephropathic cystinosis. *Arch Ophthalmol* **108**(5):689–693.

80 Cantani A, Giardini O, Ciarnella Cantani A (1983). Nephropathic cystinosis: ineffectiveness of cysteamine therapy for ocular changes. *Am J Ophthalmol* **95**(5):713–714.

81 Macsai MS, Schwartz TL, Hinkle D, *et al*. (2001). Tyrosinemia type II: nine cases of ocular signs and symptoms. *Am J Ophthalmol* **132**(4):522–527.

82 Cotran PR, Bajart AM (1992). Congenital corneal opacities. *Int Ophthalmol Clin* **32**(1): 93–105.

83 Momtchilova M, *et al*. (2000). [Congenital corneal anesthesia in children: diagnostic and therapeutic problems.] *J Fr Ophthalmol* **23**(3): 245–248.

84 Malik AN, Hildebrand GD, Sekhri R, *et al*. (2008). Bilateral macular scars following intrauterine herpes simplex virus type 2 infection. *J AAPOS* **12**(3):305–306.

85 Corey L, Whitley RJ, Stone EF, *et al*. (1988). Difference between herpes simplex virus type 1 and type 2 neonatal encephalitis in neurological outcome. *Lancet* **1**(8575–6):1–4.

86 Jeffries DJ (1991). Intra-uterine and neonatal herpes simplex virus infection. *Scand J Infect Dis Suppl* **80**:21–26.

87 Kimberlin DW (2007). Management of HSV encephalitis in adults and neonates: diagnosis, prognosis and treatment. *Herpes* **14**(1):11–16.

88 Graper C, Milne M, Stevens MR (1996). The traumatic saddle nose deformity: etiology and treatment. *J Craniomaxillofac Trauma* **2**(1):37–49; discussion 50–51.

89 Kirk RW (2005). Syphilitic interstitial keratitis. In: *Cornea*. MGM Jay, H Krachmer, EJ Holland (eds). Elsevier Mosby, Philadelphia, pp. 1133–1159.

90 O'Neill JF (1998). The ocular manifestations of congenital infection: a study of the early effect and long-term outcome of maternally transmitted rubella and toxoplasmosis. *Trans Am Ophthalmol Soc* **96**:813–879.

91 Deluise VP, CoboVM, Chandler D (1983). Persistent corneal edema in the congenital rubella syndrome. *Ophthalmology* **90**(7):835–839.

92 Roush SW, Murphy TV (2007). Historical comparisons of morbidity and mortality for vaccine-preventable diseases in the United States. *JAMA* **298**(18):2155–2163.

CHAPTER 8
References

1 Cross HE, Jensen AD (1973). Ocular manifestations in the Marfan's syndrome and homocystinuria. *Am J Ophthalmol* **75**(3):405–420.

2 Karr DJ, Scott WE (1986). Visual acuity results following treatment of persistent hyperplastic primary vitreous. *Arch Ophthalmol* **104**(5):662–667.

3 Pollard ZF (1997). Persistent hyperplastic primary vitreous: diagnosis, treatment and results. *Trans Am Ophthalmol Soc* **95**:487–549.

4 Wilson ME, Buckley EG, Kivlin JD, *et al*. (2001). Childhood cataracts and other pediatric lens disorders. In: *Basic and Clinical Science Course Section 6: Pediatric Ophthalmology and Strabismus*. The Foundation of the American Academy of Ophthalmology, San Francisco, ch 22, pp. 238–250.

5 Wright KW (2003). Lens abnormalities. In: *Pediatric Ophthalmology and Strabismus*, 2nd edn. KW Wright, PH Spiegel (eds). Springer-Verlag, New York, ch 27, pp. 450–480.

6 Nelson LB, Calhoun JH, Simon JW, *et al*. (1985). Progression of congenital anterior polar cataracts in childhood. *Arch Ophthalmol* **103**(12):1842–1843.

7 Krill AE, Woodbury G, Bowman JE (1969). X-chromosomal-linked sutural cataracts. *Am J Ophthalmol* **68**(5):867–872.

8 Litt M, Carrero-Valenzuela R, LaMorticella DM, *et al*. (1997). Autosomal dominant cerulean cataract is associated with a chain termination mutation in the human beta-crystalline gene CRYBB2. *Hum Mol Genet* **6**(5):665–668.

9 Caputo AR, Wagner RS, Reynolds DR, *et al*. (1989). Down syndrome. Clinical review of ocular features. *Clin Pediatr* **28**(8):355–358.

10 Stambolian D (1988). Galactose and cataract. *Surv Ophthalmol* **32**(5):333–349.

11 Tripathi AC, Cibis GW, Tripathi BJ (1986). Pathogenesis of cataracts in patients with Lowe's syndrome. *Ophthalmology* **93**(8):1046–1051.

12 Johnston SS, Nevin NC (1976). Ocular manifestations in patients and female relatives of families with oculocerebrorenal syndrome of Lowe. *Birth Defects* **12**(3):569–577.

13 Colville DJ, Savige J (1997). Alport syndrome. A review of the ocular manifestations. *Ophthal Genet* **18**(4):161–173.

14 Wilson ME, Trivedi RH, Biber JM, *et al*. (2006). Anterior capsule rupture and subsequent cataract formation in Alport syndrome. *J AAPOS* **10**(2):182–183.

15 Machuca-Tzili L, Brook D, Hilton-Jones D (2005). Clinical and molecular aspects of the myotonic dystrophies: a review. *Muscle Nerve* **32**(1):1–18.

16 Sher NA, Letson RD, Desnick RJ (1979). The ocular manifestations in Fabry's disease. *Arch Ophthalmol* **97**(4):671–676.

17 Claridge KJ, Gibberd FB, Sidey MC (1992). Refsum disease: the presentation and ophthalmic aspects of Refsum disease in a series of 23 patients. *Eye* **6**(Pt 4):371–375.

18 Herron BE (1976). Wilson's disease (hepatolenticular degeneration). *Ophthal Sem* **1**(1):63–69.

19 Happle R (1979). X-linked dominant chondrodysplasia punctata. Review of literature and report of a case. *Hum Genet* **53**(1):65–73.

20 Arbisser AI, Murphree AL, Carcia CA, *et al*. (1976). Ocular findings in mannosidosis. *Am J Ophthalmol* **82**(3):465–471.

21 Alward WL (2000). Axenfeld–Reiger syndrome in the age of molecular genetics. *Am J Ophthalmol* **130**(1):107–115.

22 Fraumeni JF, Glass AG (1968). Wilm's tumor and aniridia. *J Am Med Assoc* **206**(4):825–828.

23 Miller RW, Fraumeni JF, Manning MD (1964). Association of Wilms' tumor with aniridia, hemi-hypertrophy and other congenital malformations. *New Engl J Med* **270**:922–927.

24 Nelson LB, Spaeth GL, Nowinski TS, *et al*. (1984). Aniridia: a review. *Surv Ophthalmol* **28**(6):621–642.

25 De Wilde GA, Meire FM (1991). The Hallermann–Streiff syndrome. *Bull Soc Belge d'Ophthalmol* **241**:71–75.

26 Johns KJ, Feder RS, Hamill MB, *et al*. (2001). Embryology. In: *Basic and Clinical Science Course Section 11: Lens and Cataract*. The Foundation of the American Academy of Ophthalmology, San Francisco, ch 4, pp. 21–39.

27 Givens KD, Lee DA, Jones T, *et al*. (1993). Congenital rubella syndrome: ophthalmic manifestations and associated systemic disorders. *Br J Ophthalmol* **77**(6):358–363.

28 Lambert SR, Lynn MJ, Reeves R, *et al*. (2006). Is there a latent period for the surgical treatment of children with dense bilateral congenital cataracts? *J AAPOS* **10**(1):30–36.

29 Birch EE, Stager DR (1996). The critical period for surgical treatment of dense, congenital, unilateral cataracts. *Invest Ophthalmol Vis Sci* **37**(8):1532–1538.

30 Rogers BL, Tishler CL, Tsou BH, *et al.* (1981). Visual acuities in infants with congenital cataracts operated on prior to 6 months of age. *Arch Ophthalmol* **99**(6):999–1003.

31 Wright KW, Matsumoto E, Edelman PM (1992). Binocular fusion and stereopsis associated with early surgery for monocular congenital cataracts. *Arch Ophthalmol* **110**(11):1607–1609.

32 Pandey SK (2005). Evaluation of visually significant cataracts. In: *Pediatric Cataract Surgery: Techniques, Complications, and Management*. ME Wilson, RH Trivedi, SK Pandey (eds). Lippincott, Williams & Wilkins, Philadelphia, ch 5, pp. 23–26.

33 Trivedi RH, Wilson ME (2005). Posterior capsulotomy and anterior vitrectomy for the management of pediatric cataracts. In: *Pediatric Cataract Surgery: Techniques, Complications, and Management*. ME Wilson, RH Trivedi, SK Pandey (eds). Lippincott, Williams & Wilkins, Philadelphia, ch 16, pp. 83–92.

34 Wilson ME, Trivedi RH (2007). Choice of intraocular lens for pediatric cataract surgery: survey of AAPOS members. *J Catar Refrac Surg* **33**(9):1666–1668.

35 Fan DS, Rao SK, Yu CB, *et al.* (2006). Changes in refraction and ocular dimensions after cataract surgery and primary intraocular lens implantation in infants. *J Catar Refract Surg* **32**(7):1104–1108.

36 Ashworth JL, Maino AP, Biswas S, *et al.* (2007). Refractive outcomes after primary intraocular lens implantation in infants. *Br J Ophthalmol* **91**(5):596–599.

37 Eibschitz-Tsimhoni M, Archer SM, Del Monte MA (2007). Intraocular lens power calculation in children. *Surv Ophthalmol* **52**(5):474–482.

38 Wallace DK, Chandler DL, Beck RW, *et al.* (2007). Treatment of bilateral refractive amblyopia in children three to less than 10 years of age. *Am J Ophthalmol* **144**(4):487–496.

CHAPTER 9
Bibliography

Barkan O (1942). Operation for congenital glaucoma. *Am J Ophthalmol* **25**:552.

Beck AD, Freedman SF, Kammer J, *et al.* (2003). Aqueous shunt devices compard with trabeculectomy with mitomycin-C for children in the first two years of life. *Am J Ophthalmol* **136**:994–1000.

Carter BC, Plager DA, Neely DE, *et al.* (2007). Endoscopic diode laser cyclophotocoagulation in the management of aphakic and pseudophakic glaucoma in children. *J AAPOS* **11**(1):34–40.

DeLuise VP, Anderson DR (1983). Primary infantile glaucoma (congenital glaucoma). *Surv Ophthalmol* **28**:1–18.

Dickens CJ, Hoskins HD Jr (1994). Developmental glaucoma. In: *The Eye in Infancy*, 2nd edn. SJ Isenberg (ed). Mosby, St. Louis.

Egbert JE, Wright MM, Dahlhauser KF, *et al.* (1995). A prospective study of ocular hypertension and glaucoma after pediatric cataract surgery. *Ophthalmology* **102**(7):1098–1101.

Enyedi LB, Freedman SF (2001). Safety and efficacy of brimonidine in children with glaucoma. *J AAPOS* **5**(5):281–284.

Enyedi LB, Freedman SF (2002). Latanoprost for the treatment of pediatric glaucoma. *Surv Ophthalmol* **47**(1 Suppl):S129–S132.

Freedman SF, Walton DS (2005). Glaucoma in infants and children. In: *Harley's Pediatric Ophthalmology*, 5th edn. LB Nelson, SE Olitsky (eds). Lippincott, Williams and Wilkins, Philadelphia.

Hoskins HD Jr, Kass M (eds) (1989). *Becker-Shaffer's Diagnosis and Therapy of the Glaucomas*, 6th edn. Mosby, St. Louis.

Kirwan JF, Shah P, Khaw PT (2002). Diode laser cyclophotocoagulation: role in the management of refractory pediatric glaucomas. *Ophthalmology* **109**(2):316–323.

Mandal AK, Gothwal VK, Bagga H, *et al.* (2003). Outcome of surgery on infants younger than 1 month with congenital glaucoma. *Ophthalmology* **110**:1909–1915.

Mandal AK, Netland PA (eds) (2006). *The Pediatric Glaucomas*. Elsevier, Philadelphia.

Mendocino ME, Lynch MG, Drack A, *et al.* (2000). Long-term surgical and visual outcomes in primary congenital glaucoma: 360° trabeculotomy versus goniotomy. *J AAPOS* **4**:205–210.

Minckler DS, Baerveldt G, Heuer DK, *et al.* (1987). Clinical evaluation of the Oculab tono-pen. *Am J Ophthalmol* **104**:168–173.

Molteno ACB (1973). Children with advanced glaucoma treated by drainage implants. *S Afr Arch Ophthalmol* **1**:55–61.

Muir KW, Jin J, Freedman SF (2004). Central corneal thickness and its relationship to intraocular pressure in children. *Ophthalmology* **111**:220–223.

Pensiero S, DaPozza S, Perissutti P, *et al.* (1992). Normal intraocular pressure in children. *J Pediatr Ophthalmol Strabismus* **29**:79–84.

Rajaraman RT, Kimura Y, Li S, *et al.* (2006). Retrospective case review of pediatric patients with uveitis treated with infliximab. *Ophthalmology* **113**:308–314.

Shields MB, Buckley EG, Klintworth GK, *et al.* (1985). Axenfeld–Rieger syndrome. A spectrum of developmental disorders. *Surv Ophthalmol* **29**:387–409.

Wagle NS, Freedman SF, Buckley EG, *et al*. (1998). Long-term outcome of cyclocryotherapy for refractory pediatric glaucoma. *Ophthalmology* **105**:1921–1927.

Walton DS (1995). Pediatric aphakic glaucoma: a study of 65 patients. *Trans Am Ophthalmol Soc* **93**:403–413.

Walton DS (2000). Glaucomas. In: *Pediatric Ophthalmology: a Clinical Guide*. PF Gallin (ed). Thieme, New York, 232–240.

Zaidman GW, Flanagan JK, Furey CC (2007). Long term visual prognosis in children after corneal transplant surgery for Peters anomaly type 1. *Am J Ophthalmol* **144**:104–108.

Zimmerman TJ, Kooner KS, Morgan KS (1983). Safety and efficacy of timolol in pediatric glaucoma. *Surv Ophthalmol* **28**:262–264.

CHAPTER 10
References

1 Tarkkanen A, Laatikainen L (1983). Coat's disease: clinical, angiographic, histopathological findings and clinical management. *Br J Ophthalmol* **67**(11):766–776.

2 Manschot WA, de Bruijn WC (1967). Coats's disease: definition and pathogenesis. *Br J Ophthalmol* **51**(3):145–157.

3 Woods AV, Duke JR (1963). Coats's disease. 1. Review of the literature, diagnostic criteria, clinical findings, and plasma lipid studies. *Br J Ophthalmol* **47**:385–412.

4 Fernandes BF, Odashiro AN, Maloney S, *et al*. (2006). Clinical-histopathological correlation in a case of Coats' disease. *Diagn Pathol* **1**:24.

5 Lambert SR, Taylor D, Kriss A (1989). The infant with nystagmus, normal appearing fundi, but an abnormal ERG. *Surv Ophthalmol* **34**(3):173–186.

6 Weleber RG (2002). Infantile and childhood retinal blindness: a molecular perspective (The Franceschetti Lecture). *Opthalmic Genet* **23**(2):71–97.

7 Fazzi E, Signorini SG, Scelsa B, *et al*. (2003). Leber's congenital amaurosis: an update. *Eur J Paediatr Neurol* **7**(1):13–22.

8 Michaelides M, Hunt DM, Moore AT (2004). The cone dysfunction syndromes. *Br J Ophthalmol* **88**(2):291–297.

9 Koenekoop RK (2003). The gene for Stargardt disease, ABCA4, is a major retinal gene: a mini-review. *Ophthalmic Genet* **24**(2):75–80.

10 Zhang K, Nguyen TH, Crandall A, *et al*. (1995). Genetic and molecular studies of macular dystrophies: recent developments. *Surv Ophthalmol* **40**(1):51–61.

11 Fishman GA, Stone EM, Grover S, *et al*. (1999). Variation of clinical expression in patients with Stargardt dystrophy and sequence variations in the ABCR Gene. *Arch Ophthalmol* **117**:504–510.

12 Spaide RF, Noble K, Morgan A, *et al*. (2006). Vitelliform macular dystrophy. *Ophthalmology* **113**(8):1392–1400.

13 Zhang K, Nguyen TH, Crandall A, *et al*. (1995). Genetic and molecular studies of macular dystrophies: recent developments. *Surv Ophthalmol* **40**(1):51–61.

14 Petrukhin K, Koisti MJ, Bakall B, *et al*. (1998). Identification of the gene responsible for Best macular dystrophy. *Nat Genet* **19**(3):241–247.

15 Goldberg MF (1997). Persistent fetal vasculature (PFV): an integrated interpretation of signs and symptoms associated with persistent hyperplastic primary vitreous (PHPV). LIV Edward Jackson Memorial Lecture. *Am J Ophthalmol* **124**(5):587–626.

16 Silbert M, Gurwood AS (2000). Clinical review: persistent hyperplastic primary vitreous. *Clin Eye Vision Care* **12**(3–4):131–137.

17 Mullner-Eidenbock A, Amon M, Moser E, *et al*. (2004). Persistent fetal vasculature and minimal fetal vascular remnants: a frequent cause of unilateral congenital cataracts. *Ophthalmology* **111**(5):906–913.

18 Anteby I, Cohen E, Karshai I, *et al*. (2002). Unilateral hyperplastic primary vitreous: course and outcomes. *J AAPOS* **6**:92–99.

19 Sikkink SK, Biswas S, Parry NR, *et al*. (2007). X-linked retinoschisis: an update. *Med Genet* **44**(4):225–232. Epub Dec 2006.

20 Oetting WS, Fryer JP, Shriram S, *et al*. (2003). Oculocutaneous albinism type 1: the last 100 years. *Pigment Cell Res* **16**(3):307–311.

21 Wolf AB, Rubin SE, Kodsi SR (2005). Comparison of clinical findings in pediatric patients with albinism and different amplitudes of nystagmus. *J AAPOS* **9**(4):363–368.

22 Adams NA, Awadein A, Tom HS (2007). The retinal ciliopathies. *Ophthalmic Genet* **28**(3):113–125.

CHAPTER 11
References

1 Cassidy J, Kivlin J, Lindsley C, Nocton J (2006). Ophthalmologic examinations in children with juvenile rheumatoid arthritis. *Pediatrics* **117**(5):1843–1845.

2 Smith JA, Mackensen F, Sen HN, *et al*. (2009). Epidemiology and course of disease in childhood uveitis. *Ophthalmology* **116**(8):1544–1551, 1551.e1.

3 Hoover DL, Khan JA, Giangiacomo J (1986). Pediatric ocular sarcoidosis. *Survey Ophthalmology* **30**:215–228.

4 Cunningham ET Jr (2001). Diagnosis and management of herpetic anterior uveitis. *Ophthalmology* **107**:2129–2130.

5 Womack LW, Liesegang TJ (1983). Complications of herpes zoster ophthalmicus. *Arch Ophthalmol* **101**:42–45.

6 Bloch-Michel E, Nussenblatt RB (1987). International Uveitis Study Group recommendations for the evaluation of intraocular inflammatory disease. *Am J Ophthalmol* **103**:234–235.

7 Malinowski SM, Pulido JS, Folk JC (1993). Long-term visual outcome and complications associated with pars planitis. *Ophthalmology* **100**:818–824.

8 Bosch-Driessen LE (2002). Ocular toxoplasmosis: clinical features and prognosis of 154 patients. *Ophthalmology* **109**(5):869–878.

9 Felberg NT, Shields JA, Federman JL (1981). Antibody to *Toxocara canis* in the aqueous humor. *Arch Ophthalmol* **99**:1563–1564.

10 Winter FC (1955). Sympathetic uveitis: a clinical and pathologic study of the visual result. *Am J Ophthalmol* **39**:340–347.

11 Murphree AL, Villalance JG, Deegan WF III (1996). Chemotherapy plus local treatment in the management of intraocular retinoblastoma. *Arch Ophthalmol* **114**:1348–1356.

12 Rosenthal AR (1983). Ocular manifestation of leukemia. A review. *Ophthalmology* **90**:899–905.

CHAPTER 12
References

1 Phillips PH, Brodsky MC (2002). Congenital optic nerve abnormalities. In: *Pediatric Ophthalmology and Strabismus*, 2nd edn, K Wright, PH Spiegel (eds). Springer, Berlin.

2 Bradford GM, Kutschke PJ, Scott WE (1992). Results of amblyopia therapy in eyes with unilateral structural abnormalities. *Ophthalmology* **99**(10):1616–1621.

3 Hoyt CS, Billson FA (1986). Optic nerve hypoplasia: changing perspectives. *Aus NZ J Ophthalmol* **14**:325–331.

4 Brodsky MC, Glasier CM, Pollock SC, *et al*. (1990). Optic nerve hypoplasia: identification by magnetic resonance imaging. *Arch Ophthalmol* **108**:562–567.

5 Frisen L, Holmegaard L (1975). Spectrum of optic nerve hypoplasia. *Br J Ophthalmol* **62**:7–15.

6 De Morsier G (1956). Etudes sur les dysraphies cranio-encephaliques. III. Agenesis du septum lucidum avec malformation du tractus optique. La dysplasie septo-optique. *Schweizer Archiv fur Neurol Psych* **77**(1–2):267–292.

7 Brodsky MC, Glasier CM (1993). Optic nerve hypoplasia: clinical significance of associated central nervous system abnormalities on magnetic resonance imaging. *Arch Ophthalmol* **111**:66–74.

8 Phillips PH, Spear C, Brodsky MC (2001). Magnetic resonance diagnosis of congenital hypopituitarism in children with optic nerve hypoplasia. *J AAPOS* **5**(5):275–280.

9 Sorkin JA, Davis PC, Meacham LR (1996). Optic nerve hypoplasia: absence of posterior pituitary bright signal on magnetic resonance imaging correlates with diabetes insipidus. *Am J Ophthalmol* **122**(5):717–723.

10 Brodsky MC (1991). Septo-optic dysplasia: a reappraisal. *Sem Ophthalmol* **6**:227–232.

11 Lambert SR, Hoyt CS, Narahara MH (1987). Optic nerve hypoplasia. *Surv Ophthalmol* **32**(1):1–9.

12 Arslanian SA, Rothfus WE, Foley TP, *et al*. (1984). Hormonal, metabolic, and neuroradiologic abnormalities associated with septo-optic dysplasia. *Acta Endocrinol* **107**:282–288.

13 Izenberg N, Rosenblum M, Parks JS (1984). The endocrine spectrum of septo-optic dysplasia. *Clinical Pediatr* **23**(11):632–636.

14 Margalith D, Tze WJ, Jan JE (1985). Congenital optic nerve hypoplasia with hypothalamic-pituitary dysplasia. *Am J Dis Child* **139**(4):361–366.

15 Brodsky MC, Conte FA, Taylor D, *et al*. (1997). Sudden death in septo-optic dysplasia. Report of 5 cases. *Arch Ophthalmol* **115**(1):66–70.

16 Jacobson L, Hellström A, Flodmark O (1997). Large cups in normal-sized optic discs: a variant of optic nerve hypoplasia in children with periventricular leukomalacia. *Arch Ophthalmol* **115**(10):1263–1269.

17 Brodsky MC (2001). Periventricular leukomalacia: an intracranial cause of pseudoglaucomatous cupping. *Arch Ophthalmol* **119**(4):626–627.

18 Kim RY, Hoyt WF, Lessell S, *et al*. (1989). Superior segmental optic hypoplasia. A sign of maternal diabetes. *Arch Ophthalmol* **107**(9):1312–1315.

19 Brodsky MC, Schroeder GT, Ford R (1993). Superior segmental optic hypoplasia in identical twins. *J Clin Neuro-Ophthalmol* **13**(2):152–154.

20 Pollock S (1988). The morning glory disc anomaly: contractile movement, classification, and embryogenesis. *Documenta Ophthalmol Adv Ophthalmol* **65**:439–460.

21 Kindler P (1970). Morning glory syndrome: unusual congenital optic disc anomaly. *Am J Ophthalmol* **69**:376–384.

22 Beyer WB, Quencer RM, Osher RH (1982). Morning glory syndrome: a functional analysis including fluorescein angiography, ultrasonography, and computerized tomography. *Ophthalmology* **89**:1362–1364.

23 Haik BG, Greenstein SH, Smith ME, *et al*. (1984). Retinal detachment in the morning glory disc anomaly. *Ophthalmology* **91**(12):1638–1647.

24 Mafee MF, Jampol LM, Langer BG, *et al*. (1987). Computed tomography of optic nerve colobomas, morning glory anomaly, and colobomatous cyst. *Radiol Clin North Am* **25**(4):693–699.

25 Savell J, Cook JR (1976). Optic nerve colobomas of autosomal-dominant heredity. *Arch Ophthalmol* **94**:395–400.

26 Francois J (1968). Colobomatous malformations of the ocular globe. *Int Ophthalmol Clin* **8**:797–816.

27 Gopal L, Badrinath SS, Kumar KS, *et al*. (1996). Optic disc in fundus coloboma. *Ophthalmology* **103**(12):2120–2127.

28 Lin CC, Tso MO, Vygantas CM (1984). Coloboma of optic nerve associated with serous maculopathy: a clinicopathologic correlative study. *Arch Ophthalmol* **102**(11):1651–1654.

29 Pagon RA (1981). Ocular coloboma. *Surv Ophthalmol* **25**(4):223–236.

30 Brown GC, Tasman W (1983). *Congenital Anomalies of the Optic Disc*. Grune & Stratton, New York.

31 Hodgkins P, Lees M, Lawson J, *et al*. (1998). Optic disc anomalies and frontonasal dysplasia. *Br J Ophthalmol* **82**(3):290–293.

32 Apple DJ, Rabb MF, Walsh PM (1982). Congenital anomalies of the optic disc. *Surv Ophthalmol* **27**:3–41.

33 Young SE, Walsh FB, Knox DL (1976). The tilted disk syndrome. *Am J Ophthalmol* **82**(1):16–23.

34 Keane JR (1977). Suprasellar tumors and incidental optic disc anomalies: diagnostic problems in two patients with hemianopic temporal scotomas. *Arch Ophthalmol* **95**(12):2180–2183.

35 Osher RH, Schatz NJ (1979). A sinister association of the congenital tilted disc syndrome with chiasmal compression. In: *Neuro-ophthalmology Focus*. JL Smith (ed). Masson, New York, pp. 112–123.

36 Taylor D (1982). Congenital tumors of the anterior visual pathways. *Br J Ophthalmol* **66**:455–463.

37 Hittner HM, Borda RP, Justice J (1981). X-linked recessive congenital stationary night blindness, myopia, and tilted discs. *J Pediatr Ophthalmol Strabismus* **18**:15–20.

38 Stefko ST, Campochiaro P, Wang P, *et al*. (1997). Dominant inheritance of optic pits. *Am J Ophthalmol* **124**(1):112–113.

39 Lincoff H, Lopez R, Kreissig I, *et al*. (1988). Retinoschisis associated with optic nerve pits. *Arch Ophthalmol* **106**(1):61–67.

40 Brown GC, Shields JA, Goldberg RE (1980). Congenital pits of the optic nerve head. II. Clinical studies in humans. *Ophthalmology* **87**(1):51–65.

41 Lincoff H, Yannuzzi L, Singerman L, *et al*. (1993). Improvement in visual function after displacement of the retinal elevations emanating from optic pits. *Arch Ophthalmol* **111**(8):1071–1079.

42 McDonald HR, Schatz H, Johnson RN (1992). Treatment of retinal detachment associated with optic pits. *Int Ophthalmol Clin* **32**(2):35–42.

43 Phillips PH, Repka MX, Lambert SR (1998). Pseudotumor cerebri in children. *J AAPOS* **2**:33–38.

CHAPTER 13
References

1 MacEwen CJ (2005). The lacrimal system. In: *Pediatric Ophthalmology and Strabismus*, 3rd edn. D Taylor, C Hoyt (eds). Elsevier Saunders, Edinburgh, ch 31, pp. 285–294.

2 Robb R (1994). Tearing abnormalities. In: *The Eye in Infancy*, 2nd edn. S Isenberg (ed). Mosby, St. Louis, ch 29, pp. 248–253.

3 Schnall BM, Christian CJ (1996). Conservative treatment of congenital dacryocele. *J Pediatr Ophthalmol Strabismus* **33**:219–222.

4 Becker BB (2006). The treatment of congenital dacryocystocele. *Am J Ophthalmol* **142**:835–838.

5 Paysse EA, Coats DK, Bernstein JM, *et al*. (2000). Management and complications of congenital dacryocele with concurrent intranasal mucocele. *J AAPOS* **4**:46–53.

6 Farrer RS, Mohammed TL, Hahn FJ (2003). MRI of childhood dacryocystocele. *Neuroradiology* **45**:259–261.

7 D'Addario V, Pinto A, Anfossi A, *et al*. (2001). Antenatal sonographic diagnosis of dacryocystocele. *Acta Ophthalmol Scand* **79**:330–331.

8 Peterson RA, Robb RM (1978). The natural course of congenital obstruction of the nasolacrimal duct. *J Pediatr Ophthalmol Strabismus* **15**:246–250.

9 Katowitz JA, Welsh MG (1997). Timing of initial probing and irrigation in congenital nasolacrimal duct obstruction. *Ophthalmology* **94**:698–705.

10 Becker BB, Berry FD, Koller H (1996). Balloon catheter dilatation for treatment of congenital nasolacrimal duct obstruction. *Am J Ophthalmol* **121**:304–309.

11 Engel JM, Hichie-Schmidt C, Khammar A, *et al*. (2007). Monocanalicular silastic intubation for the initial correction of congenital nasolacrimal duct obstruction. *J AAPOS* **11**:183–186.

12 Tien AM, Tien DR (2006). Bilateral congenital lacrimal sac fistulae in a patient with ectodactyly-ectodermal dysplasia-clefting syndrome. *J AAPOS* **10**(6):577–578.

13 Birchansky LD, Nerad JA, Kerster RC, *et al*. (1990). Management of congenital lacrimal sac fistula. *Arch Ophthalmol* **108**:388–390.

14 Dunnington JH (1954). Congential alacrima in familial autonomic dysfunction. *Trans Am Ophthalmol Soc* **52**:23–33.

15 Brooks BP, Kleta R, Caruso RC, *et al*. (2004). Triple-A syndrome with prominent ophthalmic features and a novel mutation in the AAAS gene: a case report. *BMC Ophthalmol* **4**:7.

16 Kim SH, Hwang S, Kweon S, *et al*. (2005). Two cases of lacrimal gland agenesis in the same family – clinicoradiologic findings and management. *Can J Ophthalmol* **40**:502–505.

17 Merayo-Lloves J, Baltatzis S, Foster CS (2001). Epstein–Barr virus dacryoadenitis resulting in keratoconjunctivitis sicca in a child. *Am J Ophthalmol* **132**:922–923.

18 Mottow-Lippa L, Jakobiec FA, Smith M (1981). Idiopathic inflammatory orbital pseudotumor in childhood. *Ophthalmology* **88**(6):565–574.

CHAPTER 14
References

1 Dortzbach RK, Sutula FC (1980). Involutional blepharoptosis. A histopathological study. *Arch Ophthalmol* **98**(11):2045–2049.

2 Niemi KM, Kanerva L, Kuokkanen K, *et al*. (1994). Clinical, light and electron microscopic features of recessive congenital ichthyosis type I. *Br J Dermatol* **130**(5):626–633.

3 Kohn R, Romano PE (1971). Blepharoptosis, blepharophimosis, epicanthus inversus, and telecanthus – a syndrome with no name. *Am J Ophthalmol* **72**(3):625–632.

4 Shorr N, Seiff SR (1986). Central retinal artery occlusion associated with periocular corticosteroid injection for juvenile hemangioma. *Ophthalmic Surg* **17**(4):229–231.

5 McKinley SH, Yen MT, Miller AM, *et al*. (2007). Microbiology of pediatric orbital cellulitis. *Am J Ophthalmol* **144**(4):497–501.

CHAPTER 15
References

1 Abderhalden E (1903). Familiare cystindiathese. *Z Physiol Chem* **38**:557–561.

2 Gahl WA, Bahsan N, Tietze F, *et al*. (1982). Cystine transport is defective in isolated leukocyte lysosomes from patients with cystinosis. *Science* **217**:1263–1265.

3 Jonas AJ, Smith ML, Schneider JA (1982). ATP-dependent lysosomal cystine efflux is defective in cystinosis. *J Biol Chem* **257**:13185–13188.

4 Town M, Jean G, Cherqui S, *et al*. (1998). A novel gene encoding an integral membrane protein is mutated in nephrogenic cystinosis. *Nature Genetics* **18**(4):319–324.

5 Broyer M (2006). Cystinosis. In: *Inborn Metabolic Diseases*, 4th edn. J Fernandes, JM Saudubray, G van den Berghe, JH Walter (eds). Springer Medizin Verlag, Heidelberg, pp. 531–538.

6 Gahl WA, Thoene JG, Schneider JA (2002). Cystinosis. *NEJM* **347**:111–121.

7 Schneider JA, Bradley K, Seegmiller JE (1967). Increased cystine in leukocytes from individuals homozygous and heterozygous for cystinosis. *Science* **157**:1321–1322.

8 Burki E (1941). Uber die cystinkrankheit unter besorderer beruck sichtigung des augenbefundes. *Ophthalmologica* **101**:257–272.

9 Gahl WA, Kuehl EM, Iwata F, *et al*. (2000). Corneal crystals in nephrogenic cystinosis: natural history and treatment with cysteamine eyedrops. *Mol Genet Metab* **71**:100–120.

10 Tsilou E, Rubin BI, Reed G, *et al*. (2006). Nephropathic cystinosis: posterior segment manifestations and effects of cysteamine therapy. *Ophthalmology* **113**:1002–1009.

11 Dureau P, Broyer M, Difer JL (2003). Evolution of ocular manifestations in nephropathic dystinosis: a long-term study of a population treated with cysteamine. *J Pediatr Ophthalmol Strabismus* **40**:142–146.

12 Katz B, Melles RB, Swenson MR, *et al*. (1990). Photic sneeze reflex in nephropathic cystinosis. *Br J Ophthalmol* **74**:706–708.

13 Elder MJ, Austin CL (2003). Recurrent corneal erosion in cystinosis. *J Pediatr Ophthalmol Strabismus* **40**:142–146.

14 Wong VG, Lietman PS, Seegmiller JE (1967). Alterations of pigment epithelium in cystinosis. *Arch Ophthalmol* **77**:361–369.

15 Tsilou E, Zhou M, Gahl W, *et al*. (2007). Ophthalmic manifestations and histopathology of infantile nephropathic cystinosis. *Surv Ophthalmol* **52**:97–105.

16 Marfan AB (1896). Un cas de deformation congenitales des quatre members plus prononcee aux extremities characterisee par l'allongement des os avec un certain degree d'amincissement. *Bull Mem Soc Med Hop* (Paris) **13**:220.

17 Pyertiz PE, McKusick VA (1979). The Marfan syndrome: diagnosis and management. *NEJM* **300**:772–777.

18 DePaepe A, Devereux RB, Dietz HC, *et al*. (1996). Revised diagnostic criteria for the Marfan syndrome. *Am J Med Genet A* **62**:417–426.

19 American Academy of Pediatrics (1996). Health supervision for children with Marfan syndrome. American Academy of Pediatrics Committee on Genetics. *Pediatrics* **98**:978–982.

20 Maumenee IH (1981). The eye in the Marfan syndrome. *Trans Am Ophthalmol Soc* **79**:684–733.

21 Wheatley HM, Traboulsi EI, Flowers BE, *et al*. (1995). Immunohistochemical localization of fibrillin in human ocular tissues and relevance to Marfan syndrome. *Arch Ophthalmol* **113**:103–109.

22 Traboulsi EI (2006). *A Compendium of Inherited Disorders and the Eye*. Oxford University Press, Oxford.

23 Traboulsi EL, Whittum-Hudson JA, *et al*. (2000). Microfibril abnormalities of the lens capsule in patients with Marfan syndrome and ectopia lentis. *Ophthalmic Genet* **21**:9–15.

24 Sachdev NH, DiGirolamo ND, McCluskey RJ, *et al*. (2002). Lens dislocation in Marfan syndrome and potential role of matrix metalloproteinases in fibrillin degradation. *Arch Ophthalmol* **120**:833–835.

25 Kim SY, Choung HK, Kim SJ, *et al.* (2008). Long term results of lensectomy in children with ectopia lentis. *J Pediatr Ophthalmol Strabismus* **45**:13–19.

26 Siganos DS, Siganos CS, Popescu CN, *et al.* (2000). Clear lens extraction and intraocular lens implantation in Marfan's syndrome. *J Catar act Refract Surg* **26**:781–784.

27 Dureau P, de Laage de Meux P, Edelson C, *et al.* (2006). Iris fixation of foldable intraocular lenses for ectopia lentis in children. *J Catar act Refract Surg* **332**:1109–1114.

28 Carson NA, Neill DW (1962). Metabolic abnormalities detected in a survey of mentally backward individuals in Northern Ireland. *Arch Dis Child* **37**:505–513.

29 Mudd SH, Finkelstein JD, Irreverre F, *et al.* (1964). Homocystinuria: an enzymatic defect. *Science* **143**:1443–1445.

30 Mudd SH, Skovby F, Levy HL, *et al.* (1985). The natural history of homocystinuria due to cystathionine β-synthase deficiency. *Am J Hum Genet* **37**(1):1–31.

31 Barber GW, Spaeth GL (1969). The successful treatment of homocystinuria with pyridoxine. *J Pediatr* **75**:463–478.

32 Freeman JM, Finkelstein JD, Mudd SH, *et al.* (1972). Homocystinuria presenting as reversible 'schizophrenia'. A new defect in methionine metabolism with reduced methylene-tetrahydrofolate reductase activity. *Pediatr Res* **6**:423.

33 Fowler B (1998). Genetic defects of folate and cobalamin metabolism. *Eur J Pediatr* **157**(2Suppl):S60–S66.

34 Rosenblatt DS, Fowler B (2006). Disorders of cobalamin and folate transport and metabolism. In: *Inborn Metabolic Diseases* 4th edn. J Fernandes, JM Saudubray, G van den Berghe, JH Walter (eds). Springer Medizin Verlag, Heidelberg, pp. 341–356.

35 Nelson LB, Maumenee IH (1975). Ectopia lentis. *Surv Ophthalmol* **27**:143–160.

36 Ramsey MD, Dickson DH (1975). Lensfringe in homocystinuria. *Br J Ophthalmol* **59**:338–342.

37 Harrison DA, Mullaney PB, Mesfer SA (1998). Management of ophthalmic complications of homocystinuria. *Ophthalmology* **105**:1886–1890.

38 Burke JP, O'Keefe M, Bowell R, Naughten ER (1989). Ocular complications in homocystinuria: early and late treated. *Br J Ophthalmol* **73**(6):427–431.

39 Ozdek S, Bahceci UA, Gnol M (2005). Postoperative secondary glaucoma and anterior staphyloma in a patient with homocystinuria. *J Pediatr Ophthalmol Strabismus* **42**:243–246.

40 Kayser B (1902). Ueber einen fall von angeborener grublicher verfarbung der kornea. *Klin Monatsbl Augenheilk* **40**:22.

41 Fleischer B (1903). Zwei witerere falle von grublicher verfarbung der kornea. *Klin Monatsbl Augenheilk* **41**:489.

42 Wilson SAK (1912). Progressive lenticular degeneration: a familial nervous disease associated with cirrhosis of the liver. *Brain* **34**:295.

43 Bull PC, Thomas GR, Rommens JM, *et al.* (1993). The Wilson disease gene is a putative copper transporting P-type ATPase similar to the Menkes gene. *Nat Genet* **5**:327–337.

44 Prashanth LK, Taly AB, Sinha S, *et al.* (2004). Wilson's disease: diagnostic errors and clinical implications. *J Neurol Neurosurg Psychiatry* **75**:907–909.

45 Das SK, Ray K (2006). Wilson's disease: an update. *Nature Clin Prac Neurol* **2**:482–493.

46 Roberts EA, Schilsky ML (2008). Diagnosis and treatment of Wilson disease: an update. *Hepatology* **47**:2089–2111.

47 Anderson W (1898). A case of angiokeratoma. *Brit J Dermatol* **10**:113.

48 Fabry J (1898). Ein beitrag zur kenntnis der purpura haemorrhagica nodularis (purpura papulosa hemorrahagica hebrae). *Arch Dermatol Syph* **43**:187.

49 MacDermot KD, Homes A, Miners AH (2001). Anderson–Fabry disease: clinical manifestations and impact of disease in a cohort of 60 obligate carrier females. *J Med Genet* **38**:769–775.

50 International Fabry Disease Study Group (2004). Long-term safety and efficacy of enzyme replacement therapy for Fabry disease. *Am J Hum Genet* **75**:65–74.

51 Sodi A, Loannidis AS, Mehta A, *et al.* (2007). Ocular manifestations of Fabry's disease: data from the Fabry Outcome Survey. *Br J Ophthalmol* **91**:210–214.

52 Glorieux FH (2008). Osteogenesis imperfecta. *Best Prac Res Clin Rheumatol* **22**:85–100.

53 Sillence DO, Senn A, Danks DM (1979). Genetic heterogeneity in osteogenesis imperfecta. *J Med Genet* **16**:101–116.

54 Szilvássy J, Jóri J, Czigner J, *et al.* (1998). Cochlear implantation in osteogenesis imperfecta. *Acta Otorhinolaryngol Belg* **52**:253–256.

55 Speiser PW, Clarson CL, Eugster EA, *et al.* (2005). Bisphosphonate treatment of pediatric bone disease. *Ped Endocr Rev* **3**:87–96.

56 Chan CC, Green R, de la Cruz SC, *et al.* (1982). Ocular findings in osteogenesis imperfecta congenita. *Arch Ophthalmol* **100**:1459–463.

57 Sillence D, Butler B, Latham M, *et al.* (1993). Natural history of blue sclerae in osteogenesis imperfecta. *Am J Med Genet* **45**:183–186.

58 Evereklioglu C, Madenci E, Bayazit YA, *et al.* (2002). Central corneal thickness is lower in osteogenesis imperfecta and negatively correlates with the presence of blue sclera. *Ophthalmic Physiol Opt* **22**:511–515.

59 Ganesh A, Jenny C, Geyer J, *et al.* (2004). Retinal hemorrhages in type I osteogenesis imperfecta after minor trauma. *Ophthalmology* **111**:1428–1431.

60 Pirouzian A, O'Halloran H, Scher C, *et al.* (2007). Traumatic and spontaneous scleral rupture and uveal prolapse in osteogenesis imperfecta. *J Pediatr Ophthalmol Strabismus* **44**:315–317.

61 Neufeld EF, Muenzer J (2001). The mucopolysaccharidoses. In: *The Metabolic and Molecular Bases of Inherited Disease*, 8th edn. CA Scriver, A Beaudet, W Sly, *et al.* (eds). McGraw-Hill, New York, pp. 3421–3452.

62 Clarke LA (2008). The mucopolysaccharidoses: a success of molecular medicine. *Expert Rev Mol Med* **10**:e1.

63 Rohrback M, Clarke JT (2007). Treatment of lysosomal storage disorders; progress with enzyme replacement therapy. *Drugs* **67**:2697–2716.

64 Orchard PJ, Blazar BR, Wagner J, *et al.* (2007). Hematopoietic cell therapy for metabolic disease. *J Pediatr* **151**:340–346.

65 Krivit W, Sung JH, Shapiro EG, *et al.* (1995). Microglia: the effector cell for reconstitution of the central nervous system following bone marrow transplantation for lysosomal and peroxisomal storage diseases. *Cell Transplant* **4**:385–392.

66 Connell P, McCreery K, Doyle A, *et al.* (2008). Central corneal thickness and its relationship to intraocular pressure in MPS-1 following bone marrow transplantation. *J AAPOS* **12**:7–10.

67 Collins ML, Traboulsi EI, Maumenee IH (1990). Optic nerve head swelling and optic atrophy in the systemic MPS. *Ophthalmology* **97**:1445–1449.

68 Pitz S, Ogun O, Bajbouj M, *et al.* (2007). Ocular changes in patients with MPSI receiving enzyme replacement therapy. *Arch Ophthalmol* **125**:1353–1356.

69 Herrick JB (1910). Peculiar elongated and sickle-shaped red blood corpuscles in a case of severe anemia. *Arch Intern Med* **6**:517–521.

70 Williams TN, Mwangi TW, Wambua S, *et al.* (2005). Sickle cell trait and the risk of *Plasmodium falciparum* malaria and other childhood diseases. *J Infect Dis* **192**:178–186.

71 Frenette PS, Atweh GF (2007). Sickle cell disease: old discoveries, new concepts, and future promise. *J Clin Invest* **117**:850–858.

72 Gladwin MT, Sachdev V, Jison ML, *et al.* (2004). Pulmonary hypertension as a risk factor for death in patients with sickle cell disease. *New Engl J Med* **350**:886–895.

73 Bonds DR (2005). Three decades of innovation in the management of sickle cell disease: the road to understanding the sickle cell disease clinical phenotype. *Blood Rev* **19**:99–110.

74 Pinto FO, Roberts I (2008). Cord blood stem transplantation for haemoglobinopathies. *Br J Haematol* **141**:309–324.

75 Kimmel AS, Magargal LE, Maizel R, *et al.* (1987). Proliferative sickle cell retinopathy under age 20: a review. *Ophthalmolic Surg* **18**:126–128.

76 Henry M, Driscoll MC, Miller M, *et al.* (2004). Psuedotumor cerebri in children with sickle cell disease. *Pediatrics* **113**:265–269.

77 Nasrullah A, Derr NC (1997). Sickle cell trait as a risk factor for secondary hemorrhage in children with traumatic hyphema. *Am J Ophthalmol* **123**:783–790.

78 Grønskov K, Ek J, Brondum-Nielsen K (2007). Oculocutaneous albinism. *Orphanet J Rare Dis* **2**:43–51.

79 Wei ML (2006). Hermansky–Pudlak syndrome: a disease of protein trafficking and organelle function. *Pigment Cell Res* **19**:19–42.

80 Introne W, Boissy R, Gahl W (1999). Clinical, molecular, and cell biological aspects of Chediak–Higashi syndrome. *Mol Genet Metab* **68**:283–303.

81 Eapen M, DeLaat CA, Baker KS, *et al.* (2007). Hematopoietic cell transplantation for Chediak–Higashi syndrome. *Bone Marrow Transplant* **39**:411–415.

82 Seo JH, Yu YS, Kim JH, *et al.* (2007). Correlation of visual acuity with foveal hypoplasia grading by OCT in albinism. *Ophthalmology* **114**:1547–1551.

83 Kelly JP, Weiss AH (2006). Topographical retinal function in oculocutaneous albinism. *Am J Ophthalmol* **141**:1156–1157.

84 Guo S, Reinecke RD, Fendick M (1989). Visual pathway abnormalities in albinism and infantile nystagmus: VECPs and stereoacutiy measurements. *J Pediatr Ophthalmol Strabismus* **26**:97–104.

85 Kutzbach BR, Summers CG, Holleschau AM, MacDonald JT (2008). Neurodevelopment in children with albinism. *Ophthalmology* **115**(10):1805–1808, 1808.e1-2. Epub 2008 Apr 28.

86 Anderson J, Lavoie J, Merrill K, *et al.* (2004). Efficacy of spectacles in persons with albinism. *J AAPOS* **8**:515–520.

87 Anderson JR (1953). Causes and treatment of congenital eccentric nystagmus. *Br J Ophthalmol* **37**(5):267–281.

88 Dell'Osso LF (1998). Extraocular muscle tenotomy, dissection and suture: a hypothetical therapy for congenital nystagmus. *J Pediatr Ophthalmol Strabismus* **35**:232–233.

89 Hertle RW, Dell'Osso LF, FitzGibbon EJ, *et al.* (2004). Horizontal rectus muscle tenotomy in patients with infantile nystagmus syndrome: a pilot study. *J AAPOS* **8**:539–548.

90 Wang ZI, Dell'Osso LF, Tomsak RL (2007). Combining recessions with tenotomy, improved visual function and decreased oscillopsia and diplopia in acquired downbeat nystagmus and horizontal infantile nystagmus. *J AAPOS* **11**:135–141.

91 Mets MB, Chhabra MS (2008). Eye manifestations of intrauterine infections and their impact on childhood blindness. *Surv Ophthalmol* **53**:95–111.

CHAPTER 16
References

1 Shields JA, Shields CL (2008). *Intraocular Tumors. An Atlas and Textbook*, 2nd edn. Lippincott, Williams & Wilkins, Philadelphia.

2 Shields JA, Shields CL (2008). *Eyelid, Conjunctival and Orbital Tumors. An Atlas and Textbook*, 2nd edn. Lippincott, Williams and Wilkins, Philadelphia.

3 Shields JA, Shields CL (1992). Systemic hamartomatoses ('phakomatoses'). In: *Intraocular Tumors. A Text and Atlas*. JA Shields, CL Shields (eds). WB Saunders, Philadelphia, pp. 513–539.

4 Bourneville D (1880). Sclereuse tubereuse des circonvolution cerebrales. Idiote et epilepsie hemiplegique. *Arch Neurol* (Paris) **1**:81–91.

5 Kwiatkowski DJ, Short MP (1994). Tuberous sclerosis. *Arch Dermatol* **130**:348–354.

6 Lucchese NJ, Goldberg MF (1981). Iris and fundus pigmentary changes in tuberous sclerosis. *J Pediatr Ophthalmol Strabismus* **18**:45–46.

7 Lagos JC, Gomez MR (1967). Tuberous sclerosis. Reappraisal of a clinical entity. *Mayo Clin Proc* **42**:26–49.

8 Reed WB, Nickel WR, Campion G (1963). Internal manifestations of tuberous sclerosis. *Arch Dermatol* **87**:715–728.

9 Shields JA, Eagle RC Jr, Shields CL, *et al.* (2005). Aggressive retinal astrocytomas in 4 patients with tuberous sclerosis complex. The first John Dickerson Lecture. *Arch Ophthalmol* **123**:856–863.

10 Brasfield RD, Das Gupta TK (1972). Von Recklinghausen's disease: a clinicopathological study. *Ann Surg* **175**:86–104.

11 von Recklinghausen FD (1882). Uber die multiplen fibrome der haut und ihre beziehungen zu den neurrommen. Festschr feier fundfund-zwanzigjahrigen. *Best Path Inst*. A Hirschwald, Berlin.

12 Kaiser-Kupfer MI, Freidlin V, Dariles MB, *et al.* (1989). The association of posterior capsular lens opacities with bilateral acoustic neuromas in patients with neurofibromatosis type 2. *Arch Ophthalmol* **107**:541–544.

13 Lewis RA, Riccardi VM (1981). Von Recklinghausen neurofibromatosis. Incidence of iris hamartoma. *Ophthalmology* **88**:348–354.

14 Shields JA, Shields CL, Lieb WE, *et al.* (1990). Multiple orbital neurofibromas unassociated with von Recklinghausen's disease. *Arch Ophthalmol* **108**:80–83.

15 Shields JA, Sanborn GE, Kurz GH, *et al.* (1981). Benign peripheral nerve tumor of the choroid. *Ophthalmology* **88**:1322–1329.

16 Wiznia RA, Freedman JE, Mancini AD, *et al.* (1978). Malignant melanoma of the choroid in neurofibromatosis. *Am J Ophthalmol* **86**:684–687.

17 Lewis RA, Gerson LP, Axelson KA, *et al.* (1984). Von Recklinghausen neurofibromatosis II. Incidence of optic gliomata. *Ophthalmology* **91**:929–935.

18 Von Hippel E Jr (1895). Vorstellung eines patienten mit einem sehr ungewohnlichen aderhautleiden. *Ber Versamml Ophthalmol Gesellsch*, Stuttgart **24**:269–280.

19 Lindau A (1926). Studien uber kleinhirncystein. Bau, pathogenese und beziehungen zur angiomatose retinae. *Acta Pathol Microbiol Scand* **3**(1Suppl):1–28.

20 Laatikainen L, Immonen I, Summanen P (1989). Peripheral retinal angiomalike lesion and macular pucker. *Am J Ophthalmol* **108**:563–566.

21 Hardwig P, Robertson DM (1984). Von Hippel–Lindau disease: a familial, often lethal, multi-system phakomatosis. *Ophthalmology* **91**:263–270.

22 Shields CL, Shields JA, Barrett J, *et al.* (1995). Vasoproliferative tumors of the ocular fundus. Classification and clinical manifestations in 103 patients. *Arch Ophthalmol* **113**:615–623.

23 Gass JD, Braunstein R (1980). Sessile and exophytic capillary angiomas of the juxtapapillary retina and optic nerve head. *Arch Ophthalmol* **98**:1790–1797.

24 Singh AD, Shields CL, Shields JA (2001). Major review: Von Hippel–Lindau disease. *Surv Ophthalmol* **46**:117–142.

25 Chan CC, Vortmeyer AO, Chew EY, *et al.* (1999). VHL gene deletion and enhanced VEGF gene expression detected in the stromal cells of retinal angioma. *Arch Ophthalmol* **117**:625–630.

26 Sturge WA (1879). A case of partial epilepsy apparently due to a lesion of one of the vasomotor centres of the brain. *Trans Clin Soc (Lond)* **12**:162–167.

27 Weber FP (1922). Right-sided hemihypertrophy resulting from right-sided congenital spastic hemiplegia with a morbid condition of the left side of the brain revealed by radiogram. *J Neurol Psycho-pathol (Lond)* **37**:301–311.

28 Stevenson RF, Morin JD (1975). Ocular findings in nevus flammeus. *Can J Ophthalmol* **10**:136–139.

29 Shields CL, Shields JA, De Potter P (1995). Patterns of indocyanine green video angiography of choroidal tumours. *Br J Ophthalmol* **79**:237–245.

30 Witschel H, Font RL (1976). Hemangioma of the choroid. A clinicopathologic study of 71 cases and a review of the literature. *Surv Ophthalmol* **20**:415–431.

31 Wyburn-Mason R (1943). Arteriovenous aneurysm of midbrain and retina, facial naevi and mental changes. *Brain* **66**:163–203.

32 Archer DM, Deutman A, Ernest JT, *et al*. (1973). Arteriovenous communications of the retina. *Am J Ophthalmol* **75**:224–241.

33 Gass JD (1971). Cavernous hemangioma of the retina. A neuro-oculocutaneous syndrome. *Am J Ophthalmol* **71**:799–814.

34 Goldberg RE, Pheasant TR, Shields JA (1979). Cavernous hemangioma of the retina. A four-generation pedigree with neurocutaneous manifestations and an example of bilateral retinal involvement. *Arch Ophthalmol* **97**:2321–2324.

35 Thangappan A, Shields CL, Gerontis CC, *et al*. (2007). Iris cavernous hemangioma associated with multiple cavernous hemangiomas in the brain, kidney, and skin. *Cornea* **26**:481–483.

36 Sarraf D, Payne AM, Kitchen ND, *et al*. (2000). Familial cavernous hemangioma: An expanding ocular spectrum. *Arch Ophthalmol* **118**:969–973.

37 Couteulx SL, Brezin AP, Fontaine B, *et al*. (2002). A novel KRIT1/CCM1 truncating mutation in a patient with cerebral and retinal cavernous angiomas. *Arch Ophthalmol* **120**:217–218.

38 Shields JA, Shields CL, Eagle RC Jr, *et al*. (1997). Ocular manifestations of the organoid nevus syndrome. *Ophthalmology* **104**:549–557.

CHAPTER 17
References
1 Good WV, Jan JE, DeSa L, *et al*. (1994). Cortical visual impairment in children. *Surv Ophthalmol* **38**:351–364.

2 Good WV, Jan JE, Burden SK, *et al*. (2001). Recent advances in cortical visual impairment. *Dev Med Child Neurol* **43**:56–60.

3 Hertle RW, Yang D (2006). Clinical and electrophysiological effects of extraocular muscle surgery on patients with infantile nystagmus syndrome (INS). *Semin Ophthalmol* **21**:103–110.

4 Kiblinger GD, Wallace BS, Hines M, *et al*. (2007). Spasmus nutans-like nystagmus is often associated with underlying ocular, intracranial, or systemic abnormalities. *J Neuro-ophthalmol* **27**:118–122.

5 Gottlob I, Wizov SS, Reinecke RD (1995). Spasmus nutans. A long-term follow-up. *Invest Ophthalmol Vis Sci* **36**:2768–2771.

6 Mahoney NR, Liu GT, Menacker SJ, *et al*. (2006). Pediatric Horner syndrome: etiologies and roles of imaging and urine studies to detect neuroblastoma and other responsible mass lesions. *Am J Ophthalmol* **142**:651–659.

7 Walton KA, Buono LM (2003). Horner syndrome. *Curr Opin Ophthalmol* **14**:357–363.

8 Harris CM, Shawkat F, Russell-Eggitt I, *et al*. (1996). Intermittent horizontal saccade failure ('ocular motor apraxia') in children. *Br J Ophthalmol* **80**:151–158.

9 Mullaney P, Vajsar J, Smith R, *et al*. (2000). The natural history and ophthalmic involvement in childhood myasthenia gravis at the hospital for sick children. *Ophthalmology* **107**:504–510.

10 Ellis FD, Hoyt CS, Ellis FJ, *et al*. (2000). Extraocular muscle responses to orbital cooling (ice test) for ocular myasthenia gravis diagnosis. *J AAPOS* **4**:271–281.

CHAPTER 18
References
1 Shields CL, Shields JA (2007). Conjunctival tumors in children. *Curr Opin Ophthalmol* **18**:351–360.

2 Shields JA, Shields CL (1992). *Intraocular Tumors. A Text and Atlas*. WB Saunders, Philadelphia.

3 Shields JA, Shields CL (2008). *Eyelid, Conjunctival, and Orbital Tumors. An Atlas and Textbook*, 2nd edn. Lippincott, Williams and Wilkins, Philadelphia.

4 Shields JA, Shields CL (2008). *Intraocular Tumors. An Atlas and Textbook*, 2nd edn. Lippincott, Williams and Wilkins, Philadelphia.

5 Shields JA (1989). *Diagnosis and Management of Orbital Tumors*. WB Saunders, Philadelphia.

6 Shields JA, Parsons HM, Shields CL, *et al*. (1991). Lesions simulating retinoblastoma. *J Pediatr Ophthalmol Strabismus* **28**:338–340.

7 Shields JA, Shields CL (2002). Review: Coats disease. The 2001 LuEsther Mertz Lecture. *Retina* **22**:80–91.

8 De Potter P, Shields JA, Shields CL (1994). *MRI of the Eye and Orbit*. Lippincott, Philadelphia.

9 Mills DM, Tsai S, Meyer DR, *et al*. (2006). Pediatric ophthalmic computed tomographic scanning and associated cancer risk. *Am J Ophthalmol* **142**:1046–1053.

10 Shields CL, Mashayekhi A, Luo CK, *et al*. (2004). Optical coherence tomography in children. Analysis of 44 eyes with intraocular tumors and simulating conditions. *J Pediatr Ophthalmol Strabismus* **41**(6):338–344.

11 O'Hara BJ, Ehya H, Shields JA, *et al*. (1993). Fine needle aspiration biopsy in pediatric ophthalmic tumors and pseudotumors. *Acta Cytologica* **37**:125–130.

12 Shields CL, Shields JA (2008). Forget me nots in the care of children with retinoblastoma. *Sem Ophthalmol* **23**(5):324–334.

13 Epstein J, Shields CL, Shields JA (2003). Trends in the management of retinoblastoma; evaluation of 1,196 consecutive eyes during 1974–2001. *J Pediatr Ophthalmol Strabismus* **40**:196–203.

14 Marr BP, Shields CL, Shields JA (2005). Tumors of the eyelids. In: *Duane's Foundations of Clinical Ophthalmology*, 3rd edn. WS Tasman, EA Jaeger (eds). Lippincott, Willliams and Wilkins, Philadelphia, ch3, pp. 1–12.

15 Haik BG, Karcioglu ZA, Gordon RA, *et al*. (1994). Capillary hemangioma (infantile periocular hemangioma). Review. *Surv Ophthalmol* **38**:399–426.

16 Taylor SF, Cook AE, Leatherbarrow B (2006). Review of patients with basal cell nevus syndrome. *Ophthal Plast Reconstr Surg* **22**:259–265.

17 Farris SR, Grove AS, Jr (1996). Orbital and eyelid manifestations of neurofibromatosis: a clinical study and literature review. *Ophthal Plast Reconstr Surg* **12**:245–259.

18 Shields JA, Kiratli H, Shields CL, *et al*. (1994). Schwannoma of the eyelid in a child. *J Pediatr Ophthalmol Strabismus* **31**:332–333.

19 Shields CL, Shields JA (2004). Tumors of the conjunctiva and cornea. *Surv Ophthalmol* **49**:3–24.

20 Grossniklaus HE, Green WR, Luckenbach M, *et al*. (1987). Conjunctival lesions in adults. A clinical and histopathologic review. *Cornea* **6**:78–116.

21 Shields CL, Shields JA, White D, *et al*. (1986). Types and frequency of lesions of the caruncle. *Am J Ophthalmol* **102**:771–778.

22 Shields CL, Demirci H, Karatza EC, *et al*. (2004). Clinical survey of 1,643 melanocytic and nonmelanocytic conjunctival tumors. *Ophthalmology* **111**:1747–1754.

23 Elsas FJ, Green WR (1975). Epibulbar tumors in childhood. *Am J Ophthalmol* **79**:1001–1007.

24 Cunha RP, Cunha MC, Shields JA (1987). Epibulbar tumors in children: a survey of 282 biopsies. *J Pediatr Ophthalmol Strabismus* **24**:249–254.

25 Scott JA, Tan DT (2001). Therapeutic lamellar keratoplasty for limbal dermoids. *Ophthalmology* **108**:1858–1867.

26 Shields JA, Shields CL, Eagle RC Jr, *et al*. (1997). Ophthalmic features of the organoid nevus syndrome. *Ophthalmology* **104**:549–557.

27 Scott IU, Karp CL, Nuovo GJ (2002). Human papillomavirus 16 and 18 expression in conjunctival intraepithelial neoplasia. *Ophthalmology* **109**:542–547.

28 Sjo NC, Heegaard S, Prause JU, *et al*. (2001). Human papillomavirus in conjunctival papilloma. *Br J Ophthalmol* **85**:785–787.

29 Shields JA, Shields CL, De Potter P (1998). Surgical management of circumscribed conjunctival melanomas. *Ophthal Plast Reconstr Surg* **14**:208–215.

30 Shields JA, Shields CL, De Potter P (1997). Surgical management of conjunctival tumors. The 1994 Lynn B. McMahan Lecture. *Arch Ophthalmol* **115**:808–815.

31 Frucht-Pery J, Sugar J, Baum J, *et al*. (1997). Mitomycin C treatment for conjunctival-corneal intraepithelial neoplasia: a multicenter experience. *Ophthalmology* **104**:2085–2093.

32 Karp CL, Moore JK, Rosa RH, Jr (2001). Treatment of conjunctival and corneal intraepithelial neoplasia with topical interferon alpha-2b. *Ophthalmology* **108**:1093–1098.

33 Shields CL, Lally MR, Singh AD, *et al*. (1999). Oral cimetidine (Tagamet) for recalcitrant, diffuse conjunctival papillomatosis. *Am J Ophthalmol* **128**:362–364.

34 Shields CL, Naseripour M, Shields JA (2002). Topical mitomycin C for extensive, recurrent conjunctival-corneal squamous cell carcinoma. *Am J Ophthalmol* **133**(5):601–606.

35 Yeatts RP, Engelbrecht NE, Curry CD, *et al*. (2000). 5-Fluorouracil for the treatment of intraepithelial neoplasia of the conjunctiva and cornea. *Ophthalmology* **107**:2190–2195.

36 Singh AD, DePotter P, Fijal BA, *et al*. (1998). Lifetime prevalence of uveal melanoma in white patients with oculo (dermal) melanocytosis. *Ophthalmology* **105**:195–198.

37 Gerner N, Norregaard JC, Jensen OA, *et al*. (1996). Conjunctival naevi in Denmark 1960–1980. A 21-year follow-up study. *Acta Ophthalmol Scand* **74**:334–337.

38 Shields CL, Fasiudden A, Mashayekhi A, *et al*. (2004). Conjunctival nevi: clinical features and natural course in 410 consecutive patients. *Arch Ophthalmol* **122**:167–175.

39 Folberg R, McLean IW, Zimmerman LE (1985). Primary acquired melanosis of the conjunctiva. *Hum Pathol* **16**:136–143.

40 Shields JA, Shields CL, Mashayekhi A, *et al*. (2008). Primary acquired melanosis of the conjunctiva. Risks for progression to melanoma in 311 eyes. The 2006 Lorenz E. Zimmerman Lecture. *Ophthalmology* **115**(3):511–519.e2. Epub 2007 Sep 20.

41 Shields CL, Demirci H, Shields JA, *et al*. (2002). Dramatic regression of conjunctival and corneal acquired melanosis with topical mitomycin C. *Br J Ophthalmol* **86**:244–245.

42 Shields CL, Shields JA, Gunduz K, *et al*. (2000). Conjunctival melanoma: risk factors for recurrence, exenteration, metastasis, and death in 150 consecutive patients. *Arch Ophthalmol* **118**:1497–1507.

43 Seregard S (1998). Conjunctival melanoma. *Surv Ophthalmol* **42**:321–350.

44 Strempel I, Kroll P (1999). Conjunctival malignant melanoma in children. *Ophthalmologica* **213**:129–132.

45 Knowles DM II, Jakobiec FA (1982). Ocular adnexal lymphoid neoplasms: clinical, histopathologic, electron microscopic, and immunologic characteristics. *Hum Pathol* **123**:148–162.

46 McKelvie PA, McNab A, Francis IC, *et al*. (2001). Ocular adnexal lymphoproliferative disease: a series of 73 cases. *Clin Exp Ophthalmol* **29**:387–393.

47 Shields CL, Shields JA, Carvalho C, *et al*. (2001). Conjunctival lymphoid tumors: clinical analysis of 117 cases and relationship to systemic lymphoma. *Ophthalmology* **108**:979–984.

48 Shields CL, Shields JA (2006). Basic understanding of current classification and management of retinoblastoma. *Curr Opin Ophthalmol* **17**:228–234.

49 Rodrigues KE, Latorre Mdo R, de Camargo B. (2004). Delayed diagnosis in retinoblastoma. *J Pediatr (Rio J)* **80**:511–516.

50 Nichols KE, Houseknecht MD, Godmilow L, *et al*. (2005). Sensitive multistep clinical molecular screening of 180 unrelated individuals with retinoblastoma detects 36 novel mutations in the RB1 gene. *Hum Mutat* **25**:566–574.

51 Shields CL, Shields JA, Baez K, *et al*. (1994). Optic nerve invasion of retinoblastoma. Metastatic potential and clinical risk factors. *Cancer* **1**(73):692–698.

52 Shields CL, Shields JA, Baez KA (1993). Choroidal invasion of retinoblastoma: metastatic potential and clinical risk factors. *Br J Ophthalmol* **77**:544–548.

53 Honavar SG, Singh AD, Shields CL, *et al*. (2002). Postenucleation adjuvant therapy in high-risk retinoblastoma. *Arch Ophthalmol* **120**:923–931.

54 Kivela T (1999). Trilateral retinoblastoma: a meta-analysis of hereditary retinoblastoma associated with primary ectopic intracranial retinoblastoma. *J Clin Oncol* **17**:1829–1837.

55 De Potter P, Shields CL, Shields JA (1994). Clinical variations of trilateral retinoblastoma: a report of 13 cases. *J Pediatr Ophthalmol Strabismus* **31**:26–31.

56 Shields CL, Meadows AT, Shields JA, *et al*. (2001). Chemoreduction for retinoblastoma may prevent intracranial neuroblastic malignancy (trilateral retinoblastoma). *Arch Ophthalmol* **119**:1269–1272.

57 Karatza E, Shields CL, Flanders AE, *et al*. (2006). Pineal cyst simulating pinealoblastoma in 11 children with retinoblastoma. *Arch Ophthalmol* **124**:595–597.

58 Roarty JD, McLean IW, Zimmerman LE (1988). Incidence of second neoplasms in patients with bilateral retinoblastoma. *Ophthalmology* **95**:1583–1587.

59 Wong FL, Boice JD Jr, Abramson DH, *et al*. (1997). Cancer incidence after retinoblastoma. Radiation dose and sarcoma risk. *JAMA* **278**:1262–1267.

60 Abramson DH, Melson MR, Dunkel IJ, *et al*. (2001). Third (fourth and fifth) nonocular tumors in survivors of retinoblastoma. *Ophthalmology* **108**:1868–1876.

61 Gombos DS, Hungerford J, Abramson DH, *et al*. (2007). Secondary acute myelogenous leukemia in patients with retinoblastoma: is chemotherapy a factor? *Ophthalmology* **114**(7):1378–1383.

62 Murphree AL (2005). Intraocular retinoblastoma: the case for a new group classification. *Ophthalmol Clin North Am* **18**:41–53, viii.

63 Shields CL, Mashayekhi A, Au AK (2006). The International Classification of Retinoblastoma predicts chemoreduction success. *Ophthalmology* **113**:2276–2280.

64 Shields CL, Meadows AT, Leahey AM, *et al*. (2004). Continuing challenges in the management of retinoblastoma with chemoreduction. *Retina* **24**:849–862.

65 Shields CL, Honavar SG, Shields JA, *et al*. (2002). Factors predictive of recurrence of retinal tumor, vitreous seeds and subretinal seeds following chemoreduction for retinoblastoma. *Arch Ophthalmol* **120**:460–464.

66 Shields CL, Honavar SG, Meadows AT, *et al*. (2002). Chemoreduction plus focal therapy for retinoblastoma: factors predictive of need for treatment with external beam radiotherapy or enucleation. *Am J Ophthalmol* **133**:657–664.

67 Shields CL, Mashayekhi A, Cater J, *et al*. (2004). Chemoreduction for retinoblastoma. Analysis of tumor control and risks for recurrence in 457 tumors. *Am J Ophthalmol* **138**:329–337.

68 Shields CL, Mashayekhi A, Cater J, *et al*. (2005). Macular retinoblastoma managed with chemoreduction. Analysis of tumor control with or without adjuvant thermotherapy in 68 tumors. *Arch Ophthalmol* **123**:765–773.

69 Shields CL, Mashayekhi A, Sun H, *et al*. (2006). Iodine 125 plaque radiotherapy as salvage treatment for retinoblastoma recurrence after chemoreduction in 84 tumors. *Ophthalmology* **113**:2087–2092.

70 Shields CL, Uysal Y, Marr BP, *et al*. (2007). Experience with the polymer-coated hydroxyapatite implant following enucleation in 126 patients. *Ophthalmology* **114**:367–373.

71 Shields CL, Honavar S, Shields JA, *et al*. (2000). Vitrectomy in eyes with unsuspected retinoblastoma. *Ophthalmology* **107**:2250–2255.

72 Singh AD, Shields CL, Shields JA (2001). Major review: Von Hippel–Lindau disease. *Surv Ophthalmol* **46**:117–142.

73 Shields CL, Materin MA, Marr BP, *et al*. (2008). Resolution of exudative retinal detachment from retinal astrocytoma following photodynamic therapy. *Arch Ophthalmol* **126**(2):273–274.

74 Shields JA (1978). Melanocytoma of the optic nerve head. A review. *Int Ophthalmol* **1**:31–37.

75 Shields JA, Eagle RC Jr, Shields CL, *et al*. (1996). Congenital neoplasms of the nonpigmented ciliary epithelium. (medulloepithelioma). *Ophthalmology* **103**:1998–2006.

76 Shields CL, Honavar SG, Shields JA, *et al*. (2001). Circumscribed choroidal hemangioma. Clinical manifestations and factors predictive of visual outcome in 200 consecutive cases. *Ophthalmology* **108**:2237–2248.

77 Shields CL, Shields JA, Augsburger JJ (1988). Review: choroidal osteoma. *Surv Ophthalmol* **33**:17–27.

78 Shields CL, Furuta M, Mashayekhi A, *et al*. (2008). Clinical spectrum of choroidal nevi based on age at presentation in 3422 consecutive eyes. *Ophthalmology* **115**(3):546–552. Epub 2007 Dec 11.

79 Shields CL, Cater JC, Shields JA, *et al*. (2000). Combination of clinical factors predictive of growth of small choroidal melanocytic tumors. *Arch Ophthalmol* **118**:360–364.

80 Shields CL, Shields JA, Milite J, *et al*. (1991). Uveal melanoma in teenagers and children. A report of 40 cases. *Ophthalmology* **68**:1662–1666.

81 Shields CL, Mashayekhi A, Ho T, *et al*. (2003). Solitary congenital hypertrophy of the retinal pigment epithelium: clinical features and frequency of enlargement in 330 patients. *Ophthalmology* **110**:1968–1976.

82 Shields JA, Shields CL, Scartozzi R (2004). Survey of 1264 orbital tumors and pseudotumors. The 2002 Montgomery Lecture. Part 1. *Ophthalmology* **111**:997–1008.

83 Shields JA, Bakewell B, Augsberger JJ, *et al*. (1986). Space-occupying orbital masses in children: a review of 250 consecutive biopsies. *Ophthalmology* **93**:379–384.

84 Shields JA, Kaden IH, Eagle RC Jr, *et al*. (1997). Orbital dermoid cysts. Clinicopathologic correlations, classification, and management. The 1997 Josephine E. Schueler Lecture. *Ophthal Plast Reconstr Surg* **13**:265–276.

85 Sathananthan N, Mosely IF, Rose GE, *et al*. (1993). The frequency and clinical significance of bone involvement in outer canthus dermoid cysts. *Br J Ophthalmol* **77**:789–794.

86 Wright JE, Sullivan TJ, Garner A, *et al*. (1997). Orbital venous anomalies. *Ophthalmology* **104**:905–913.

87 Garrity JA (1997). Orbital venous anomalies. A long-standing dilemma. *Ophthalmology* **104**:903–904.

88 Boulos PR, Harissi-Dagher M, Kavalec C, *et al*. (2005). Intralesional injection of Tisseel fibrin glue for resection of lymphangiomas and other thin-walled orbital cysts. *Ophthal Plast Reconstr Surg* **21**:171–176.

89 Shields CL, Shields JA, Honavar SG, *et al*. (2001). The clinical spectrum of primary ophthalmic rhabdomyosarcoma. *Ophthalmology* **108**:2284–2292.

90 Shields JA, Shields CL (2003). Rhabdomyosarcoma. Review for the ophthalmologist. *Surv Ophthalmol* **48**:39–57.

91 Font RL, Zimmerman LE (1975). Ophthalmologic manifestations of granulocytic sarcoma (myeloid sarcoma or chloroma). The third Pan American Association of Ophthalmology and American Journal of Ophthalmology Lecture. *Am J Ophthalmol* **80**:975–990.

92 Shields JA, Stopyra GA, Marr BP, *et al*. (2003). Bilateral orbital myeloid sarcoma as initial sign of acute myeloid leukemia. *Arch Ophthalmol* **121**:138–142.

CHAPTER 19
Bibliography

Bracken MB, Shepard MJ, Collin WF, *et al*. (1990). A randomized, controlled trial of methylprednisolone or naloxone in the treatment of acute spinal cord injury. Results of the Second National Acute Spinal Cord Injury Study. *New Engl J Med* **322**(20):1405–1411.

Crouch ER Jr, Crouch ER (1999). Management of traumatic hyphema: therapeutic options. *J Pediatr Ophthalmol Strabismus* **36**:238–250.

Kivlin JD, Simons KB, Lazonitz S, *et al*. (2000). Shaken baby syndrome. *Ophthalmology* **107**(7):1246–1254.

Kunimoto DY, Kanitkar KD, Makar M, *et al*. (2004). *The Wills Eye Manual Office and Emergency Room Diagnosis and Treatment of Eye Disease*, 4th edn. Lippincott, Williams and Wilkins, Philadelphia.

Lane K, Penne RB, Bilyk JR (2007). Evaluation and management of pediatric orbital fractures in primary care setting. *Orbit* **26**(3):183–191.

Levin A (1990). Ocular manifestations of child abuse. *Ophthalmol Clin North Am* **3**:249–264.

Pierre-Kahn V, Roche O, Duneau P, *et al*. (2003). Ophthalmologic findings in suspected child abuse victims with subdural hematoma. *Ophthalmology* **110**(9):1718–1723.

Taylor D, Hoyt CS (2005). *Pediatric Ophthalmology and Strabismus*, 3rd edn. Elsevier, Edinburgh.

Index

Note: Page numbers in *italic* refer to tables or boxes

acetazolamide 128
acetylcholine receptors 242
achromatopsia 138–9
aciclovir 76
acoustic neuroma 222
adenoma sebaceum 220
adhesions 123, 125
adrenergic agonists 128
AIDS 248, 272
Alagille's syndrome 106
albinism 148–9, 210–15
Allen figures *24*
allergens 79
Allgrove syndrome 183
Alport syndrome 104, 105
amacrine cells 19
amblyopia
  ametropic 44
  anisometropic 44
  cataracts 108, 111
  classification 44
  congenital rubella 216
  diagnosis 27, 47–8
  etiology and epidemiology 43–5
  in glaucoma 116, 120
  management 48–9
  organic 45
  in ptosis 187
  strabismic 44
  visual deprivation 45
American Academy of Pediatrics (AAP) 31
aminoglycosides *72*
Ancyclostoma duodenale 82
aneurysm, intracranial 58
angiofibroma 220, 221
angiotensin-converting enzyme (ACE) 156

angle kappa 29
angle surgery 120, 128, 129
anhidrosis 240
aniridia 106, 124
anisometropia 32, 44, 48, 108
ankyloblepharon 186
annulus of Zinn 14
anomalous head positions (AHPs) 214
anophthalmia 186
anterior chamber 18
  hemorrhage (hyphema) 126, 157, 282–3
  maldevelopment 119
anterior segment
  anatomy 17–19, 66, 67
  dysgenesis syndromes 106
  embryogenesis 86
anterior segment (iridocorneal) angle 18
anterior uveitis 126, 155–7, *155*
antibiotic resistance *72*, 73
antibiotic/steroid combinations *72*, 82
antihistamines, and tear production 183
antioxidant therapy 41–2
aphakia 98, 110, 111
apraclonidine 128
arginine 150
Ascaris lumbricoides 82
ash leaf sign 220, 221
Ashkenazi Jewish populations 94
asthma 80
astigmatism, corneal dermoid 88, 89
astrocytic hamartoma, retinal 218–20, 266, 267

astrocytoma
  optic nerve 224
  paraventricular 220, 221
  pilocytic 224, 272, 273
atopic keratoconjunctivitis (AKC) 78, 79
atropine 49
attention deficit hyperactivity disorder (ADHD) 214
aura, migraine 237
autorefraction 32
Axenfeld–Rieger syndrome 106, 123
azithromycin *72*

β-hemolytic streptococci 70
bacitracin *72*
bacterial conjunctivitis 69–73
balloon dacryoplasty 181
band keratopathy 156
Bardet–Biedl syndrome 149–50
basal cell carcinoma 248
basal cell nevus syndrome 190
Best's disease 142–3
beta blockers, topical 128
bevacizumab 42
bimatoprost 128
birth trauma 88–9, 117
birth weight, and ROP 34, 38
bisphosphonates 202
black sunburst 209
blepharitis 183, 189–90
blepharoptosis 187–8, 248, 249
blepharospasm 116, 189
blindness, healthcare priority 33
BLOCK-ROP Trial 42
blow-out fracture 286, 287
blue nevus 248

blue-cone monochromatism 138
Brazil 259
brimonidine 128
brinzolamide 128
Brown's syndrome 62
Bruch's membrane 20, 209
Bruckner Test 23, *24*, *25*, 108
Burkitt's lymphoma 272

café au lait spots 122, 224, 225
canalicular system 178
    injury 276, *277*
Candida albicans 82
carbonic anhydrase inhibitors 128
cataracts 100–3
    anterior polar 100, *101*
    cerulean (blue-dot) 102
    'Christmas tree' 105
    complete 102, *103*
    congenital rubella 216
    diagnosis 108
    etiology 104–7
    JIA-associated uveitis 156
    lamellar 100, *101*
    management 108–11
    nuclear 100
    persistent fetal vasculature 144, 145
    posterior polar 100
    prognosis 112
    subcapsular 102, *103*
    'sunflower' 200
    sutural 102, *103*
    traumatic 284
    visual significance 108
cats 158
cavernous hemangioma, retina 232, 265
ceftriaxone 84
cellulitis, orbit 191
central nervous system (CNS) malformations 164, 166
ceramide trihexosidase 201
chalazion 13, 190
CHARGE association 169
Chediak–Higashi syndrome 149, 210, *213*
chemical injuries 83–4, 281
chemosis, conjunctival 79
chemotherapy 262–3, *263*, 272
child abuse 289

chlamydial infections 74, 83–4, *83*
chloramphenicol *72*
'chloroma' (granulocytic sarcoma) 272
'chocolate cysts' 257
choriocapillaris 20
choristomas 249–52, *250*
    complex 252
    epibulbar complex 233
    lacrimal gland 252
choroid 152
choroidal freckles/nevi 222, *223*, 268, 269
choroidal hemangioma 230–1, 266
choroidal osteoma 266, 267
ciliary body 18–19, 152
    medulloepithelioma 266, 267
ciliary flush 126, 152, 153
ciliopathies 149–50
cimetidine, oral 253
ciprofloxacin *72*
Coats' disease 132–4, 264
'cobblestone' papillae 80, 81
cocaine solution 240
collagen synthesis, disorders 202
coloboma
    associated syndromes 169
    eyelid 186–7
    lens 98
    optic disc 169
color vision testing 30
commotio retinae 284, 285
cone-rod dystrophy 150
congenital hereditary endothelial dystrophy (CHED) 89, 118
congenital hereditary stromal dystrophy (CHSD) 90
congenital hypertrophy of retinal pigment epithelium (CHRPE) 270
congenital stationary night blindness (CSNB) 136–7, 170
conjunctiva 18, 66
    complex choristoma 233
    follicles 74, 75
    injection 70, 74, 75
    tumors 244, 245, 249–58, *250*
conjunctival intraepithelial neoplasia (CIN) 253–4

conjunctivitis 68–9
    algorithm for differential diagnosis 68
    allergic 78–9, 192
    bacterial 69–73
    giant papillary 77
    hemorrhagic 74, 75
    herpes 76
    types *69*
    viral 74–5
conjunctivitis–otitis media syndrome 71
Conradi syndrome 105
contact lens
    astigmatism 89
    conjunctivitis 70, 71, 77
    corneal abrasion 280
    position on globe 66
copper transport, disorder 200
corectopia 123
cornea 17
    birth trauma 88–9
    cystine crystals 194–5
    development 86
    edema 22, 153
    enlargement in glaucoma 117, 119
    keratic precipitates 153
    scarring 117
    structure/thickness 17
    trauma/abrasion 280–1
    ulcer 70, 71, 80–1
corneal opacity
    congenital 86–90
    glaucoma 117, 118, 129
    infectious disease 95–6
    metabolic disease 91–5
corneal transplantation 87
cortical visual impairment 236
corticosteroids
    cataract formation 106, 107
    dacryoadenitis 184
    ophthalmic drops *72*, 76, 82
Corynebacterium diptheriae 70
cover test 28–9, 53
    alternate 29
cranial nerve palsy
    fourth 16, 59–60
    sixth 60
    third 58–9
cranial nerves, eyelid function 186
cross cover test *24*, *25*
cross-fixation 26

Cryo-ROP Study 38
cryotherapy 253, 256
cryptophthalmos 186
cycloablation 130
cyclopentolate 49
cystathionine beta synthase (CBS) deficiency 198
cystinosis 94–5, 194–5
cytokines, vasoactive 33–4, 42

dacryoadenitis 184
dacryocele 178–9
dacryocystitis 178
dacryoplasty, balloon 181
dacryostenosis, congenital 69
de Morsier's syndrome 164
dendrites, corneal 76
dental anomalies 123
dermoid cyst 271
dermoid tumors 88, 251
dermolipoma 251
Descemet's membrane 17, 86
    deposits in Wilson's disease 200
    rupture 119
    snail track opacity 90
    tears 88
developing countries 259
diabetes mellitus 104, 166, 167
dissociated vertical deviation (DVD) 55
dog-bite trauma 276, 277
dorzolamide 128
double elevator palsy (monocular elevation deficiency) 62–3
Down's syndrome 104
drusen 176
Duane's syndrome 61
ductions, testing 29–30, 62, 192
dye disappearance test 180
dysautonomia, familial (Riley–Day syndrome) 183
dysostosis multiplex 204

Early Treatment of Retinopathy of Prematurity (ET-ROP) Study 36, 41
ecchymosis 276
ectopia lentis 98–9, 196, 197, 198, 199
ectropion 189
eczema 80

electro-oculogram (EOG) 142
electroretinography (ERG) 134, 135, 138, 142, 147
embryology 86, 144
endocrine abnormalities 166, 167
enhanced S-cone syndrome 136
enophthalmitis 159
enophthalmos 286
entropion 189
enzyme replacement therapy 204, 206, 207
eosinophilic granuloma 272
epiblepharon 189
epicanthal folds 188
epiphora 116, 152, 180
erythromycin 72, 84
esotropia 26, 64
    accommodative 56–7
    congenital 54, 54
euryblepharon 188
exotropia 57
extraocular muscles 14–17
    functions 15
eye
    defense mechanisms 69
    exposure 188
    structural diagram 67
eye movements, binocular 29
'eye popping' 189
eye shield 278, 279, 282
eyelashes
    matting 70
    pediculosis 189–90
eyelids 186
    anatomy 12–13
    coloboma 186–7
    foreign bodies 276, 277
    herpes simplex 191
    retraction 188–9
    trauma 192, 276–7
    tumors 190–1, 244, 245, 246–9

Fabry's disease 94, 104, 201
fascia bulbi (Tenon's capsule) 66
fibrillin 196
fibrogliosis 232
fine-needle aspiration biopsy (FNAB) 245
fixation testing 23, 26, 47
flare, anterior chamber 154

flashlight test 23
fluorescein angiography 133, 227
fluorescein staining 281
fluoroquinolones 72, 73
folinic acid 158
follicles, conjunctival 74, 75
forced duction testing 62, 192
forceps injury 117
foreign bodies
    cornea 281
    eyelid 276, 277
    intraocular 278, 279
    intraorbital 288
forme fruste 218
fornix 18, 66
fovea 20
foveal hypoplasia 148
Fuch's coloboma (congenital tilted disc) 170–1
fundus, hypopigmentation 210, 211

galactosemia 104
α-galactosidase A 201
gamma aminobutyric acid (GABA) 45
ganglion cells 19
gatifloxacin 72
gentamicin 72
germinal matrix 236
giant papillary conjunctivitis 77
glands of Krause 13
glands of Manz 13
glands of Wolfring 13
glasses, see spectacles
glaucoma
    associated with ocular anomalies 123–5
    associated with systemic disease 121
    congenital 22, 216
    diagnosis 114–18
    filtering procedures 77
    following cataract surgery 127
    juvenile open-angle 120
    neurofibromatosis 222
    Peters anomaly 87
    primary 114–15, 119–20
    pupillary block 196
    secondary 114–15, 126–7
    signs and symptoms 114, 115, 116, 180

glaucoma (*continued*)
  Sturge–Weber syndrome
    230
  treatment 128–30
globe, open 278–9
globe retraction 61
glycosaminoglycans (GAGs)
  91, 204, 205
goblet cells, conjunctival 66
Goldenhar syndrome 88, 169,
  251
gonioscopy 157
goniotomy 120, 129, 130
gonococcal disease 83–4
Gorlin–Goltz syndrome 248
granulocytic sarcoma
  ('chloroma') 272, 273
'gray line' 66

Haab's striae 119
Haemophilus influenzae 70, 72
Hallermann–Streiff syndrome
  106
hamartoma
  astrocytic retinal 218–20,
    266, 267
  iris (Lisch nodules) 122,
    222, 223, 224
Harm's trabeculotome 130
head nodding 239
head positions, anomalous
  (AHPs) 214
head thrusting 241
head tilt 59, 239
head turn 239
headache, migraine 237
hemangioblastoma 225, 226,
  227
hemangioma
  capillary 190, 231, 246–7,
    257, 264
  cavernous 232, 265
  choroidal 230–1, 266
  retinal 264–5
hemangiomatosis
  encephalofacial cavernous
    (Sturge–Weber
    syndrome) 191, 230–1
  racemose (Wyburn–Mason
    syndrome) 229, 265
hematoma, intraretinal 208–9
hemianopia, bitemporal 170
hemorrhage
  retinal 289
  retrobulbar 288
  subconjunctival 280

heparin sulfate 91
hereditary benign
  intraepithelial dyskeratosis
    (HBID) 253
Hermansky–Pudlak syndrome
  149, 210, 213, 215
herpes simplex virus (HSV)
  76, 83, 83, 95, 157, 191
herpes zoster virus (HZV) 76,
  157
heterochromia 255
heterophoria (phoria) 29, 52
heterotropia 28–9, 52
Hirschberg corneal reflex test
  52–3
Hirschberg estimates 29
histamine release 78
history taking 22
HLA-B27 haplotype 126,
  156
homatropine 49
homocystinuria 198–9
hordeolum 190
Horner–Trantas dots 80, 81
Horner's syndrome 240–1
HOTV test 24, 26, 46
human papillomavirus 253
Hunter's syndrome (MPS II)
  92, 204, 206
Hurler's syndrome
  (MPS I-H) 92, 204, 205
Hutchinson's triad 96
hyaloid artery 144
hydroxyamphetamine drops
  240
hyperopia 56
hypersensitivity reactions 82
hyphema 126, 157, 282–3
hypoglycemia, cataracts 104
hypopituitarism 166, 167
hypopyon 154, 162
hypothyroidism 194
hypoxic ischemic injury 236

I-Cell disease (ML II) 93
immunosuppression 254
inferior oblique muscle over
  action (IOOA) 55
insulin-like growth factor-1
  (IGF-1) 34
interferon, topical 253
International Classification of
  Retinoblastoma (ICRB)
  261–2, 261
intracranial pressure (ICP),
  raised 60, 174

intraepithelial neoplasia,
  conjunctival (CIN) 253–4
intraocular lens (IOL)
  109–10, 111
  Marfan's syndrome 197
  multifocal 111
  traumatic cataract 284, 285
intraocular pressure (IOP)
  elevation 114, 180
  measurement 118
  orbital injury 288
iridocorneal angle 18
iridocorneal endothelial
  (ICE) syndrome 106
iridodenesis 196
iridodialysis 282, 283, 285
iris 18
  atrophy 157, 199
  congenital defects 123
  Lisch nodules 122, 222,
    223, 224
  nodules 156, 157
  scarring (synechiae) 154
  transillumination 210, 211,
    212–13
irrigation, ocular surface 281
Ishihara testing 30
isotretinoin 183

Joubert syndrome 149, 150
juvenile idiopathic arthritis
  (JIA) 126, 155–6
juvenile pilocytic astrocytoma
  (optic nerve glioma) 224,
  272, 273

Kaposi's sarcoma 248
Kayser–Fleischer ring 200
keratic precipitates 153
keratitis 70, 71, 191
keratoconjunctivitis,
  phlyctenular 82
keratopathy, band 156
Krimsky light reflex testing 53

lacerations
  conjunctiva 280
  eyelid 276–7
lacrimal glands 13, 178
  choristoma 252
lacrimal sac 14
  fistula 182
lacrimal system 13–14
  massage 179, 181
  see also nasolacrimal duct
lagophthalmos 188

lamina cribosa 17–18
Langerhan's cell histiocytosis
272
laser therapy 40, 130
latanaprost 128
Laurence–Moon syndrome
150
Lea symbols *24*, 26, 27, 46
Leber's congenital amaurosis
(LCA) 134–5, 150
lens
anatomy and development
98
dislocation/subluxation
(ectopia lentis) 98–9,
196, 197, 198, 199, 284
lenticonus 99, 104, 105
leukemia 162, 258, 270
leukocoria 23, 108, 244, 245
levator palpebrae muscles
12–13, 186, 276
levofloxacin *72*
lid retraction, pathologic
188–9
light reflex testing 29–30,
52–3
limbus 18
linear sebaceous nevus
syndrome 169
lipofuscin 140
Lisch nodules 122, 222, *223*,
268
Lowe's syndrome 104, 121
lymphadenopathy,
conjunctivitis 70
lymphangioma 272
conjunctiva 257
eyelid 191
lymphoid tumors 258
lysosomal storage disease
105

macrolide antibiotics *72*
macula 20
'egg-yolk'(vitelliform) 142,
143
granuloma in toxocariasis
159
puckering in VKH 160,
161
retinoblastoma 262, 263
scarring in toxoplasmosis
158–9
uveitic swelling 152, 153
macular degeneration 150
mannosidosis 105

Marcus–Gunn jaw-winking
syndrome 187, 188
Marfan's syndrome 98, 99,
196–7
Maroteaux–Lamy syndrome
(MPS VI A and B) 93, 204,
207
masquerade syndromes *155*,
162
mast cells, degranulation 78
maternal infections, cataract
formation 107
medications
causing cataracts 106–7
causing decreased tear
production 183
medicolegal issues, ROP 42
medulloepithelioma,
intraocular 266, 267
meibomian glands 13
chalazion 13, 190
melanocytic tumors,
conjunctival 254–6, *254*
melanocytoma, optic nerve
266, 267
melanocytosis, ocular *254*,
255
melanoma *254*, 255, 256, 258
uveal 268, *268*, 269
meningoencephalocele 178
metabolic diseases 91–5
cataracts 104–5
cystinosis 94–5, 194–5
Fabry's disease 94, 104,
201
homocystinuria 198–9
mucopolysaccharidoses
91–4, 204–5, *206–7*
tyrosinemia 95
methionine levels 198
methylene tetrahydrofolate
reductase (MTHFR)
deficiency 198
microcornea 216
microphthalmia 186, 216
microspherophagia 197
microspherophakia 99
MIDAS syndrome 87
migraine headache 237
mitomycin C 253, 256
Mittendorf's dot 144
Möbius syndrome 64
molluscum contagiosum
191–2
monocular elevation
deficiency (MED) 62–3

Moraxella catarrhalis 70
morning glory disc anomaly
168
Morquio's syndrome (MPS
IV A and B) 93, 204, *207*
moxifloxacin *72*
mucolipidosis 93–4
mucopolysaccharidoses 91–4,
204–5, *206–7*
idiopathic 93
Müller's muscle 12, 186
myasthenia gravis 242
Mycobacterium tuberculosis 82
myelination, retinal nerve
fibers 172–3
myopia 116
myotonic dystrophy 105

nasal fundus ectasia 170–1
nasolacrimal duct 14, 178
intubation 181–2
obstruction 22, 178, 179,
180–2
probing 179, 181
Neisseria spp. 70, 83–4, *83*
neural crest cells, migration
86
neurilemoma (schwannoma)
249
neuroblastoma 239, 273
neurofibroma 222, 248, 249
neurofibromatosis 122, 191,
222–5, *223*, 248, 249
neuroma, plexiform 191
nevi
conjunctival 255–6
eyelid 190, 191
melanocytic 248
pigmented *254*, 255–6
uveal 268
nevus flammeus (port-wine
stain) 191, 231, 248, 249,
266
nevus sebaceous of Jadassohn
233, 252
night blindness, congenital
stationary 136–7, 170
nystagmus 108, 170, 210,
215, 238, 239

occlusion
amblyopia therapy 48
strabismus testing 28, 29
visual acuity testing 26, 27
ocular alignment, testing *24*,
25

ocular examination 22–3
  glaucoma 117–18
ocular flutter 239
ocular motor apraxia,
  congenital 241
oculocerebrorenal syndrome
  (Lowe's syndrome) 104,
  121
oculoneurocutaneous
  syndromes (ONCS) 218
  genetics 218
  malignant potential 218
  TSC 218–21
ofloxacin *72*
open globe 278–9
ophthalmia neonatorum
  83–4, *83*
ophthalmoscopy 31
  direct 23, *24*, *25*, 31, 117
  indirect 132
opsoclonus 239
optic canal, decompression
  286
optic disc
  coloboma 169
  congenital tilted 170–1
  cupping 116
  drusen 176
  morning glory anomaly
  168
optic nerve
  hypoplasia 164–7
  melanocytoma 266, 267
  pilocytic astrocytoma
  (glioma) 224, 272, 273
  retinoblastoma 259
  trauma 286
optic neuropathy
  clinical principles 164
  unilateral 164
optic pit 172, 173
optic radiations 236
optical axis 29
optical coherence
  tomography (OCT) 210,
  245
ora serrata 19
orbicularis oculi muscle 12,
  186
orbit
  anatomy 12
  cellulitis 191
  septum 13
  trauma 12, 192, 286–8
  tumors 222, *244*, 245, 246,
  271–3

organoid nevus syndrome
  233, *234*, 252
orthophorhia 52
osseous choristoma, epibulbar
  252
osteogenesis imperfecta
  202–3
osteoma, choroidal 266, 267
otitis media, acute 71
oxygen administration,
  neonatal 33–4, 42

PanOptic ophthalmoscope 31
panuveitis 160, 161
papillae, tarsal conjunctivae
  80, 81
papilledema 174
papilloma 253
parasites, gastrointestinal 82
parents 22
pars plana 19
pars plicata 18–19
patching 48, 110, 111
Paton's lines 174
pattern-evoked potential
  (PEVP) 32
pediculosis, eyelashes 189–90
penalization 49
D-penicillamine 41
perennial allergic
  conjunctivitis (PAC) 78, 79
periventricular leukomalacia
  166
persistent fetal vasculature
  (PFV) 99, 144–5, 264
Peters anomaly 86–7, 106,
  125
'phakomatoses' 218
phlyctenulosis 82
'photic sneeze reflex' 195
photocoagulation 40
photophobia 116, 117, 129,
  195
photoscreening 32
phthisis 281
pineal cysts 260
pinealoblastoma 259–60
pink eye, *see* conjunctivitis
pituitary abnormalities 166,
  167
plaque radiotherapy 263–4
plexiform neuroma 191
Plus disease 36–7
polycoria 123
polymyxin B/trimethoprim
  sulfate *72*

port-wine stain (nevus
  flammeus) 191, 231, 248,
  249, 266
posterior polymorphous
  membrane dystrophy
  (PPMD) 90
posterior segment 19–20
posterior synechiae 154
primary acquired melanosis
  (PAM) *254*, 256
primary ciliary dyskinesia 150
proptosis 271, *272*, *273*
prostaglandin analogs 128
pseudo-Hurler dystrophy
  (ML III) 94
pseudohypopyon 162
pseudomembrane 70, 71
Pseudomonas infections 70, 71,
  83, 280
pseudopapilledema 175
pseudophakia 111
pseudoptosis 62, 63
pseudostrabismus
  (pseudoesotropia) 53
pseudotumor cerebri 174,
  209
psychosocial factors 43
ptosis
  3rd cranial nerve palsy 58,
  59
  congenital 13, 187–8
  myasthenia gravis 242
  upper and lower lids 240
pulleys 15
puncta 13, 178
pupil 18
pupillary axis 29
pupillary constriction 240–1
pupillary defects, afferent 23
pupillary dilation 23
pupillary reflex
  unequal 44
  white (leukocoria) 23, 108,
  244, 245
pupillary strands 144
pyogenic granuloma 257

racial melanosis *254*, 256
radiotherapy 258, 263–4,
  263
Random-dot-E test *24*, *25*, 31
rectus muscles 14, *15*, 16–17
red eye, *see* conjunctivitis
red reflex 23, *24*, *25*, 108
Refsum disease 105, 150
renal disease 194, 201

retina
astrocytic hamartoma
218–20, 266, 267
cavernous hemangioma
232, 265
hemangioblastoma 225,
226
normal human 20
racemose hemangioma 229,
265
structure 19–20
telangiectasia 132
traumatic injury 284–5
retinal blood vessels
excessive oxygen exposure
33–4
tortuous 201, 265
retinal detachment 20
Marfan's syndrome 197
in ROP 40–1
sickle cell disease 209
toxocariasis 159
trauma 284, 285
VKH syndrome 161
retinal dystrophies 149–50
retinal nerve fibers,
myelinated 172–3
retinal pigment epithelium
19, 20
congenital hypertrophy
(CHRPE) 270
retinitis pigmentosa (RP)
149, 150
retinoblastoma 126, 162,
259–64
classification 261–2,
261
clinical presentation 162,
244, 245
diagnosis and management
162, 246, 261–4
disorders resembling
264
genetic mutations/testing
259
metastasis 259
second cancers 260–1
'trilateral' 259–60
retinocerebellar
hemangioblastomatosis
(von-Hippel–Lindau
syndrome) 226–8
retinochoroiditis,
toxoplasmosis 159
retinopathy, 'salt and pepper'
216

retinopathy of prematurity
(ROP) 33
clinical presentation 35–8
diagnosis 38
etiology/risk factors 33–4
management/prognosis
38–41
pathophysiology 34–5
prevention 41–2
retinoschisis
traumatic 289
X-linked juvenile 146–7
retrobulbar hemorrhage 288
rhabdomyosarcoma 272, 273
Richner Hanhart syndrome
(tyrosinemia type II) 95
Riley–Day syndrome 183
rod monochromatism 138
Rose Bengal staining 76
Rothmund–Thomson
syndrome 190
rubella 96, 107, 216
Rush disease 36–7

'salmon patch' 258
salmon patch hemorrhage
208–9
Sanfilippo A syndrome 204,
206
sarcoidosis 156, 157
Scheie's syndrome (MPS I)
92, 204, 206
Schwalbe's line 18
schwannoma 222, 223, 249
sclera 17
blue 202, 203
hydration 17
trauma 278
sclerocornea 87
scopolamine (hyoscine) 49
scotoma 158–9
scintillating 237
seasonal allergic conjunctivitis
(SAC) 78, 79
seborrheic blepharitis 189
Senior–Loken syndrome 150
septo-optic dysplasia (de
Morsier's syndrome) 164
Seton implant 130
shaking injury 289
shield ulcer 80–1
sialidosis (ML I) 93
sickle cell disease 208–9, 282
sickle cell trait 209
silver nitrate 83–4
Sjögren's syndrome 183

skin macules, depigmented
220, 221
Sly's syndrome (MPS VII) 93,
204, 207
small leucine-rich
proteoglycan (SLRP) 136
sneezing, photic 195
Snellen charts 24, 26, 46
socioeconomic factors 43
spasmus nutans 239
spectacles
accommodative esotropia
56
aphakic 110, 111
spherophakia
(microspherophakia) 99
spiral of Tillaux 14, 15
spondyloarthropathies,
juvenile 156–7
squamous cell carcinoma
253–4
squamous papilloma 253
Staphylococcus aureus 70, 73,
82
staphyloma
anterior 199
peripapillary 170, 171
Stargardt disease 140–1
stereo Fly (Titmus) test 30–1
stereoacuity, assessment 30–1
strabismus
albinism 214–15
amblyopic 44
comitant (esodeviations)
52, 54–7
definitions 52
diagnosis 28–30, 52–3
incomitant 52, 58–60
infancy 53
ocular tumors 245
surgery 55, 60
strabismus syndromes 61–4
Streptococcus pneumoniae 70,
72
Sturge–Weber syndrome 121,
191, 230–1, 248, 249, 266
subconjunctival hemorrhage
280
subretinal hemorrhage 285
substantia propria 66
sulfacetamide sodium 72
sulfisoxazole 72
sulfonamides 72
suprasellar tumors 170
sympathetic ophthalmia
160–1

synechiae, posterior/anterior 154
syphilis, congenital 96
systemic disease
  associated with ptosis 187
  glaucoma associated with 121
  retinal dystrophies 149–50
  see also metabolic disease *and individual diseases*

tarsal plates 186
tarsorrhaphy 183
tarsus 12
tearing, *see* epiphora
tears 13
  constituents 66
  decreased production 183
  drainage 13–14
telemedicine 41
Tenon's capsule (fascia bulbi) 66
teratoma 271
thermotherapy 263
'three step test' 59
thymectomy 242
thyrotoxicosis 188
Titmus (stereo Fly) test 30–1
tobramycin *72*
Togby's (corneal shield) ulcers 80–1
Tonopen 118
TORCHS titer 108
torticollis 214, 239
toxicities, cataract formation 107
toxocariasis 159
toxoplasmosis 158–9
trabeculectomy 130
trabeculitis 127
trabeculotomy 120, 129–30
trachoma inclusion conjunctivitis agent (TRIC) 84
Trantas 80, 81
trauma
  causing cataracts 1–3, 102, 106, 107, 284
  eyelid 192, 276–7
  glaucoma 126
  intraocular 282–3
  ocular surface 280–1
  optic nerve 286
  orbit 12, 192, 286–8
  retina 284–5

trauma (*continued*)
  sympathetic ophthalmia 160–1
travoprost 128
tuberous sclerosis complex (TSC) 218–21
tumbling E test *24*
tumors
  causing glaucoma 126
  conjunctival 249–58
  diagnostic approaches 245–6
  eyelids 190–1, 244, 245, 246–9
  intracranial 58
  intraocular *244*
  metastatic 259, 273
  non-neoplastic lesions simulating *250*, 258
  orbit 222, *244*, 245, 246, 271–3
tyrosinase 148
tyrosinemia 95

Usher syndrome 149
uvea 18–19, 152
uveitis 152
  anterior 126, 155–7, *155*
  classification 154, *155*
  clinical features 152–4
  glaucoma 126–7
  intermediate *155*, 158
  masquerade syndromes *155*, 162
  posterior *155*, 158–61

valve of Hasner 14, 178, 179, 181
valve of Rosenbuller 14
vascular endothelial growth factor (VEGF) 33–4
  inhibitors 42
Venereal Disease Research Laboratory (VDRL) 108
vernal keratoconjunctivitis (VKC) 77, 80–1
verruca vulgaris 192
versions 29
verticilatta, corneal 94, 201
vestibulo-oculoreflex 241
vision screening 31
visual acuity testing 23–7
  amblyopia 46, 47–8
  guidelines 23, *24–5*
visual axis 29

visual behavior assessment 47, 108
visual deprivation 45
visual development 43–4, 111
visual evoked potential 32
visual experience, abnormal 45
visual field deficits 170, 171, 174, 195
visual pathway abnormalities 210, 214
vitamin A 41, 150
vitamin E 41
vitelliform macular dystrophy type 2 (VMD2/Best's disease) 142–3
vitiligo 160, 161
vitrectomy 41, 109–10
vitreous 144
vitreous hemorrhage 289
Vogt–Koyanagi–Harada syndrome 160, 161
von Recklinghausen's syndrome, *see* neurofibromatosis
von-Hippel–Lindau syndrome (VHL) 226–8, 264

Walker–Warburg syndrome 169
wart, eyelid 192
Welch Allyn SureSight™ 32
Wilm's tumor 106
Wilson's disease 105, 200
Wyburn–Mason syndrome 229, 265

xanthogranuloma, juvenile 257
xeroderma pigmentosum 190